Small Animal **Clinical Techniques**

Small Animal **Clinical Techniques**

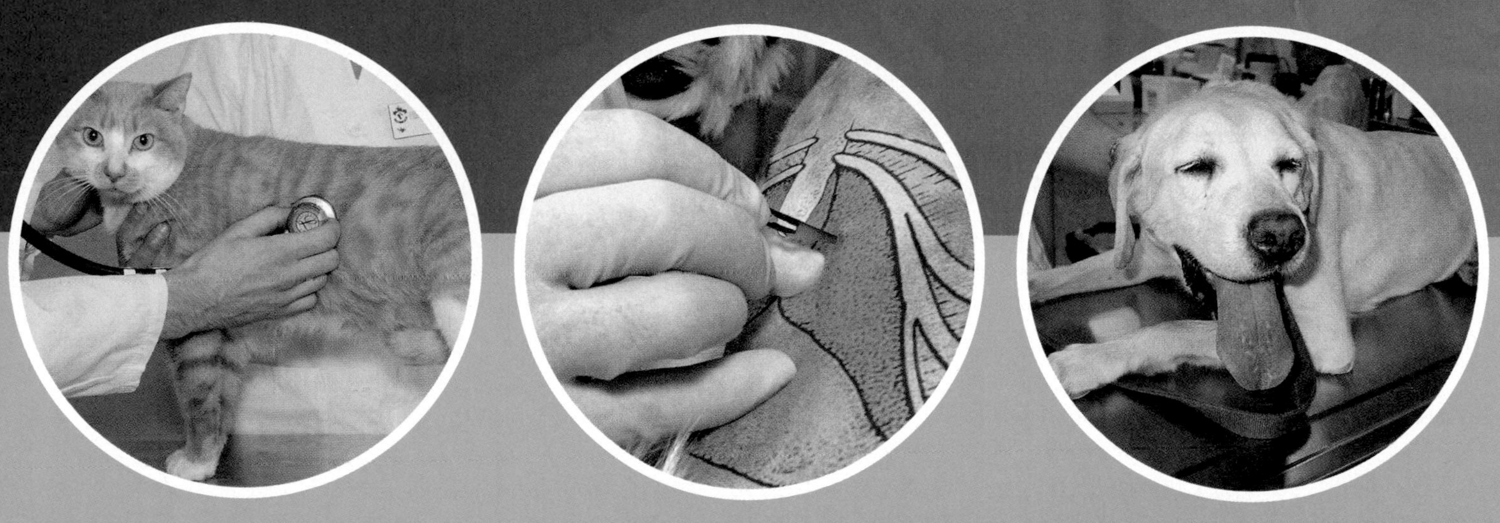

SUSAN M. TAYLOR, DVM, Diplomate ACVIM (Small Animal Internal Medicine)

Professor of Small Animal Medicine
Department of Small Animal Clinical Sciences
Western College of Veterinary Medicine
University of Saskatchewan
Saskatoon, Saskatchewan

SAUNDERS
ELSEVIER

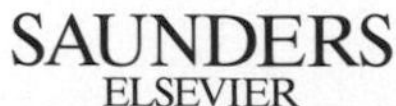

3251 Riverport Lane
St. Louis, Missouri 63043

SMALL ANIMAL CLINICAL TECHNIQUES

ISBN: 978-1-4160-5288-3

Notice

Knowledge and best practice in this field are constantly changing. As new research and experience broaden our knowledge, changes in practice, treatment, and drug therapy may become necessary or appropriate. Readers are advised to check the most current information provided (i) on procedures featured or (ii) by the manufacturer of each product to be administered, to verify the recommended dose or formula, the method and duration of administration, and contraindications. It is the responsibility of the practitioner, relying on their own experience and knowledge of the patient, to make diagnoses, to determine dosages and the best treatment for each individual patient, and to take all appropriate safety precautions. To the fullest extent of the law, neither the Publisher nor the Author assumes any liability for any injury and/or damage to persons or property arising out of or related to any use of the material contained in this book.

The Publisher

Library of Congress Cataloging in Publication Data

Taylor, Susan M.
Small animal clinical techniques / Susan M. Taylor.
p. ; cm.
Includes index.
ISBN 978-1-4160-5288-3 (pbk. : alk. paper) 1. Pet medicine–Handbooks, manuals, etc. I. Title.
[DNLM: 1. Diagnostic Techniques and Procedures–veterinary–Handbooks. 2. Cat Diseases–diagnosis–Handbooks. 3. Dog Diseases–diagnosis–Handbooks. SF 748T246s 2010]
SF981.T39 2010
636.089'6075–dc22 2009042653

Vice President and Publisher: Linda Duncan
Publisher: Penny Rudolph
Acquisitions Editor: Teri Merchant
Publishing Services Manager: Patricia Tannian
Senior Project Manager: John Casey
Designer: Amy Buxton

Printed in the United States of America

Last digit is the print number 9 8 7 6 5 4 3

To the countless beloved pets
that have allowed me to practice and perfect
these techniques on their bodies.

To the veterinary students, interns, residents, and technicians
who have taught me to be precise and clear in my teaching.

Preface

This book and the accompanying CD were designed to provide a visual guide to the diagnostic and therapeutic clinical techniques essential to small animal practice. This text is organized by body system for quick reference and describes more than 70 clinical techniques. The indications and contraindications, as well as potential complications, are listed for each technique.

I believe that in nearly every case, the "trick" to performing a technique properly and with confidence is understanding the relevant anatomy. Digital photographs and drawings provide the user with an in-depth understanding of and appreciation for important anatomical landmarks. A step-by-step guide to each technique is provided, illustrated by drawings and photographs. Some of the more challenging techniques are also illustrated on the enclosed CD:

RESPIRATORY SYSTEM
Respiratory examination
Nasal examination
Pharyngeal examination
Laryngeal examination
Transtracheal wash (small dog and large dog techniques)
Endotracheal wash
Transthoracic lung aspiration

GI SYSTEM
Oral examination
Orogastric intubation
Nasogastric intubation
Percutaneous transabdominal liver biopsy
Anal sac palpation and expression

DERMATOLOGY
Skin scraping
Cellophane tape method
Vacuuming
Bacterial culture of skin pustules
Skin biopsy
Woods lamp examination

JOINT TAPS
Arthrocentesis, including specific techniques for all joints (carpus, elbow, shoulder, hock, stifle)

URINARY SYSTEM
Cystocentesis, using both palpation and blind techniques
Urinary catheterization—Male cat
Urinary catheterization—Male dog
Urinary catheterization—Female dog
Prostatic wash

This text is designed to be used as a resource for teaching veterinary students and veterinary technician students. It may not be reasonable to expect that every veterinary professional will have an opportunity to learn and practice each of the techniques in this book before graduation, but I hope that I have made this textbook detailed enough to encourage practitioners to use these techniques with confidence on clinical patients as the opportunity arises. With the help of this textbook, inexperience or unfamiliarity with a technique should no longer be a reason for failure to provide the best treatment or collect the appropriate diagnostic sample.

I embarked on this project hoping that having a fully illustrated clinical manual and CD would help students to learn these important diagnostic techniques better while decreasing the repetitive use of research animals for demonstration purposes. Initial funding for production of a diagnostic techniques CD was made possible by the Technology Enhanced Learning Initiative of the Province of Saskatchewan, and with Elsevier's support the project was expanded to include additional techniques and this book.

ACKNOWLEDGMENTS

- Drawings and figures: Juliane Deubner, University of Saskatchewan, and Don O'Connor, St. Louis
- Video production: Wayne Giesbrecht, University of Saskatchewan
- Photography: Stewart Auchterlonie, University of Saskatchewan

Susan Meric Taylor

Contents

Venous Blood Collection

1

PROCEDURE 1-1

Jugular Venipuncture

PURPOSE

To obtain a sample of venous blood for analysis

INDICATIONS

Collection of a blood sample for clinical pathology tests

CONTRAINDICATIONS AND CONCERNS

1. Jugular venipuncture should be avoided in patients with a severe coagulopathy.
2. Proper restraint is important to prevent excessive trauma to the vein, resulting in hematoma formation.

COMPLICATIONS

1. Hemorrhage
2. Subcutaneous hematoma formation

SPECIAL ANATOMY

Jugular vein: The right and left external jugular veins are large superficial veins that lie within the jugular furrow, a groove on each side of the neck dorsolateral to the trachea.

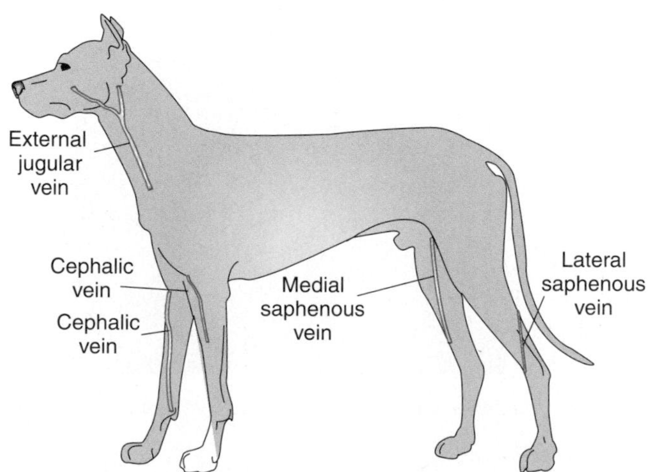

The veins accessible for collection of venous blood in dogs and cats.

EQUIPMENT

- 22- to 20-gauge, 1-inch needle
- Syringe
- 70% alcohol

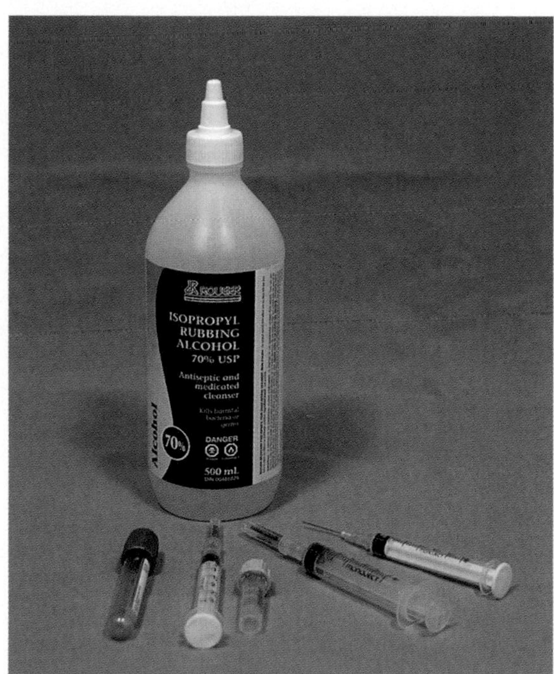

Equipment required for venipuncture in dogs and cats.

RESTRAINT

1. Small dogs and cats should be restrained on a table in sternal recumbency for jugular venipuncture. Grasp the front legs just above the carpal joints and pull the front legs off the edge of the table. Extend the animal's neck so that its nose is pointing toward the ceiling.

PROCEDURE 1-1 Jugular Venipuncture—cont'd

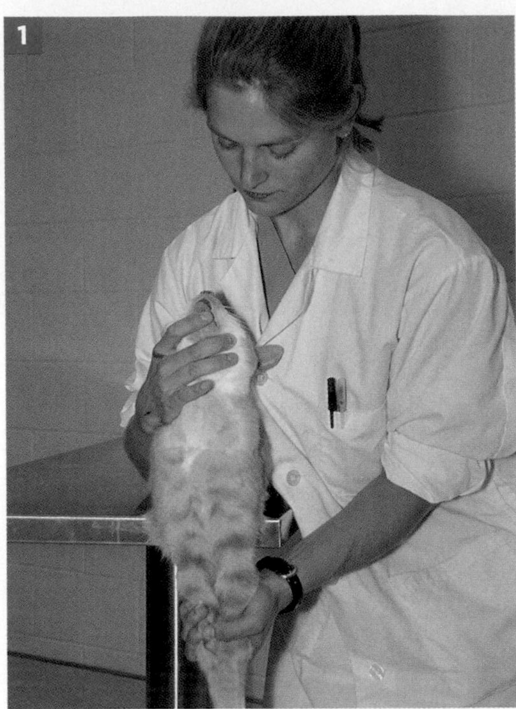

Restraining a cat for jugular venipuncture.

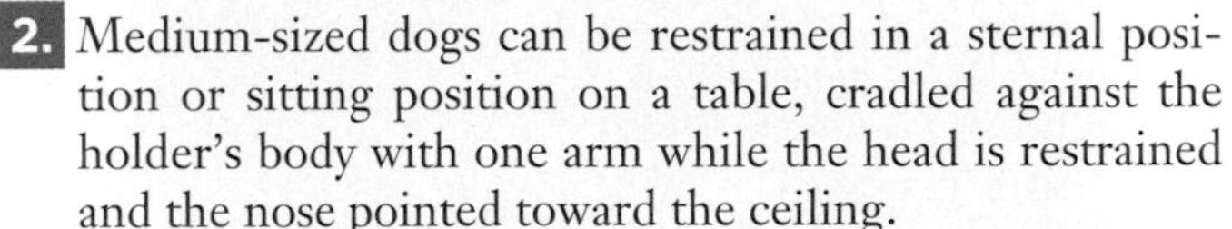

2. Medium-sized dogs can be restrained in a sternal position or sitting position on a table, cradled against the holder's body with one arm while the head is restrained and the nose pointed toward the ceiling.

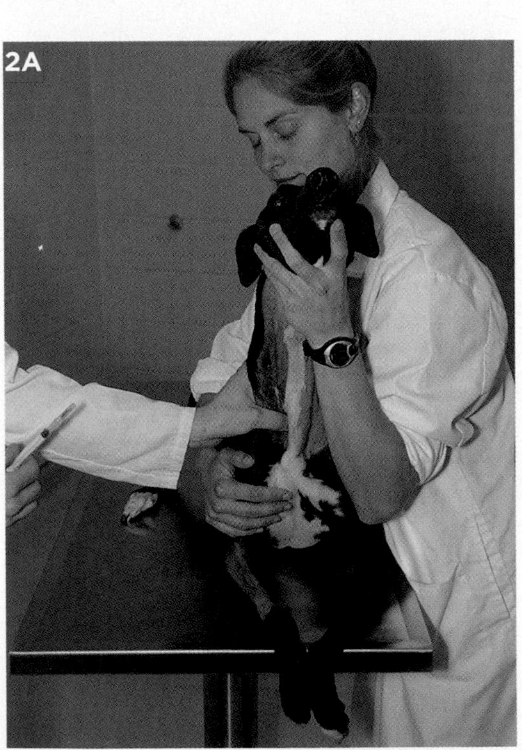

Restraining a medium-sized dog for jugular venipuncture.

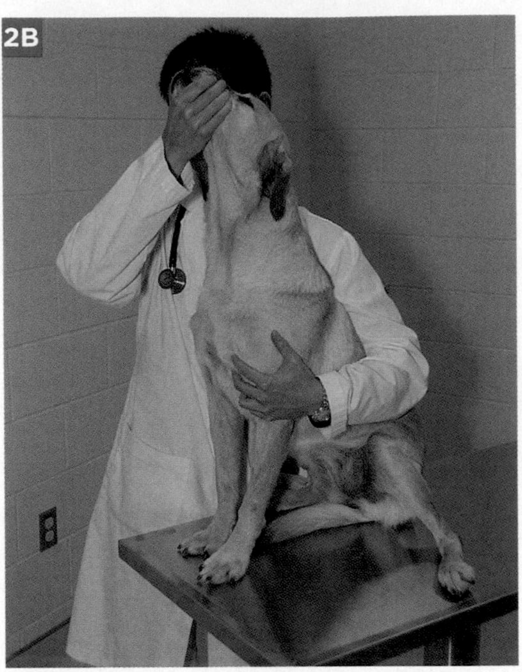

Restraining a medium-sized dog for jugular venipuncture.

3. Jugular venipuncture can be performed in large dogs while they sit on the floor, straddled by the restrainer, with the nose pointing toward the ceiling.

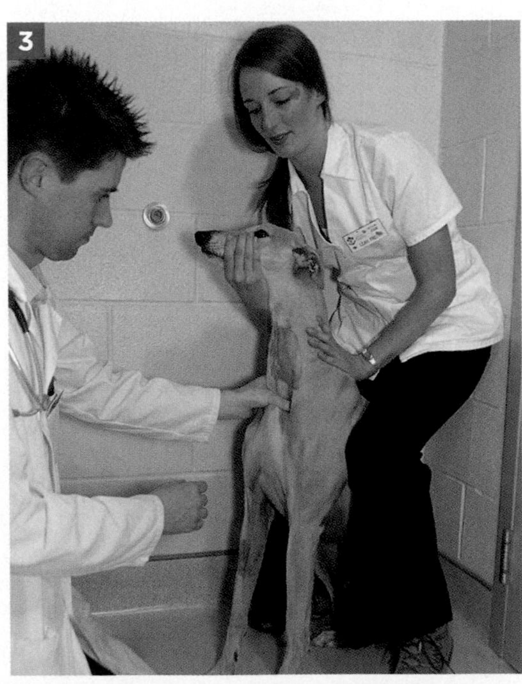

Restraining a large dog during jugular venipuncture.

TECHNIQUE

1. Anatomy

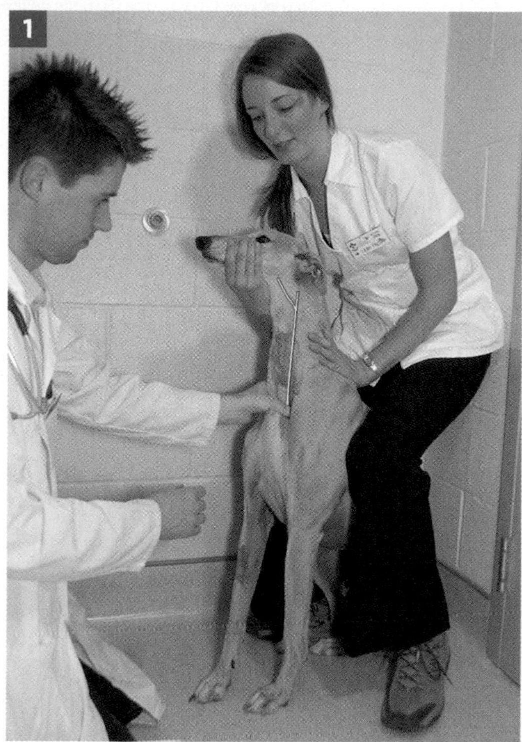

The external jugular vein is located within the jugular furrow, a groove on the side of the neck dorsolateral to the trachea.

2. Distend the vein with blood (raise the vein) by applying firm pressure at the thoracic inlet at the most ventral portion of the jugular furrow, lateral to the trachea.

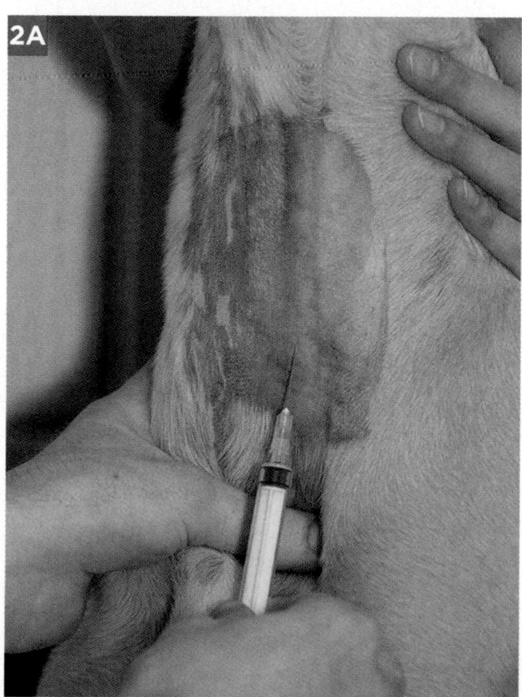

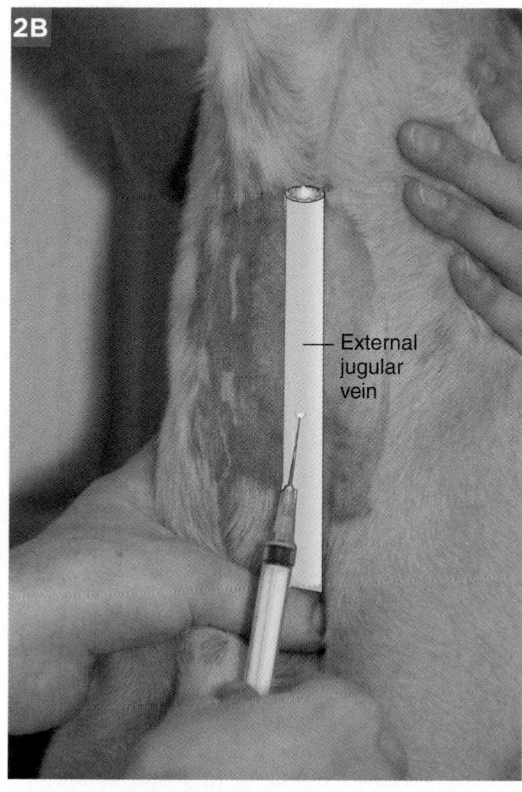

Distending the jugular vein.

3. Palpate the distended vein. If the vein cannot be seen or palpated, clip hair from a small area over the jugular furrow.

4. Apply alcohol and palpate the distended vein, tracing its path from the angle of the mandible to the thoracic inlet.

PROCEDURE 1-1 Jugular Venipuncture—cont'd

5. Insert the needle, bevel upward, at a 20- to 30-degree angle to the vein. Once the tip of the needle is in the vein, apply suction to collect the sample. If flow stops, attempt to withdraw the needle slightly to reestablish flow.

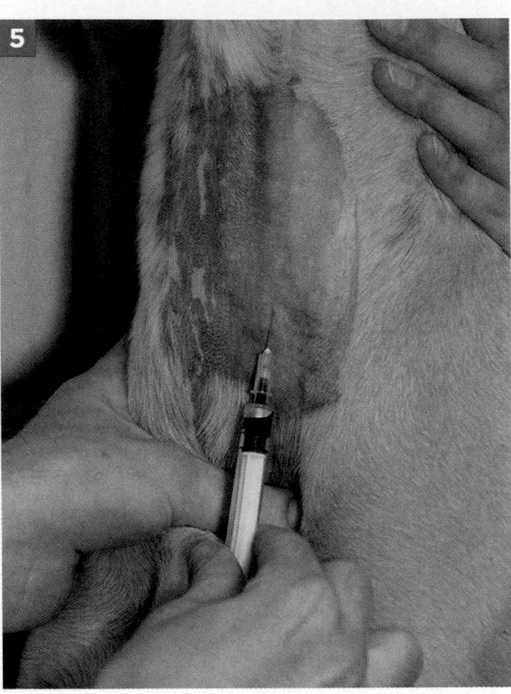

Applying suction to collect the sample.

6. Once the sample is collected, release the pressure on the vein, halt suction, and withdraw the needle from the vein. Place gentle pressure on the venipuncture site, and hold for approximately 60 seconds.

PROCEDURE 1-2

Jugular Venipuncture, Inverted Technique

PURPOSE

To obtain a sample of venous blood for analysis

INDICATIONS

Collection of a blood sample for clinical pathology tests

CONTRAINDICATIONS AND CONCERNS

1. Jugular venipuncture should be avoided in patients with a severe coagulopathy.
2. Proper restraint is important to prevent excessive trauma to the vein, resulting in hematoma formation.

COMPLICATIONS

1. Hemorrhage
2. Subcutaneous hematoma formation

SPECIAL ANATOMY

Jugular vein: The right and left external jugular veins are large superficial veins that lie within the jugular furrow, a groove on each side of the neck dorsolateral to the trachea.

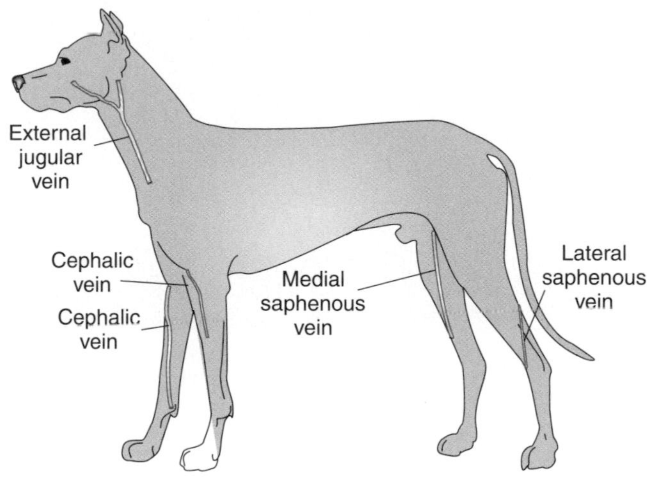

The veins accessible for collection of venous blood in dogs and cats.

EQUIPMENT

- 22- to 20-gauge, 1-inch needle
- Syringe
- 70% alcohol

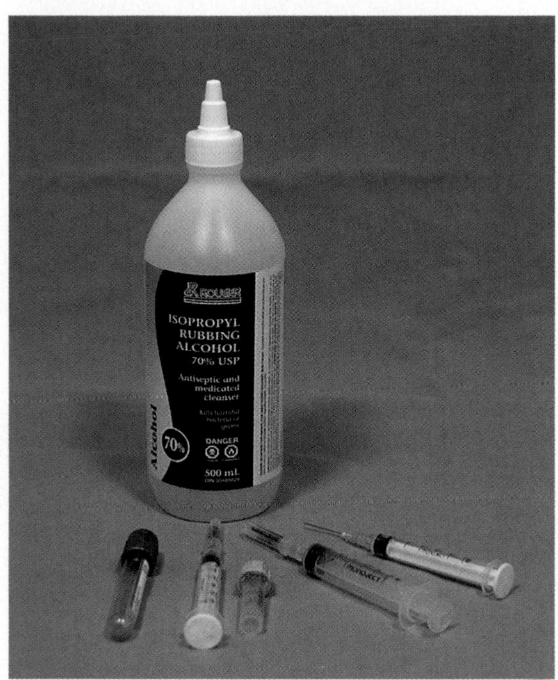

Equipment required for venipuncture in dogs and cats.

RESTRAINT

1. Some cats violently object to restraint for routine jugular venipuncture as described earlier. In these cats and in struggling young kittens and puppies, an inverted technique often is superior.
2. Place the animal in a cat bag or wrap it in a towel with only the head and neck accessible (Box 1-1).

PROCEDURE 1-2 Jugular Venipuncture, Inverted Technique—cont'd

BOX 1-1

Putting a Cat into a Cat Bag

A. Scruff the cat and place the cat on top of the open cat bag on the table.

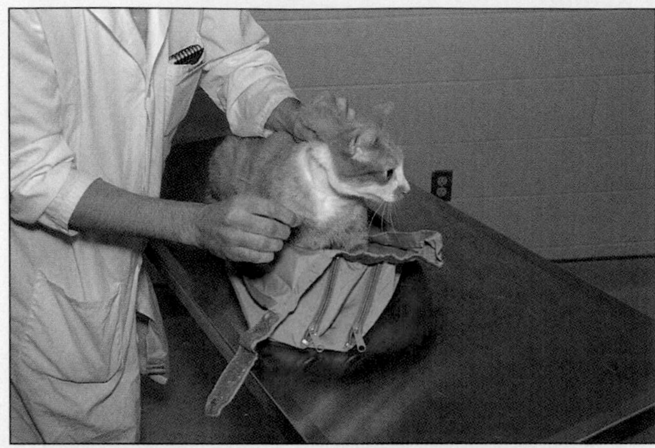

B. Fasten the Velcro band snugly around the cat's neck.

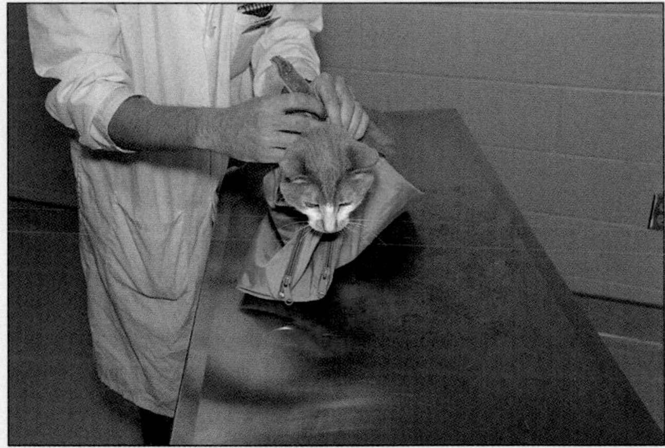

C. Grasp the cat's rear legs in one hand and curl them forward toward the cat's chest.

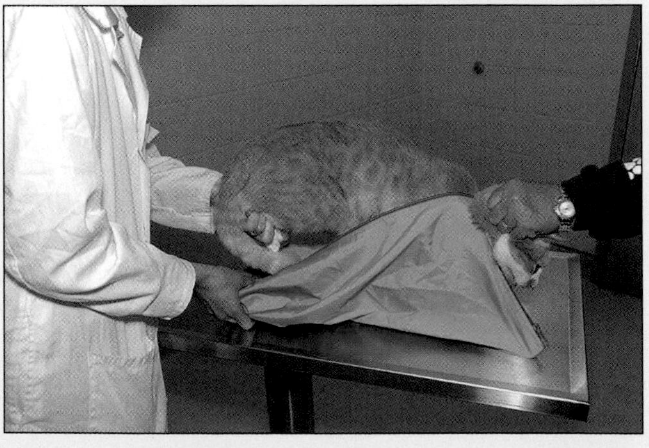

D. Zip up the back of the cat bag.

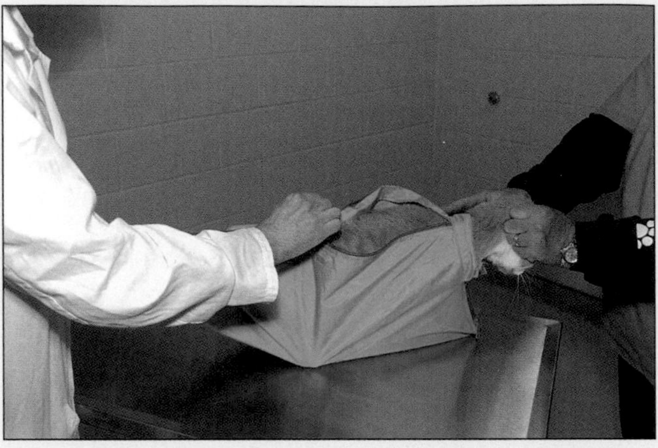

E. Cat in cat bag.

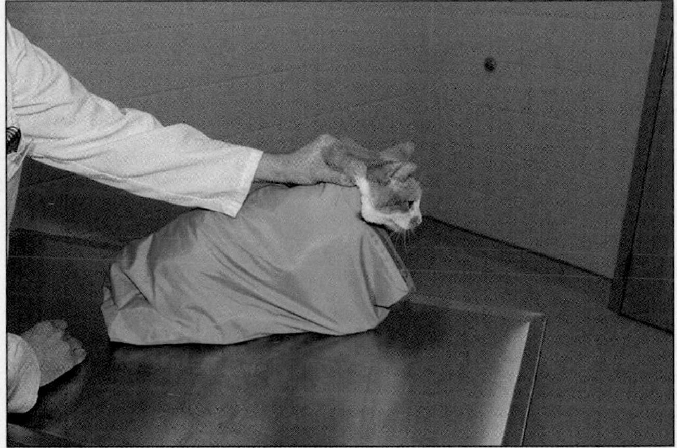

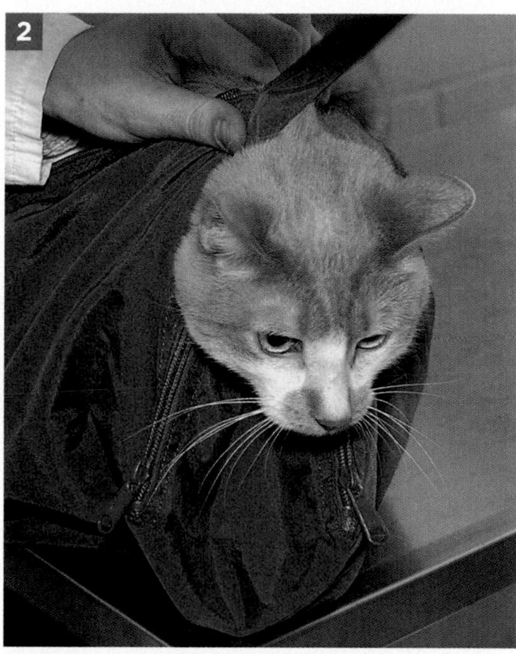

A cat restrained in a cat bag.

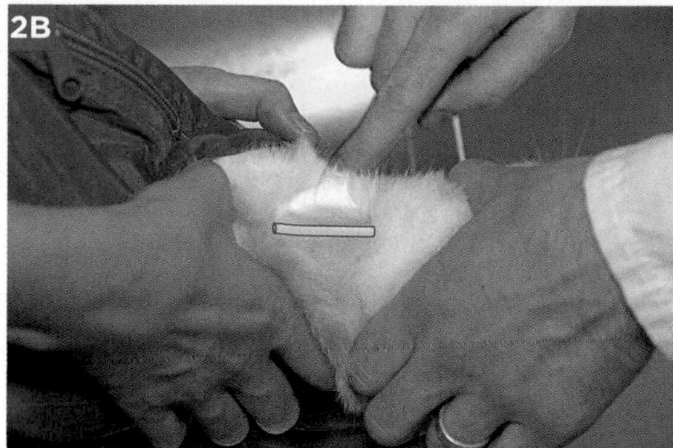

A cat restrained for inverted jugular venipuncture.

TECHNIQUE

1. Place the animal in dorsal recumbency on a table, and have the holder cradle it against their body with one arm. The holder should then compress the jugular vein in the thoracic inlet at the base of the jugular furrow, lateral to the trachea. This causes the jugular vein to distend with blood.
2. The venipuncturist should grasp the animal's head with one hand and rotate or manipulate the neck until the distended vein is visible or palpable. Clip hair from a small area over the jugular furrow if necessary, and apply alcohol.
3. Insert the needle, bevel upward, at a 20- to 30-degree angle to the vein. If the animal jumps or struggles, the venipuncturist can move with the animal because he or she has control of the head. Once the tip of the needle is in the vein, apply suction to collect the sample.
4. Once the sample is collected, have the holder release the pressure on the vein. Halt suction and withdraw the needle from the vein. Place gentle pressure on the venipuncture site, and hold for approximately 60 seconds.

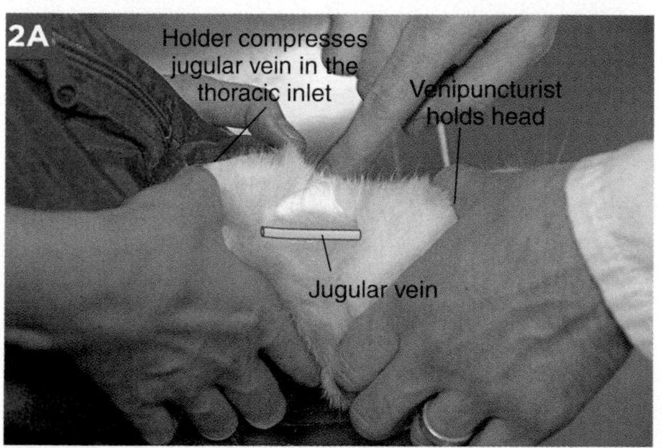

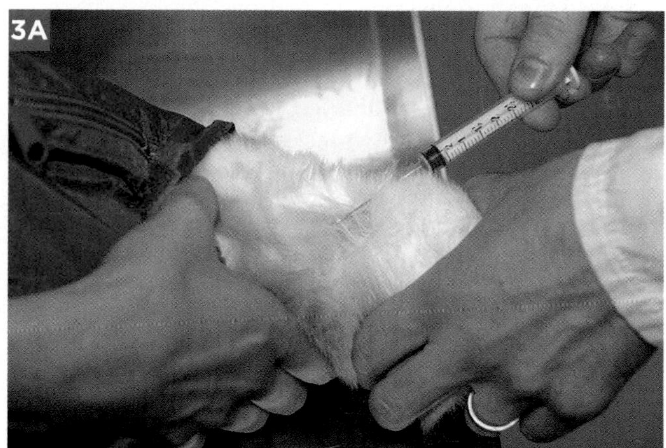

The needle is inserted bevel upward.

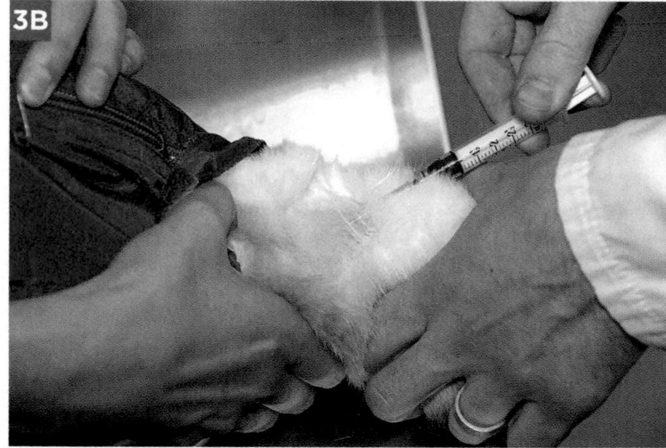

Suction is applied to collect the blood sample.

PROCEDURE 1-3

Cephalic Venipuncture

PURPOSE

To obtain a sample of venous blood for analysis

INDICATIONS

Collection of a blood sample for clinical pathology tests

CONTRAINDICATIONS AND CONCERNS

Proper restraint is important to prevent excessive trauma to the vein, resulting in hematoma formation.

COMPLICATIONS

1. Hemorrhage
2. Subcutaneous hematoma formation

SPECIAL ANATOMY

Cephalic vein: The right and left cephalic veins are superficial veins that lie on the anterior surface of the forearm, making them very accessible for venipuncture.

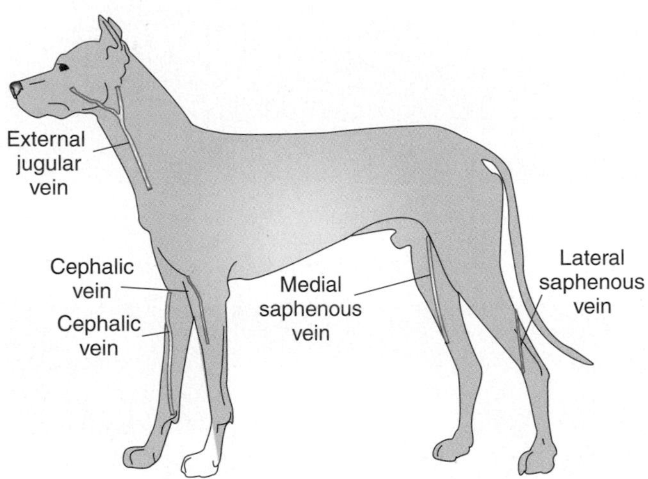

The veins accessible for collection of venous blood in dogs and cats.

EQUIPMENT

- 22- to 20-gauge, 1-inch needle
- Syringe
- 70% alcohol

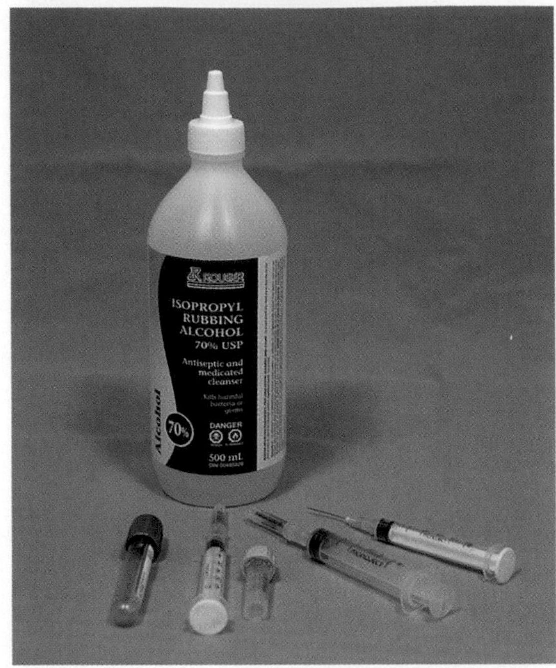

Equipment required for venipuncture in dogs and cats.

RESTRAINT

1. Place the animal in a sitting position or in sternal recumbency on a table or (for large dogs) on the floor.
2. The holder should stand on the side opposite the leg to be used, and should use one arm to restrain the animal's head by encircling the neck and turning the muzzle away from the leg to be used. The holder should use the other arm to extend the animal's front leg by holding the elbow and pushing the leg forward.

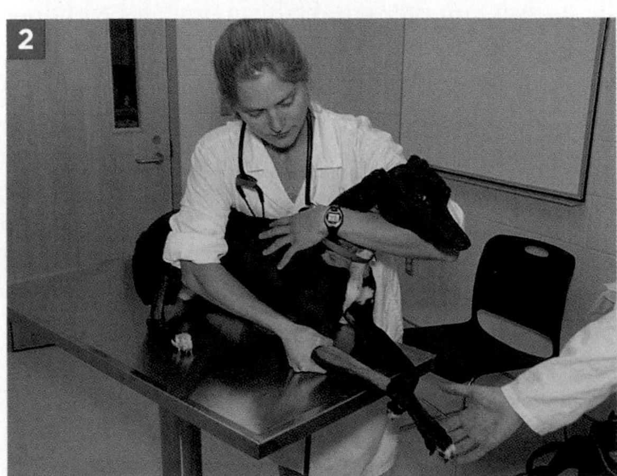

Proper restraint for cephalic venipuncture.

TECHNIQUE

1. Laterally roll and compress the cephalic vein

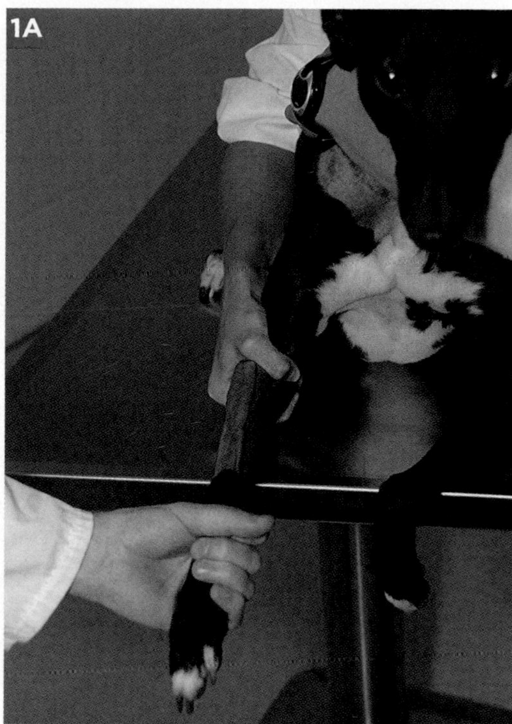

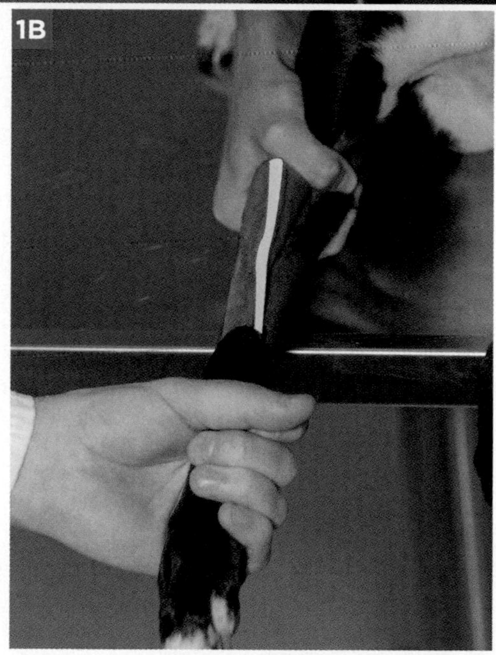

Using the thumb of the hand holding the leg, the cephalic vein is rolled laterally and compressed so that it becomes distended with blood.

2. If the vein cannot be seen or palpated, clip hair from a small area over the dorsal forearm, and apply alcohol.
3. The venipuncturist should grasp the paw to keep the leg extended. He or she should identify the distended cephalic vein and place the thumb alongside the vein to stabilize it during venipuncture.

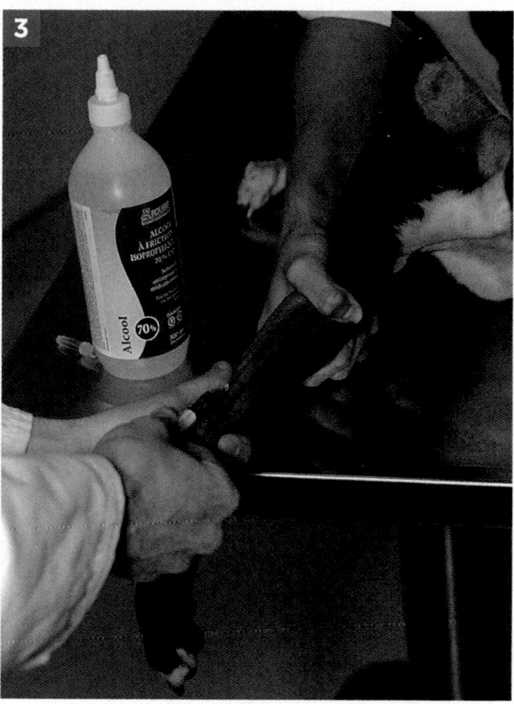

Stabilizing the cephalic vein.

4. Insert the needle, bevel upward, at a 20- to 30-degree angle to the vein. Once the tip of the needle is in the vein, apply suction to collect the sample.
5. Once the sample is collected, have the holder release the pressure on the vein. Halt suction and withdraw the needle from the vein. Place gentle pressure on the venipuncture site, and hold for approximately 60 seconds.

PROCEDURE 1-4

Lateral Saphenous Venipuncture

PURPOSE

To obtain a sample of venous blood for analysis

INDICATIONS

Collection of a blood sample for clinical pathology tests

CONTRAINDICATIONS AND CONCERNS

Proper restraint is important to prevent excessive trauma to the vein, resulting in hematoma formation.

COMPLICATIONS

1. Hemorrhage
2. Subcutaneous hematoma formation

SPECIAL ANATOMY

Lateral saphenous vein: The right and left lateral saphenous veins are small superficial veins that run diagonally across the lateral surface of the distal tibia.

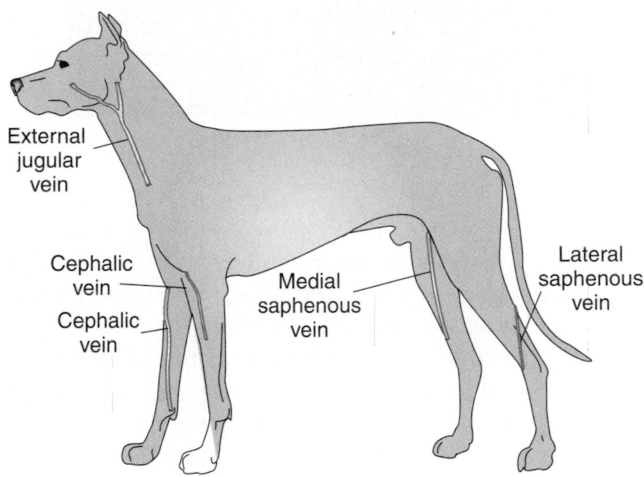

The veins accessible for collection of venous blood in dogs and cats.

EQUIPMENT

- 22- to 20-gauge, 1-inch needle
- Syringe
- 70% alcohol

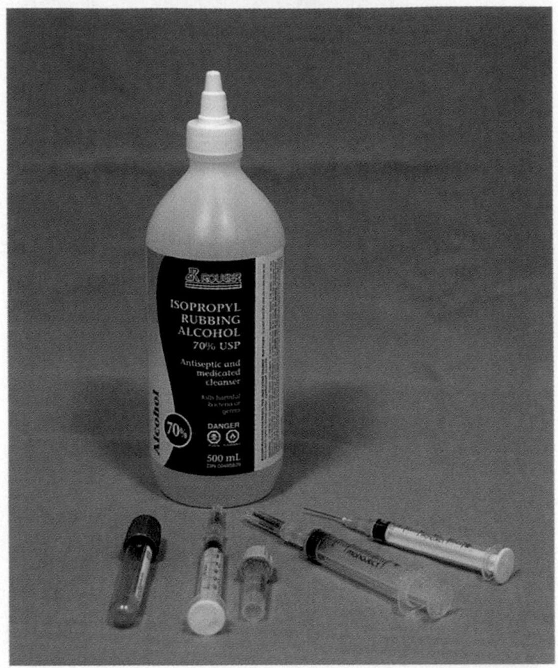

Equipment required for venipuncture in dogs and cats.

RESTRAINT

1. Restrain the animal in lateral recumbency with the legs toward the venipuncturist and the back toward the holder.
2. Have the holder restrain the animal by grasping the forelimbs with one hand and elevating them slightly off the table while applying pressure down on the neck of the patient with the same forearm. Grasp the uppermost hind leg with the other hand.

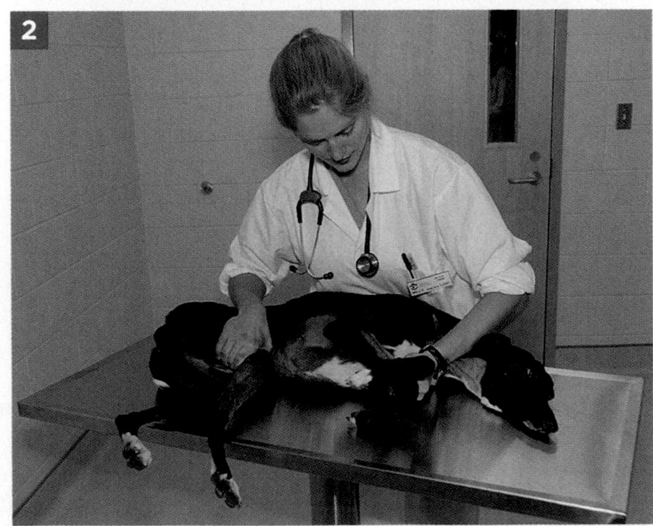

Proper restraint for lateral saphenous vein venipuncture.

TECHNIQUE

1. The holder should encircle the caudal aspect of the uppermost hind leg, applying firm pressure at the level of the stifle to compress the lateral saphenous vein and cause it to distend with blood.

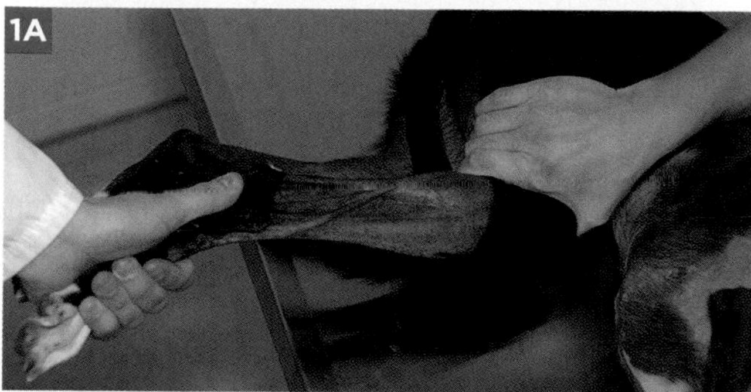

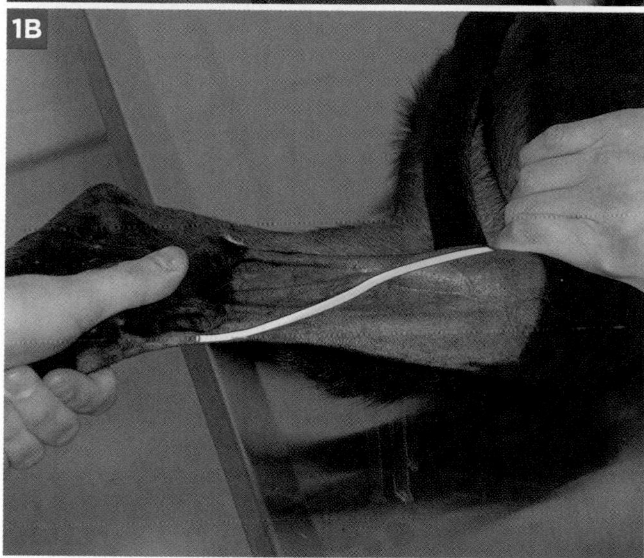

Compressing the lateral saphenous vein, causing it to distend with blood.

2. The venipuncturist should grasp the hind foot and palpate the distended vein. If the vein cannot be seen or palpated, clip hair from a small area over the vein and apply alcohol, while ensuring that the holder is compressing the vein adequately.
3. Once the vein is identified, the venipuncturist should place the thumb adjacent to the vein to stabilize it and prevent movement during venipuncture. Insert the needle, bevel upward, at a 20- to 30-degree angle to the vein. Once the tip of the needle is in the vein, apply suction to collect the sample.

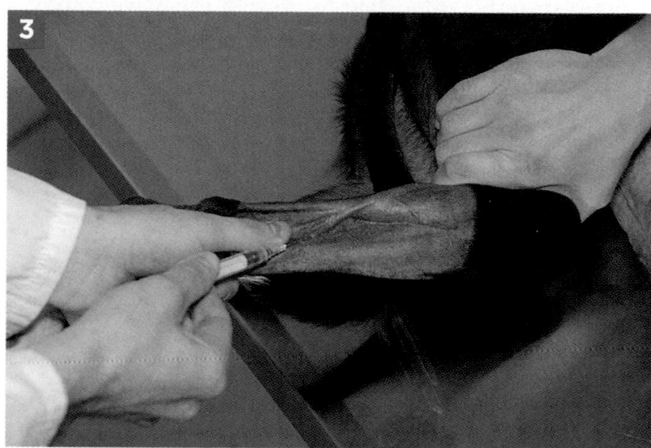

Stabilizing the lateral saphenous vein by placing the thumb adjacent to the vein during venipuncture.

4. Once the sample is collected, have the holder release pressure on the vein. Halt suction and withdraw the needle from the vein. Place gentle pressure on the venipuncture site, and hold for approximately 60 seconds.

PROCEDURE 1-5

Medial Saphenous Venipuncture

PURPOSE

To obtain a sample of venous blood for analysis

INDICATIONS

Collection of a blood sample for clinical pathology tests

CONTRAINDICATIONS AND CONCERNS

Proper restraint is important to prevent excessive trauma to the vein, resulting in hematoma formation.

COMPLICATIONS

1. Hemorrhage
2. Subcutaneous hematoma formation

SPECIAL ANATOMY

Medial saphenous vein: The right and left medial saphenous veins are very superficial veins with a long straight course up the midline of the medial surface of the rear limb, making them a preferred site for venipuncture in cats.

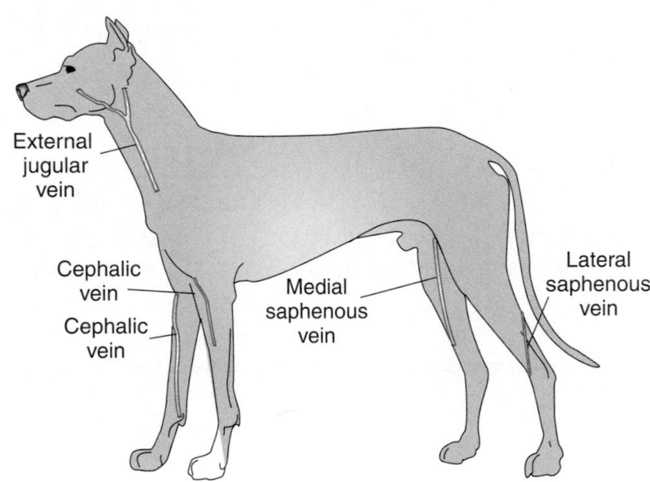

The veins accessible for collection of venous blood in dogs and cats.

EQUIPMENT

- 22- to 20-gauge, 1-inch needle
- Syringe
- 70% alcohol

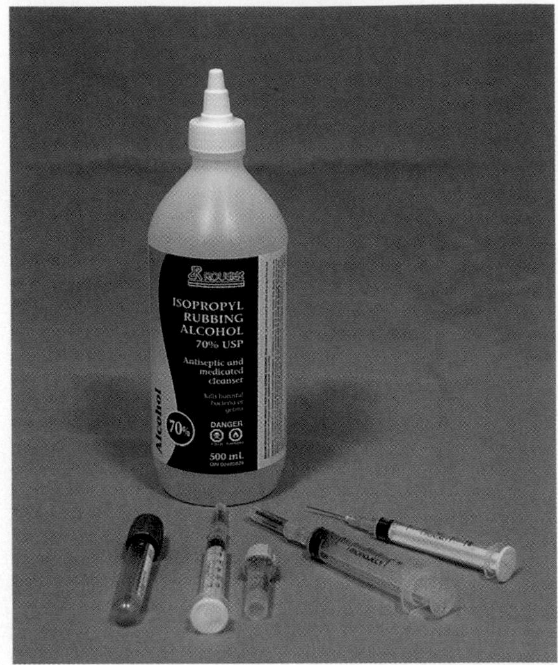

Equipment required for venipuncture in dogs and cats.

RESTRAINT

1. The medial saphenous vein is most useful in cats. Restrain the cat in lateral recumbency with the legs toward the venipuncturist and the back toward the holder.
2. Have the holder scruff and stretch the cat with one hand while retracting the uppermost hind leg with the other hand.

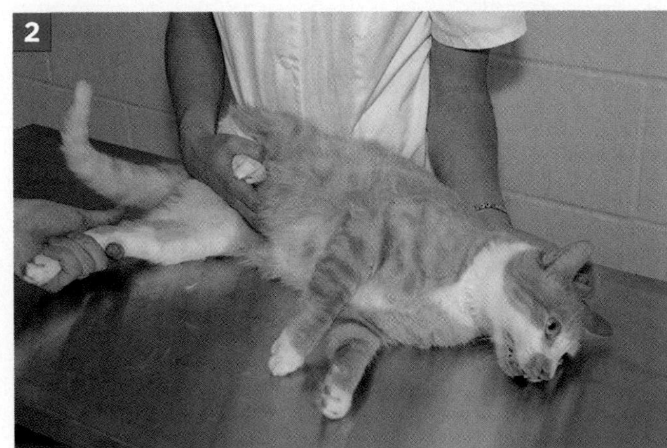

Proper restraint of a cat for medial saphenous venipuncture.

3. The venipuncturist should grasp the metatarsal region of the rear limb closest to the table and extend the leg.

TECHNIQUE

1. The holder should apply pressure in the inguinal region to occlude the medial saphenous vein and cause it to distend with blood.

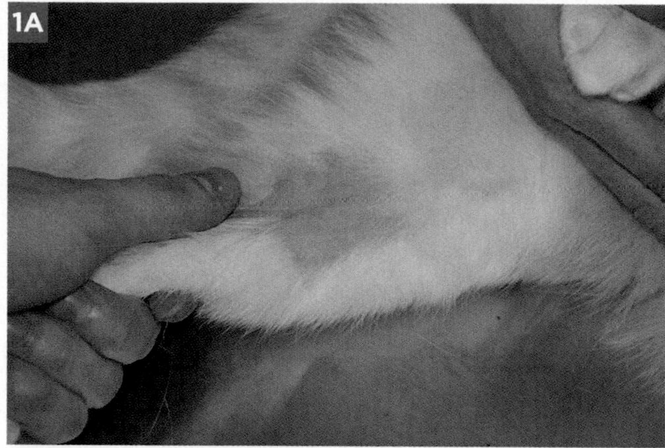

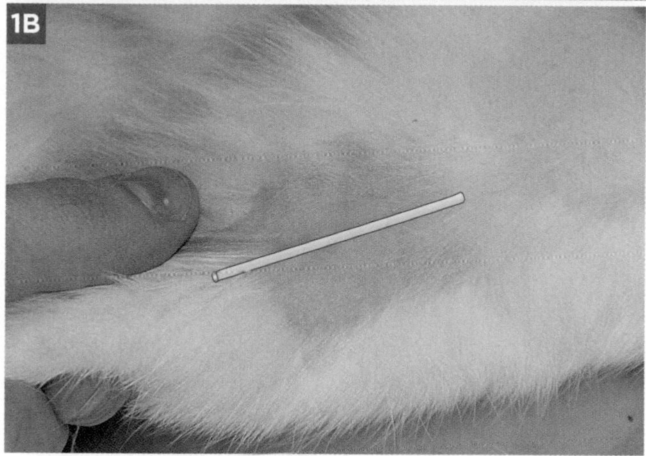

Occluding the medial saphenous vein, causing it to distend with blood.

2. The venipuncturist should observe and palpate the distended vein. If the vein cannot be seen or palpated, or if there is a heavy haircoat on the medial limb, the hair should be clipped from a small area over the vein and alcohol applied while ensuring that the holder is compressing the vein adequately.
3. Once the vein is identified, the venipuncturist should place the thumb adjacent to the vein to stabilize it and prevent movement during venipuncture.
4. Ideally attempts at venipuncture should start quite distal on the limb in case it is necessary to make more than one attempt at venipuncture.
5. While holding the leg to prevent movement and stabilizing the vein with the thumb, the needle should be inserted, bevel upward, into the vein. Once the tip of the needle is in the vein, apply very slight suction to collect the sample. This vein has a small diameter, so excessive suction will cause the vessel to collapse.

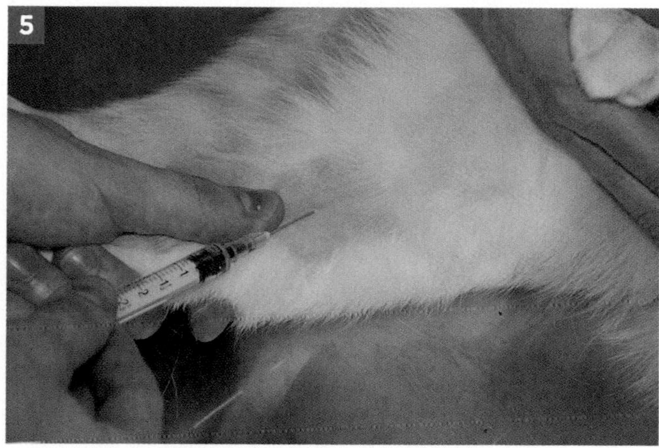

Inserting the needle, bevel upward, into the medial saphenous vein.

6. Once the sample is collected have the holder release pressure on the vein. Halt suction and withdraw the needle from the vein. Place gentle pressure on the venipuncture site, and hold for approximately 60 seconds.

Arterial Blood Collection

2

PROCEDURE 2-1

Arterial Blood Collection from the Femoral Artery

PURPOSE

To obtain a sample of arterial blood for analysis

INDICATIONS

1. To monitor respiratory function
2. To assess acid-base status in seriously ill animals
3. To assess oxygenation during the diagnostic evaluation of polycythemia

CONTRAINDICATIONS AND CONCERNS

1. Arterial puncture should be avoided in patients with significant coagulopathy or thrombocytopenia.
2. Arterial blood collection is difficult in patients with hypotension and poor perfusion, making palpation of the arterial pulse difficult.

COMPLICATIONS

1. Hematoma formation is common if pressure is not applied to the artery after sampling.
2. When air bubbles are not removed from the sample or the sample is not capped, blood gas values change as the sample equilibrates with room air.
3. Excessive heparinization of the sample reduces measured carbon dioxide content ($PaCO_2$).
4. Storage of the sample for longer than 2 to 4 hours, even on ice, can lead to erroneous results.

SPECIAL ANATOMY

The femoral artery can be palpated near the midline of the proximal medial aspect of the thigh, just cranial to the palpable pectineus muscle. This artery runs from proximal to distal, adjacent to and just anterior to the femoral vein.

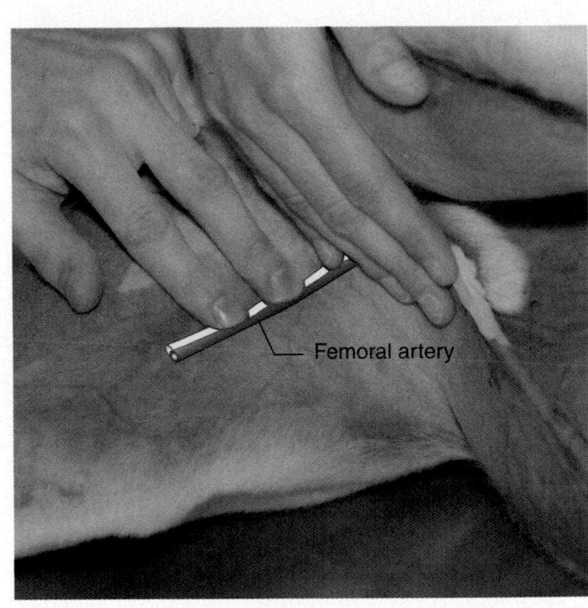

The femoral artery can be palpated near the midline of the proximal medial aspect of the thigh.

EQUIPMENT NEEDED

- 3-mL syringe
- 25- or 22-gauge needle
- Sodium heparin 1000 units/mL *or*
- Arterial blood gas syringe containing a lyophilized heparin tablet

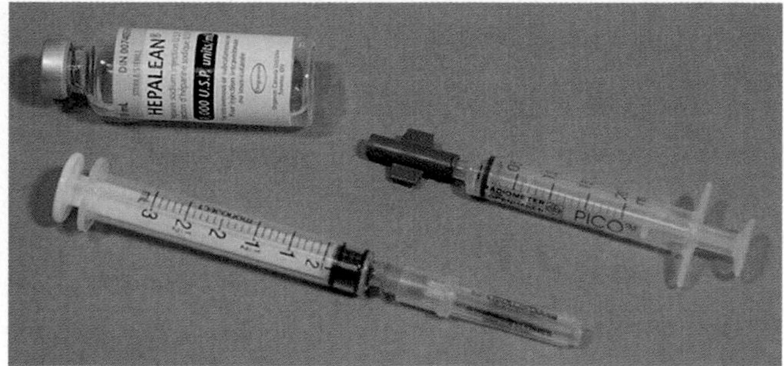

Equipment required for arterial blood collection.

PREPARATION

1. Take and record the patient's temperature if the blood gas analyzer being used adjusts for body temperature.
2. Use a pre-heparinized arterial blood gas syringe if available, or heparinize a syringe by drawing heparin (1000 units/mL) into a 3-mL syringe with a 25-gauge needle to coat the syringe, then expelling all of the heparin out of the syringe.

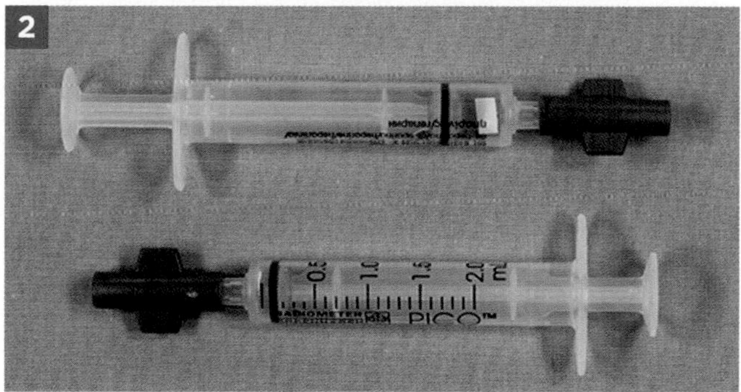

Arterial blood gas syringe containing a lyophilized heparin tablet.

TECHNIQUE

1. Restrain the patient in lateral recumbency and abduct and flex the upper rear leg to allow access to the lower limb. Extend the lower hind leg by maintaining some traction on the foot. It may be necessary for an assistant to retract folds of skin, the caudal mammary glands, or the prepuce to allow access to the inguinal region.

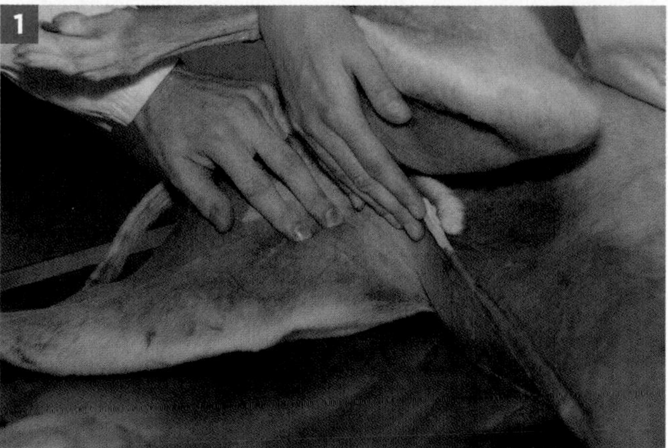

Restraint for collection of blood from the femoral artery.

2. Clip over the femoral artery if necessary and apply alcohol to the site.
3. Palpate the femoral artery as high up in the inguinal area as possible with the first and second fingers of the nondominant hand. Gently rest the fingertips against the artery so that the arterial pulse can be palpated with both fingers.

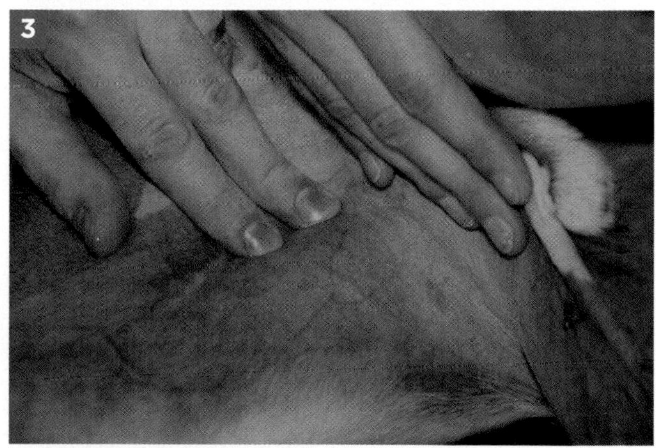

Palpating the femoral arterial pulse with the first and second fingers of the nondominant hand.

PROCEDURE 2-1 Arterial Blood Collection from the Femoral Artery—cont'd

4. Insert the needle attached to the heparinized syringe into the pulsing artery between the two fingers.

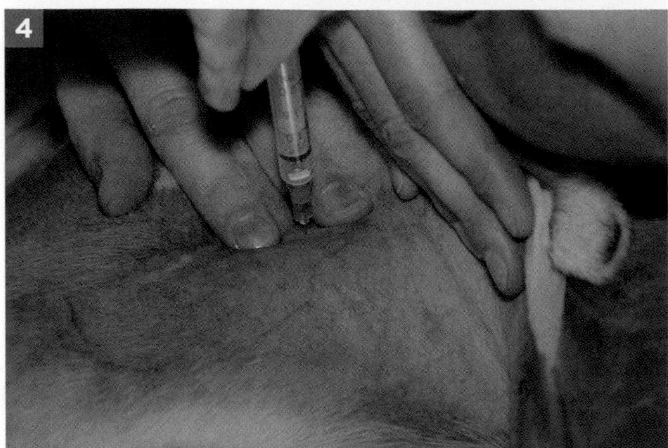

Inserting the needle into the pulsing femoral artery.

5. When the artery has been penetrated, a flash of blood will appear in the hub of the needle.

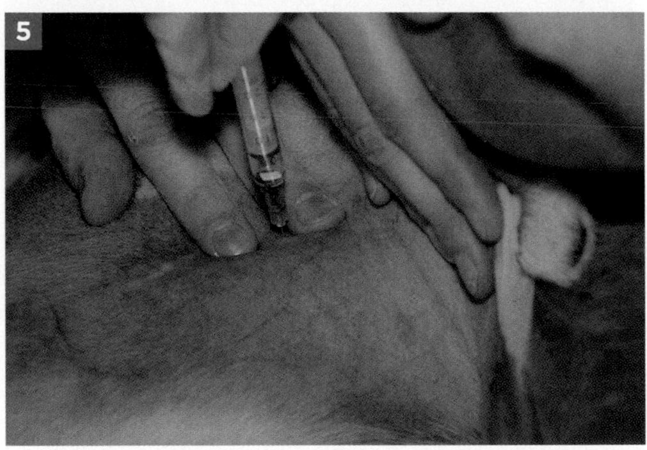

A flash of blood appears in the hub of the needle.

6. Hold the needle steady and obtain the sample by aspiration.
7. Once the sample is obtained, withdraw the needle and apply immediate direct pressure over the puncture site. Maintain pressure for 3 minutes to prevent hematoma formation.
8. Remove all air bubbles from the syringe and needle, and cap the sample in an airtight manner. Analyze the sample as soon as possible. If there will be a delay, the sample should be maintained on ice.

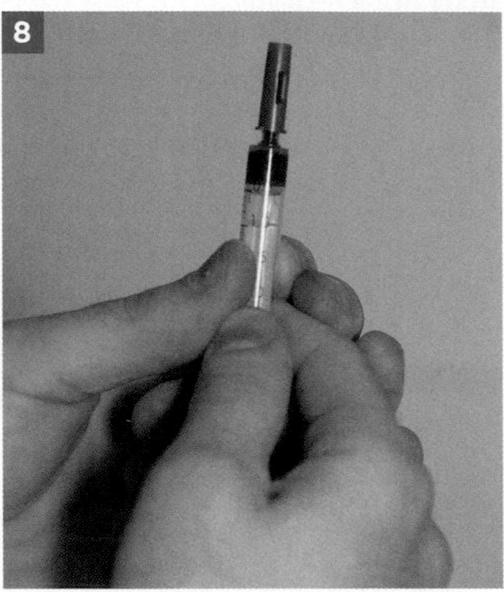

Removing air bubbles from the syringe and capping the sample in an airtight manner.

PROCEDURE 2-2

Arterial Blood Collection from the Dorsal Pedal Artery

PURPOSE

To obtain a sample of arterial blood for analysis

INDICATIONS

1. To monitor respiratory function.
2. To assess acid-base status in seriously ill animals
3. To assess oxygenation during the diagnostic evaluation of polycythemia

CONTRAINDICATIONS AND CONCERNS

1. Arterial puncture should be avoided in patients with significant coagulopathy or thrombocytopenia.
2. Arterial blood collection is difficult in patients with hypotension and poor perfusion, making palpation of the arterial pulse difficult.

COMPLICATIONS

1. Hematoma formation is common if pressure is not applied to the artery after sampling.
2. When air bubbles are not removed from the sample or the sample is not capped, blood gas values change as the sample equilibrates with room air.
3. Excessive heparinization of the sample reduces measured carbon dioxide content ($PaCO_2$).
4. Storage of the sample for longer than 2 to 4 hours, even on ice can lead to erroneous results.

SPECIAL ANATOMY

The dorsal pedal, or metatarsal, artery is located on the anterior surface of the hind leg, slightly medial to midline, over the hock and proximal metatarsals. This artery closely parallels and lies just medial to the distal course of the long digital extensor tendon, between the second and third metatarsal bones.

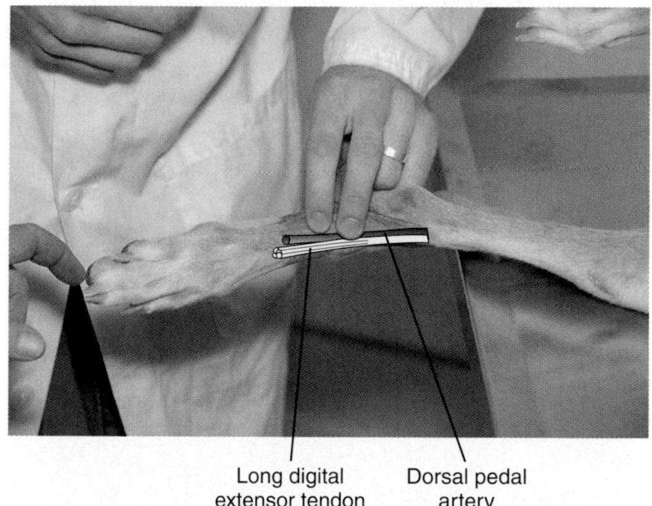

The dorsal pedal artery is located slightly medial to midline, over the hock and proximal metatarsal bones.

EQUIPMENT

- 3-mL syringe
- 25- or 22-gauge needle
- Sodium heparin 1000 units/mL *or*
- Arterial blood gas syringe containing a lyophilized heparin tablet

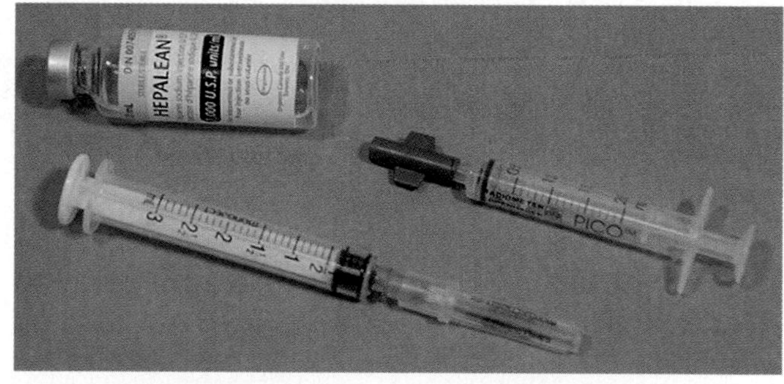

Equipment required for arterial blood collection.

PROCEDURE 2-2 Arterial Blood Collection from the Dorsal Pedal Artery—cont'd

PREPARATION

1. Take and record the patient's temperature if the blood gas analyzer being used adjusts for body temperature.
2. Use a pre-heparinized arterial blood gas syringe if available, or heparinize a syringe by drawing heparin (1000 units/mL) into a 3-mL syringe with a 25-gauge needle to coat the syringe, then expelling all of the heparin out of the syringe.

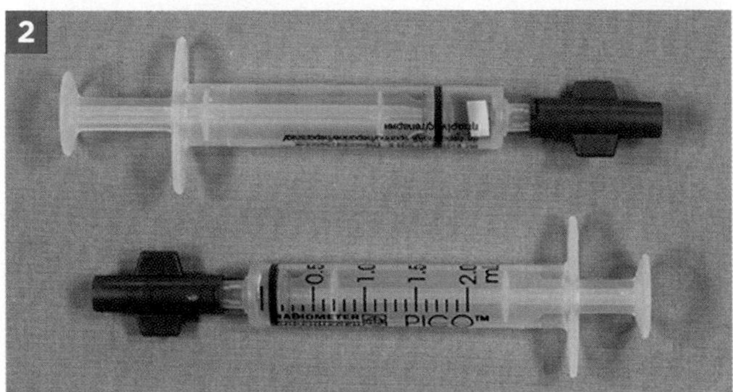

Arterial blood gas syringe containing a lyophilized heparin tablet.

TECHNIQUE

1. Restrain the patient in a comfortable position. This may be lateral or dorsal recumbency or being cradled in the holder's lap.
2. Clip over the cranial metatarsal and tarsal region and apply alcohol to the site.
3. Identify a pulse by palpation of the dorsal pedal artery just medial to the distal course of the long digital extensor tendon on the anterior surface of the metatarsal region.

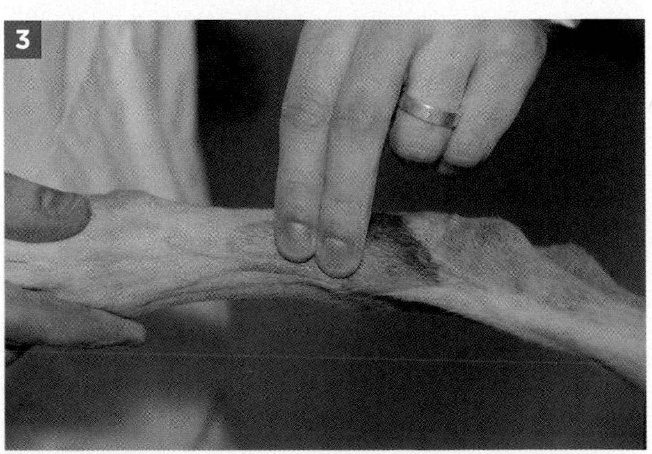

Palpating the dorsal pedal artery just medial to the distal course of the long digital extensor tendon on the anterior surface of the metatarsal region.

4. Palpate the artery with the first and second fingers of the nondominant hand, gently resting the fingertips against the artery so that the arterial pulse can be palpated with both fingers.

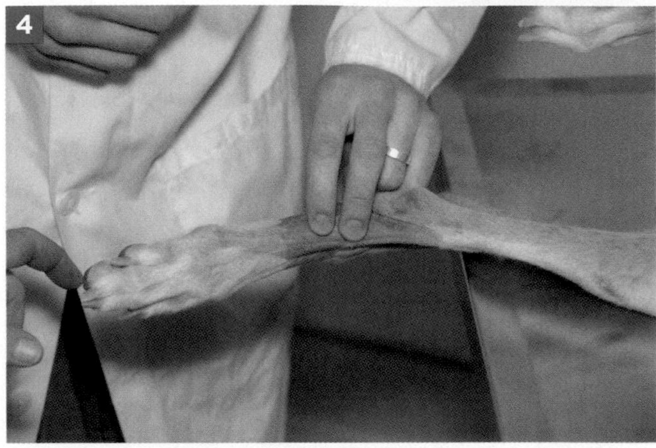

Palpate the dorsal pedal artery with the first and second fingers of the nondominant hand.

5. Insert the needle attached to the heparinized syringe into the pulsing artery between the two fingers.

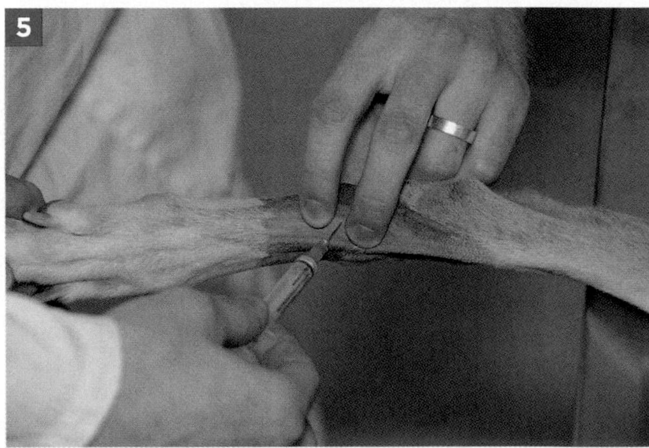

Inserting the needle into the pulsing dorsal pedal artery.

6. When the artery has been penetrated, a flash of blood will appear in the hub of the needle.

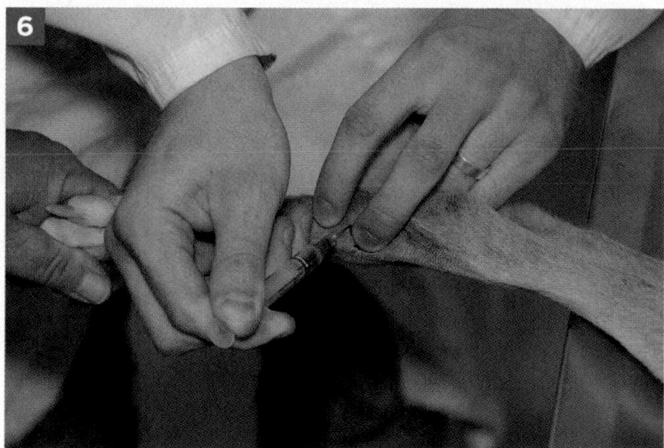

A flash of blood will appear in the hub of the needle.

7. Hold the needle steady and obtain the sample by aspiration.

8. Once the sample is obtained, withdraw the needle and apply immediate direct pressure over the puncture site. Maintain pressure for 3 minutes to prevent hematoma formation.

9. Remove all air bubbles from the syringe and needle, and cap the sample in an airtight manner. Analyze the sample as soon as possible. If there will be a delay, the sample should be maintained on ice.

Injection Techniques

3

PROCEDURE 3-1
Intravenous Injections

PURPOSE

To administer fluids, drugs, biologic preparations, or test substances by injection

INDICATIONS

Parenteral administration of drugs, biologic preparations, or test substances for treatment or diagnostic evaluation

CONTRAINDICATIONS AND CONCERNS

1. Intravenous and intramuscular injections should be avoided in patients with a severe coagulopathy.
2. To avoid potentially serious local or systemic reactions, all injectable substances should be administered only by the route recommended by the manufacturer.

SPECIAL ANATOMY

Intravenous injections are usually administered into the cephalic, lateral saphenous, or medial saphenous veins.

EQUIPMENT

- 25- to 20-gauge, 1-inch needle
- Syringe
- 70% alcohol

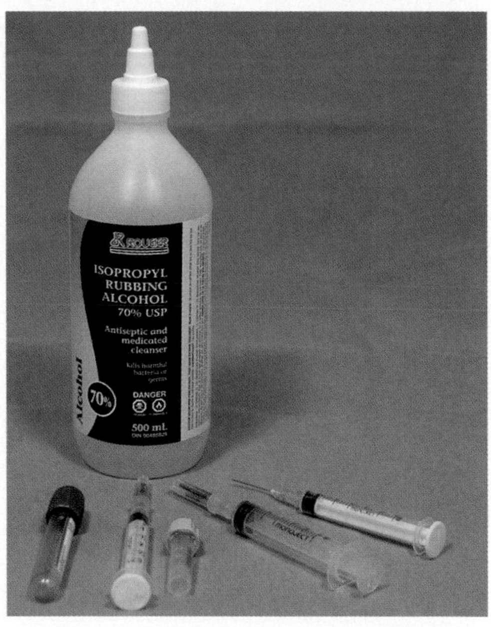

Equipment required for injections.

TECHNIQUE

1. Draw up the material to be administered into a syringe.
2. Place the animal into the appropriate position for access to the cephalic, lateral saphenous, or medial saphenous vein and restrain as described for venipuncture.
3. Follow the procedure described for blood collection from each vein and identify the distended vein.
4. Once the needle is inserted into the vein, aspirate a small amount of blood into the needle hub to confirm intravenous placement of the needle.

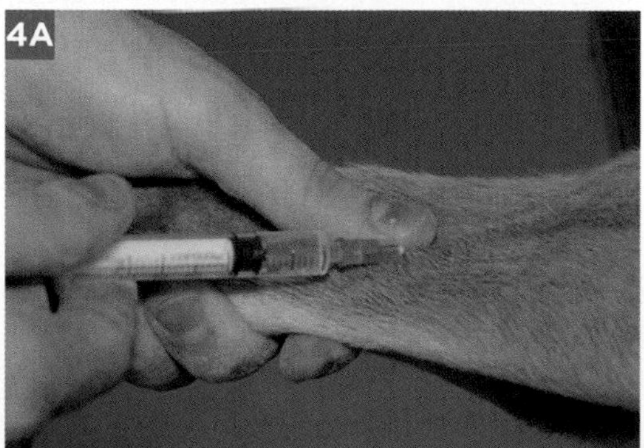

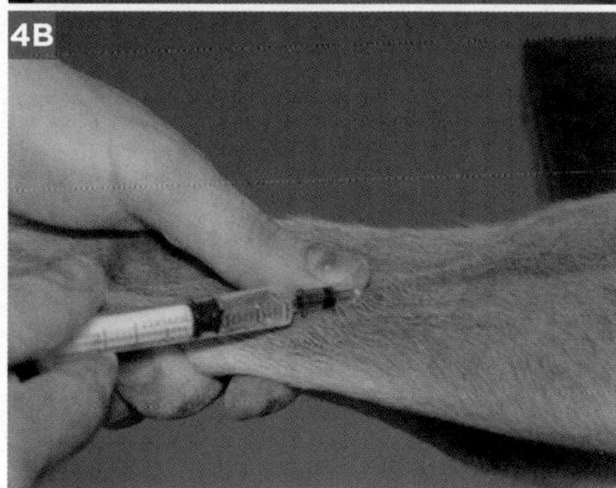

Aspirating a small amount of blood into the needle hub to confirm intravenous placement of the needle.

5. Once needle placement in the vein is confirmed, the holder should release the pressure occluding the vein, allowing injection into the vein.

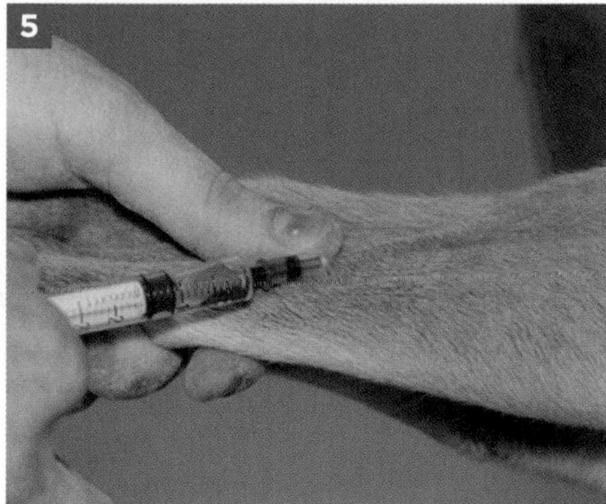

Releasing the pressure occluding the vein, allowing injection into the vein.

6. Once the injection is complete, withdraw the needle from the vein and immediately apply pressure to the venipuncture site. Maintain pressure for at least 60 seconds.
7. If needed to prevent hemorrhage, apply a light compressive bandage over the site.

PROCEDURE 3-2

Intramuscular Injections

PURPOSE

To administer fluids, drugs, biologic preparations, or test substances by injection

INDICATIONS

Parenteral administration of drugs, biologic preparations, or test substances for treatment or diagnostic evaluation

CONTRAINDICATIONS AND CONCERNS

1. Intravenous and intramuscular injections should be avoided in patients with a severe coagulopathy.
2. To avoid potentially serious local or systemic reactions, all injectable substances should be administered only by the route recommended by the manufacturer.

SPECIAL ANATOMY

Intramuscular injections can be given into the quadriceps muscle group of the anterior thigh, the semimembranosus-semitendinosus muscle group of the caudal thigh, the triceps muscle group of the caudal proximal front limb, or the lumbodorsal muscles on either side of the lumbar vertebrae. When the muscles of the thigh are used for injections, it is important to avoid needle puncture or injection into the sciatic nerve, which runs caudal to the femur.

EQUIPMENT

- 25- to 20-gauge, 1-inch needle
- Syringe
- 70% alcohol

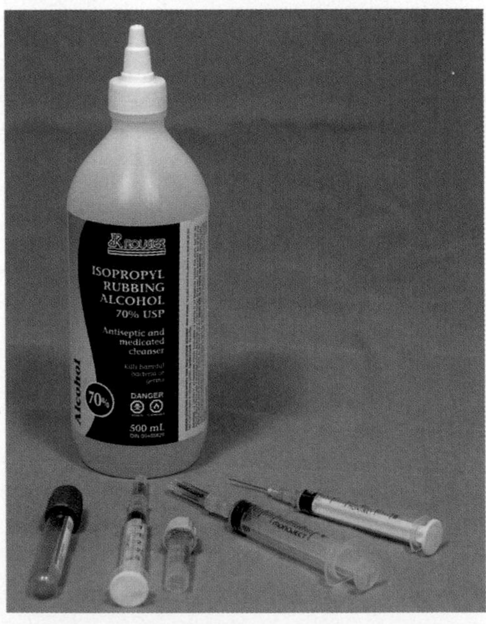

Equipment required for injections.

TECHNIQUE

1. Draw up the material to be administered into a syringe. The maximum volume that should be injected intramuscularly is 2 mL in a cat and 3 to 5 mL in a dog.
2. Restrain the animal in a standing or sitting position or in lateral recumbency. Intramuscular injections often cause some discomfort, so it is important to maintain control of the head and neck in dogs during this procedure. Cats should be scruffed and stretched as described for medial saphenous venipuncture.

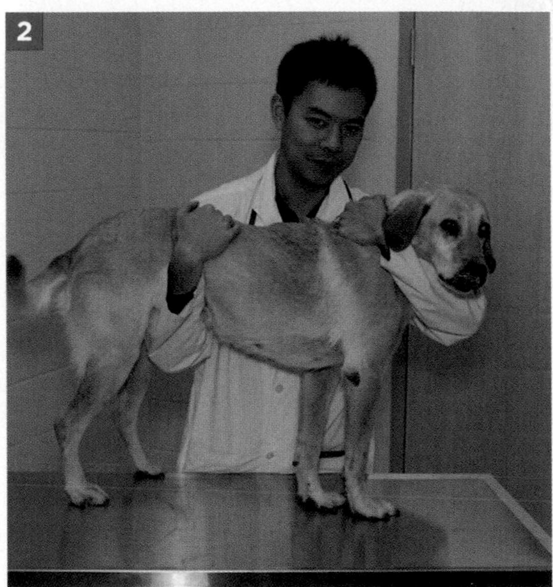

Restraint for intramuscular injection.

3. Swab the skin over the intended injection site with 70% alcohol.

4. When an injection is administered into the semimembranosus-semitendinosus (hamstring) muscle group, the thumb of the noninjecting hand should be placed in the groove just caudal to the femur, and the needle should be inserted caudal to the femur with its tip directed caudally so that even if the animal jumps or moves there is no risk of damage to the sciatic nerve.

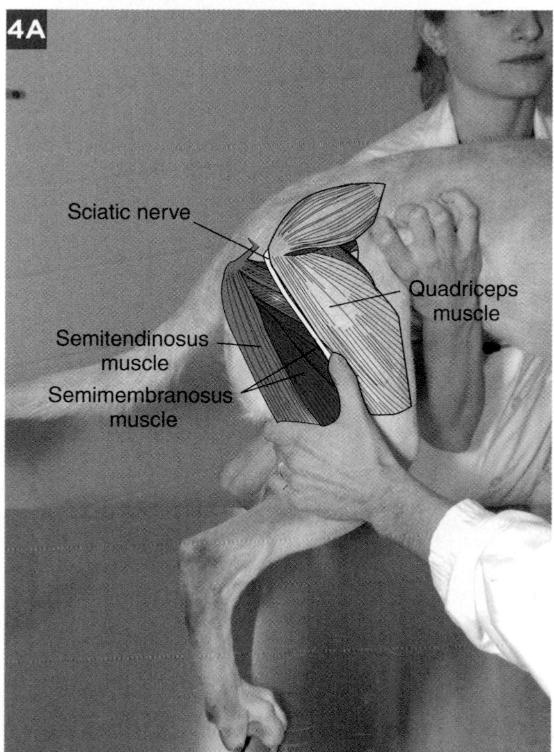

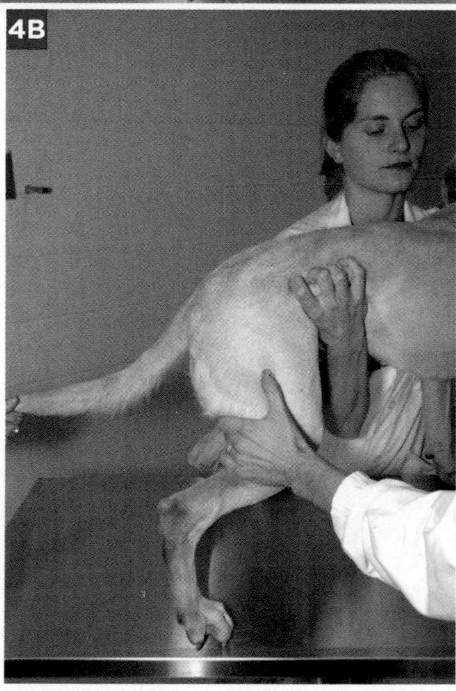

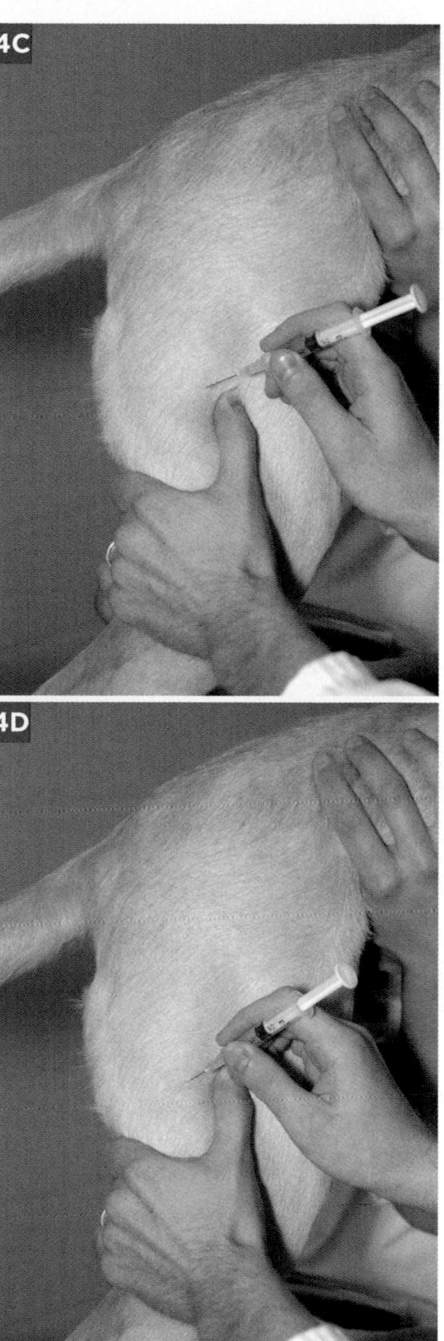

Proper technique for administering an injection into the hamstring muscles of a dog.

PROCEDURE 3-2 Intramuscular Injections—cont'd

5. When an injection is administered into the quadriceps muscle, the thumb of the noninjecting hand should be placed on the lateral femur, and the needle should be inserted cranial to the femur with its tip directed cranially.

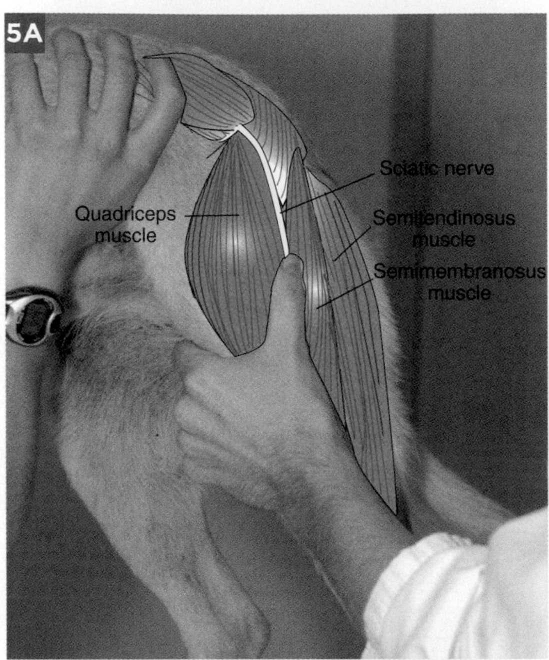

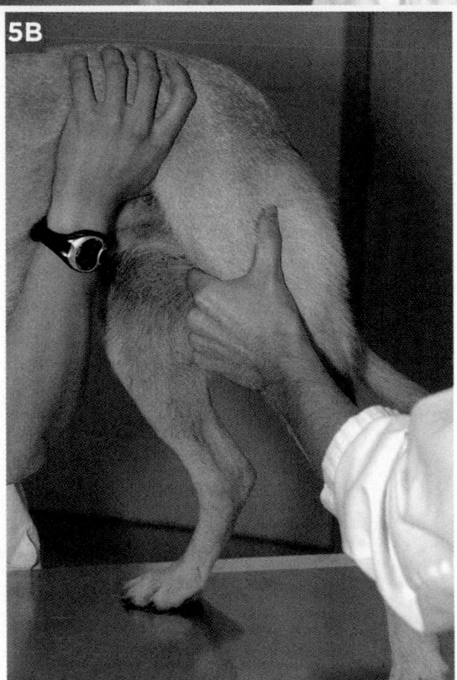

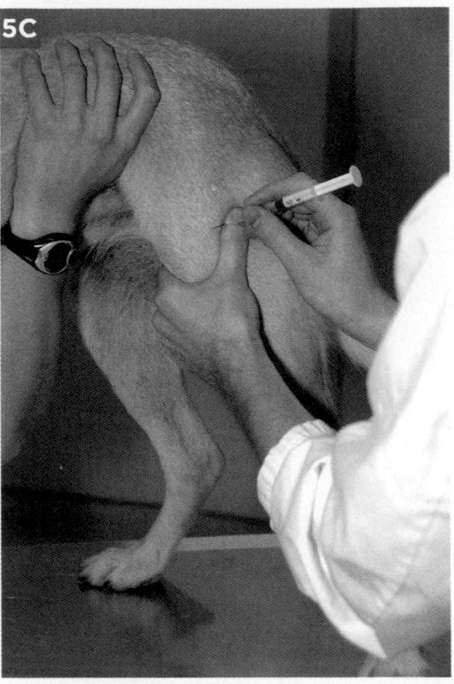

Proper technique for administering an injection into the quadriceps muscle of a dog.

6. When administering an injection into the triceps muscle group of the forelimb, the muscle belly should be grasped in the noninjecting hand, with the thumb on the humerus while the needle is inserted caudal to the humerus and directed caudally.

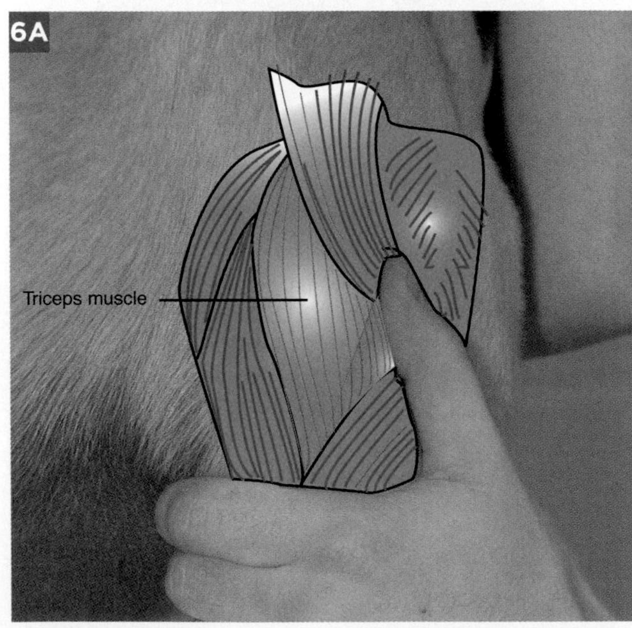

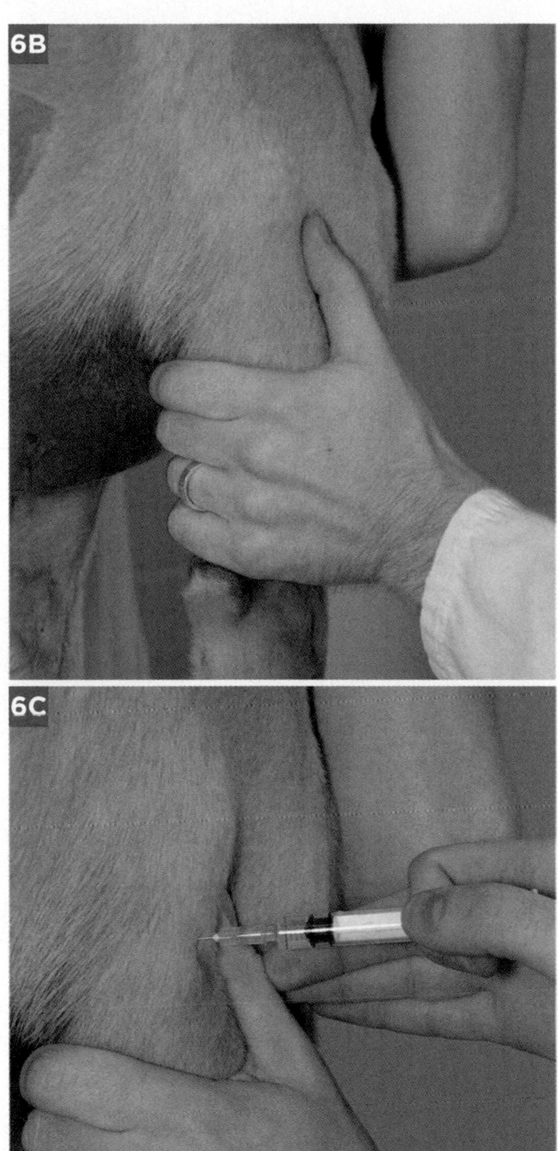

Proper technique for administering an injection into the triceps muscle of a dog.

7. When administering an injection into the lumbar muscles, select a site between the thirteenth rib and the iliac crest. Palpate the dorsal spinous processes and insert the needle 2 to 3 cm off of midline, directly into the lumbar muscles, perpendicular to the skin at that site.

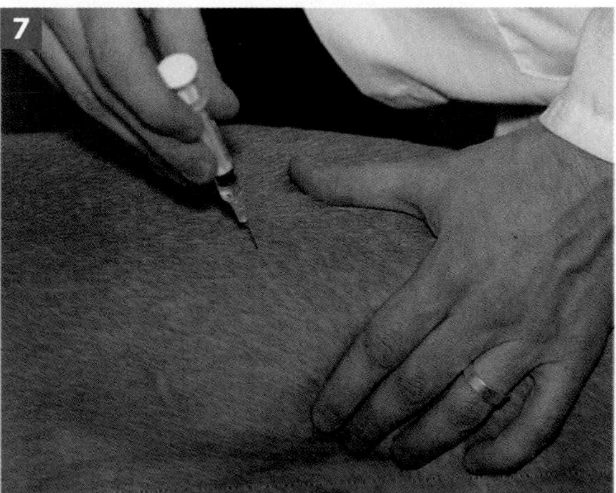

Administering an injection into the lumbar muscles of a dog.

8. Once the needle is inserted for an intramuscular injection, withdraw the plunger on the syringe to create negative pressure. If blood is aspirated, withdraw the needle and syringe and replace the needle before reinserting at another site.
9. If no blood is aspirated when negative pressure is applied, proceed with the intramuscular injection.
10. Once the injection is complete, remove the needle from the muscle and gently massage the site.

PROCEDURE 3-3

Subcutaneous Injections

PURPOSE

To administer fluids, drugs, biologic preparations, or test substances by injection

INDICATIONS

Parenteral administration of drugs, biologic preparations, or test substances for treatment or diagnostic evaluation

CONTRAINDICATIONS AND CONCERNS

To avoid potentially serious local or systemic reactions, all injectable substances should be administered only by the route recommended by the manufacturer.

SPECIAL ANATOMY

Subcutaneous injections are most often administered under the loose skin along the dorsal portion of the neck and back.

EQUIPMENT

- 25- to 20-gauge, 1-inch needle
- Syringe
- 70% alcohol

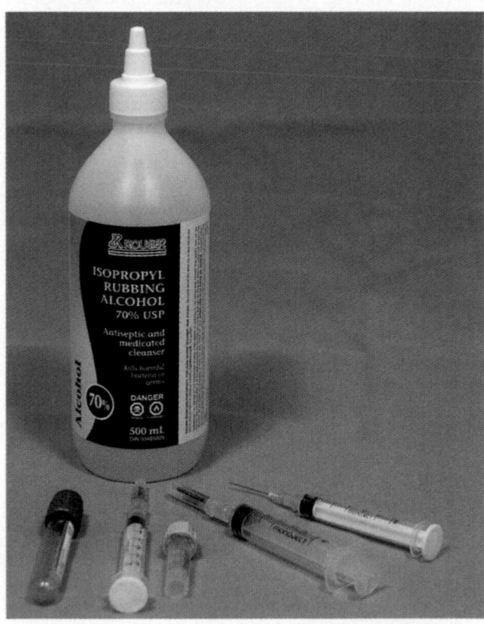

Equipment required for injections.

TECHNIQUE

1. Draw up the material to be administered into a syringe. Dogs and cats have an extensive potential subcutaneous space, so relatively large volumes of fluid (from 30 to 60 mL) can be injected at a single site. When large volumes are to be injected subcutaneously, use a flexible delivery system such as a fluid extension set to connect the needle and syringe to minimize the discomfort associated with movement of the injection apparatus once it is inserted.

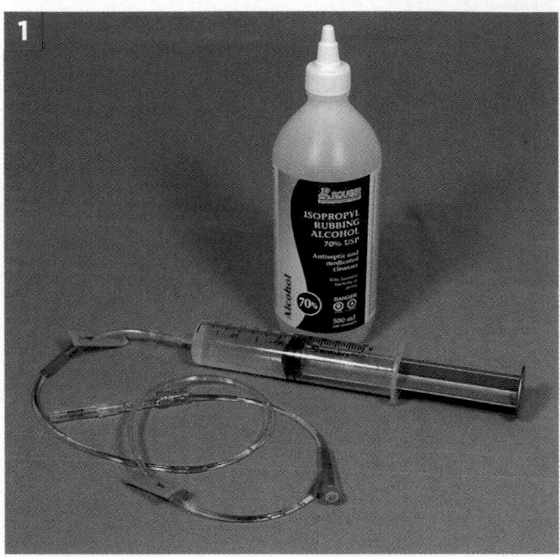

Flexible delivery system optimal for subcutaneous injection of large volumes of fluid.

2. Gently restrain the animal in a standing or sitting position or in sternal recumbency. Most dogs and cats tolerate subcutaneous injections well, so minimal restraint is required.
3. Pick up a fold of skin over the animal's neck or back and insert the needle, perpendicular to the skinfold, into the subcutaneous tissue. The needle should pass easily. If resistance is met, the needle tip should be repositioned because it is most likely intradermal or intramuscular.

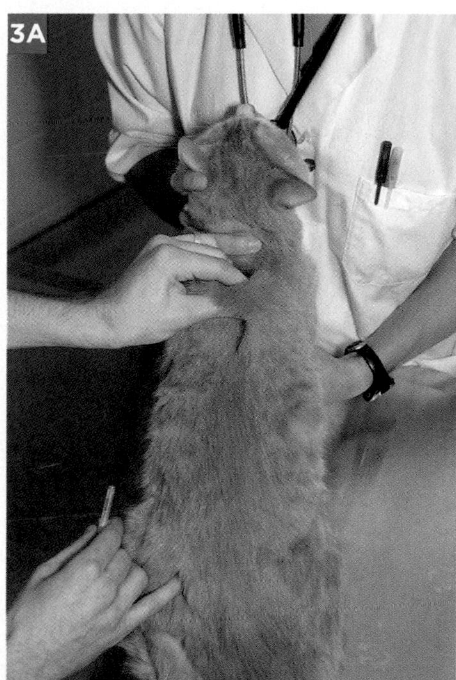

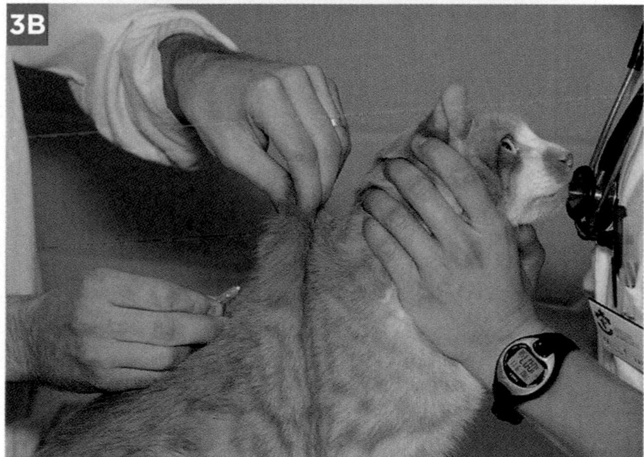

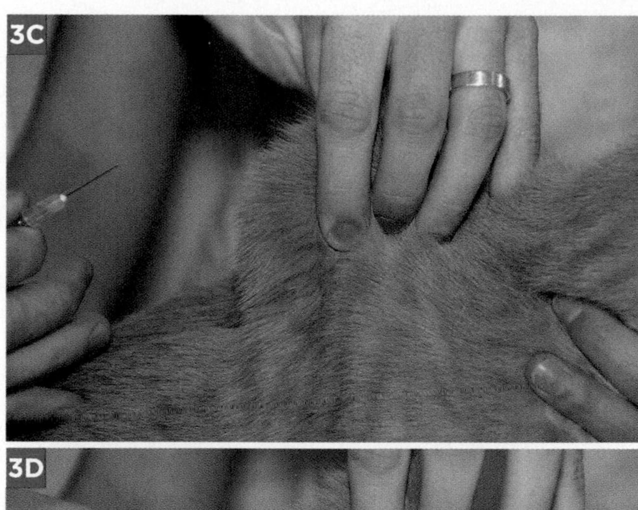

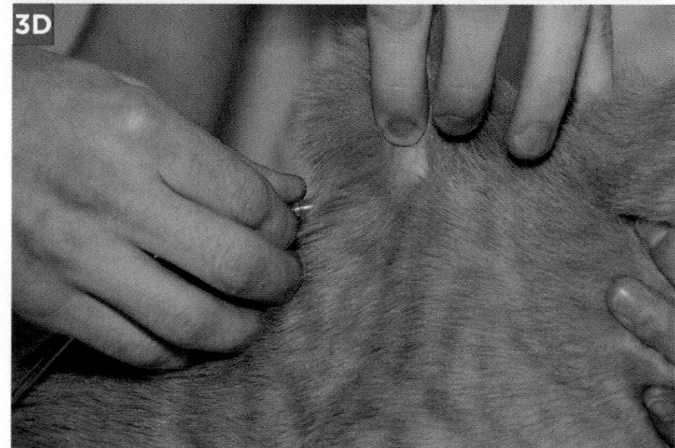

Proper technique for needle insertion for administering a subcutaneous injection in a cat.

4. Release the skinfold to let it fall back into place. This ensures that the needle tip did not penetrate both folds of skin.

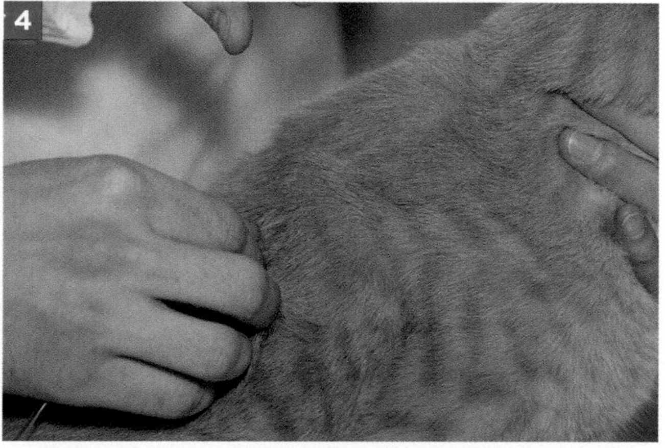

Releasing the fold of skin after needle insertion helps ensure that the injection is delivered subcutaneously.

PROCEDURE 3-1 Subcutaneous Injections—cont'd

5. Once the needle is inserted, withdraw the plunger on the syringe to create negative pressure. If blood is aspirated, withdraw the needle and syringe and replace the needle before reinserting at another site.
6. If no blood is aspirated when negative pressure is applied, proceed with the subcutaneous injection.

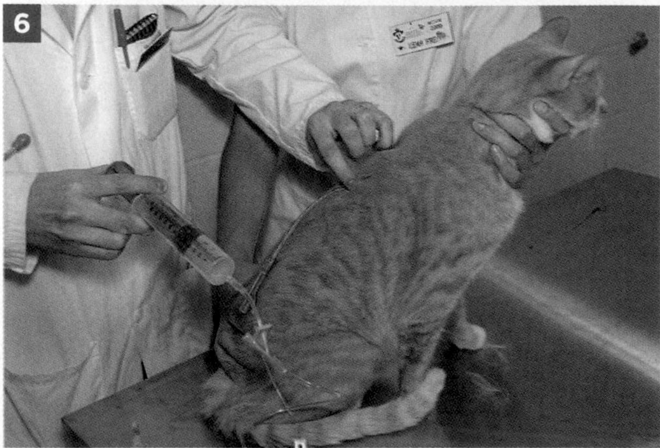

Administering subcutaneous fluids in a cat.

7. Once the injection is complete, remove the needle from the skin and gently massage the site to distribute the fluid.

Dermatologic Techniques

4

PROCEDURE 4-1
Skin Scraping

PURPOSE

To identify mites in or on the skin

INDICATIONS

Any dog or cat with alopecia, scaling, or pruritus (itchiness)

CONTRAINDICATIONS AND CONCERNS

1. No contraindications
2. This is a good test for diagnosing *Demodex* mites, but is not as sensitive for other mites. It is important to collect and evaluate numerous samples.

POSITIONING AND RESTRAINT

Adequate restraint to keep the animal still

SPECIAL ANATOMY

1. The mite you are looking for will determine the optimal site to scrape.
2. Sarcoptic mange mites are most likely to be found on pressure points like hocks and elbows as well as on the ear margins. Most affected dogs are extremely pruritic.

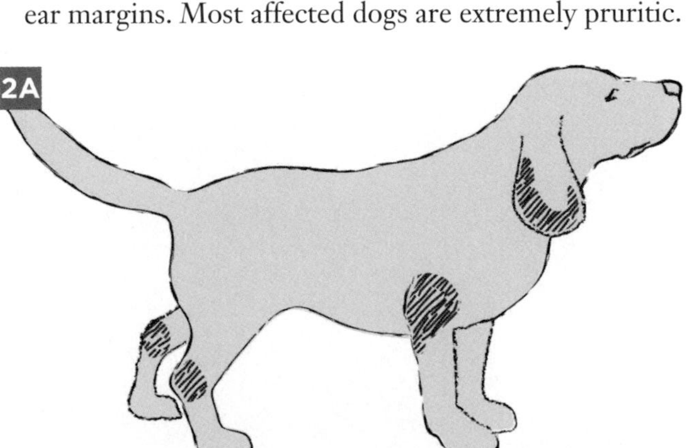

Drawing showing the most likely locations for sarcoptic mange mites.

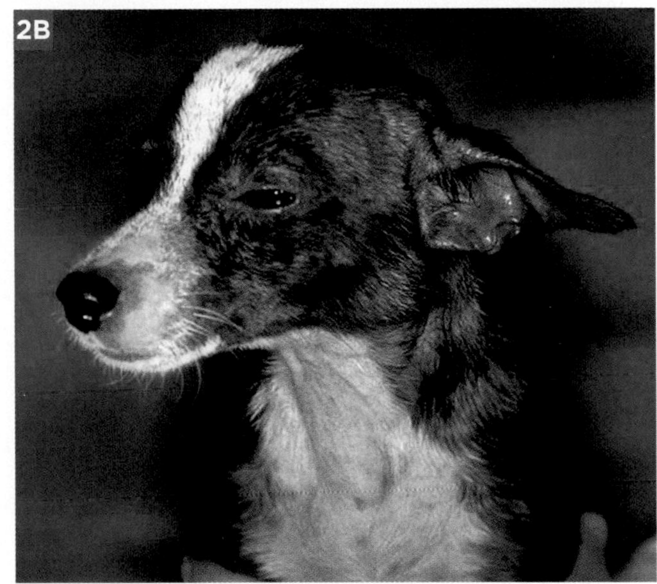

Alopecia, erythema, and excoriations in a dog with sarcoptic mange. **(Courtesy Dr. Catherine Outerbridge, University of California–Davis.)**

PROCEDURE 4-1 Skin Scraping—cont'd

3. *Demodex* mites are most likely to be found in lesions on the face and feet in dogs with focal disease, whereas generalized demodicosis can affect any location. *Demodex* mites are often deep within hair follicles, so the skin should be pinched before scraping for these mites.

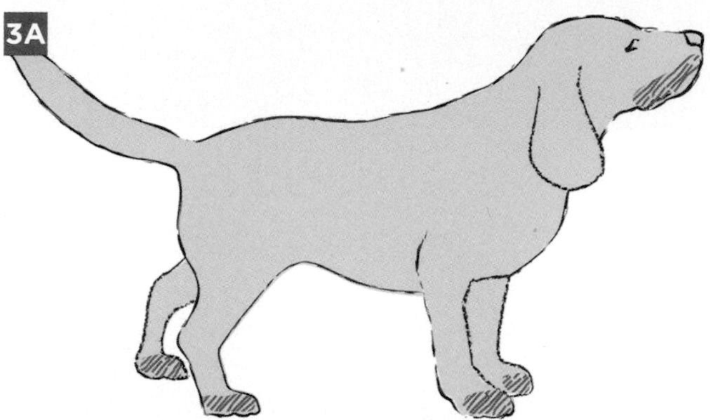

Drawing showing most likely locations for demodectic mange mites.

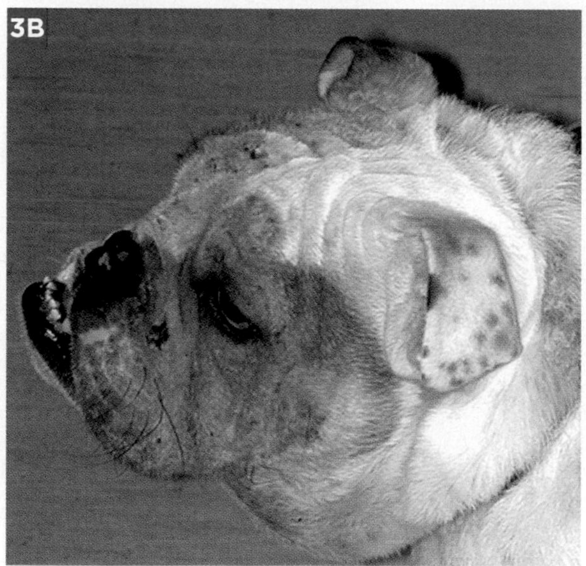

Facial erythema, scaling, and crusting in a young bulldog with *Demodex*. **(Courtesy Dr. Catherine Outerbridge, University of California–Davis.)**

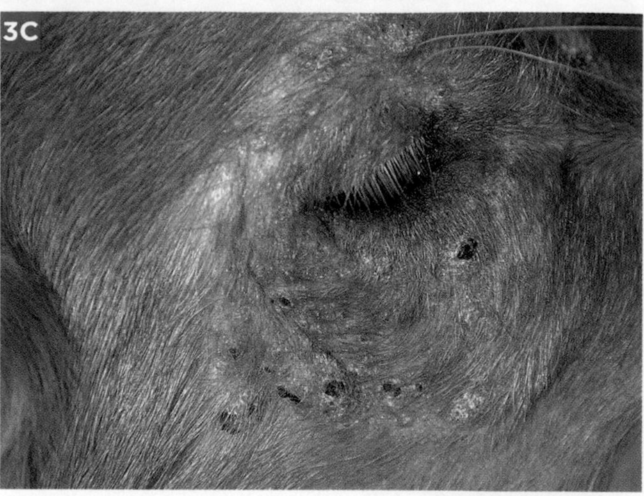

Periocular alopecia, erythema, and scaling in a Golden Retriever with *Demodex*. **(Courtesy Dr. Catherine Outerbridge, University of California–Davis.)**

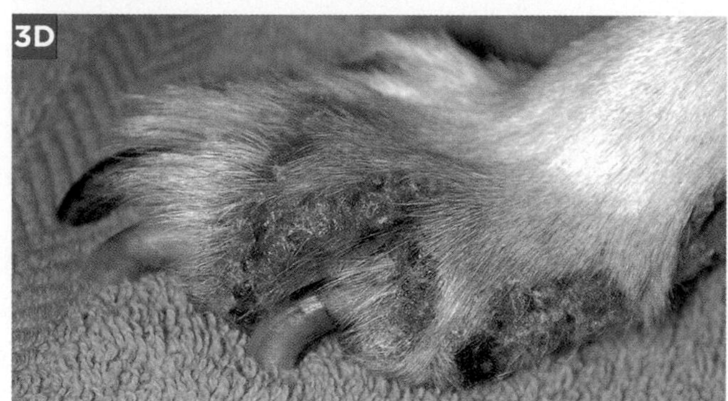

Demodex pododermatitis in a dog. **(Courtesy Dr. Catherine Outerbridge, University of California–Davis.)**

EQUIPMENT

- Clean glass slides
- Coverslips
- Mineral oil or glycerin
- Scalpel blade (use the dull end or dull the sharp edge before use)
- Microscope: use low-power objective (40×)
- Scissors to cut long hair in the region to be scraped

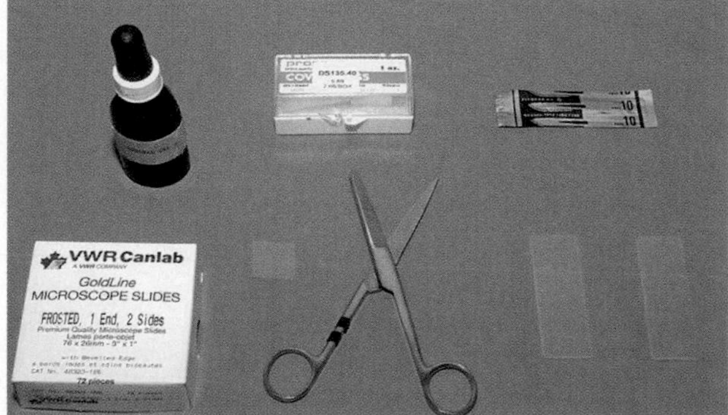

The equipment required for performing a skin scraping.

TECHNIQUE

1. If long hair surrounds the site, clip it off with scissors before doing the scraping.
2. Dip the dull end of a scalpel blade in mineral oil.

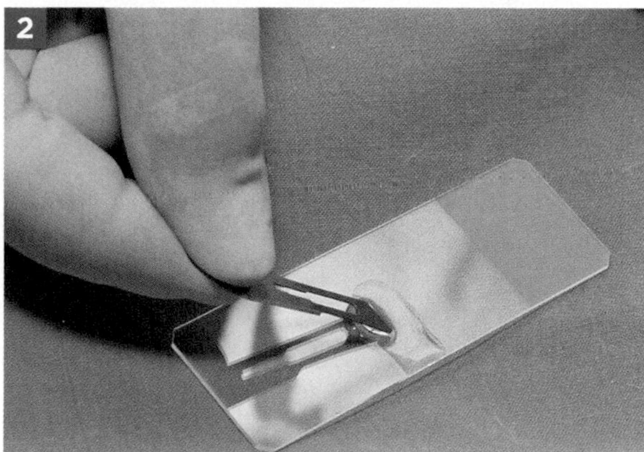

Dipping the dull end of a scalpel blade in mineral oil.

3. If you suspect *Demodex*, pinch the skin where you will scrape.

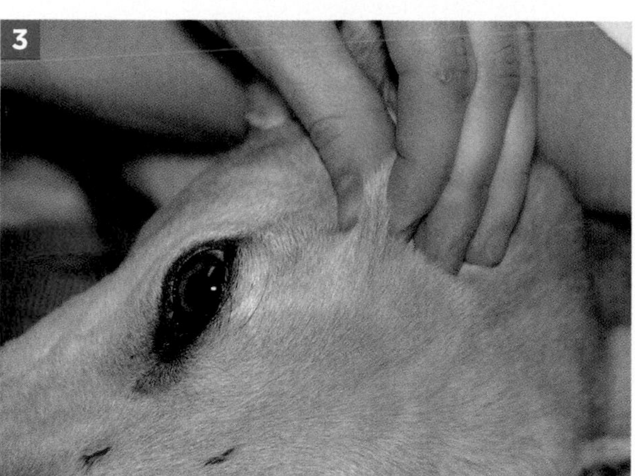

Pinching the skin before scraping.

4. Scrape the skin with the blade. Continue scraping until serum oozes and drops of capillary blood appear.

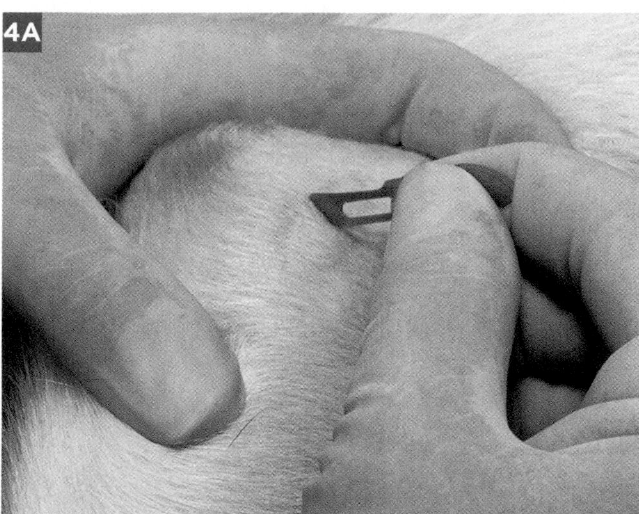

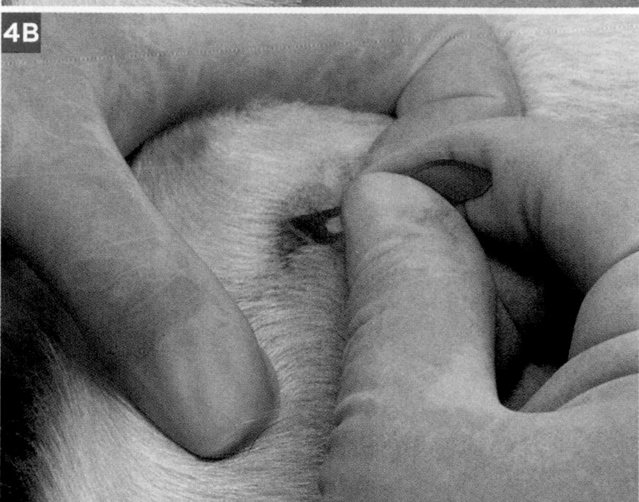

The skin is scraped until serum oozes and drops of capillary blood appear.

PROCEDURE 4-1 Skin Scraping—cont'd

5. Place the scraped material on a slide in a drop of mineral oil. Apply a coverslip and examine microscopically.

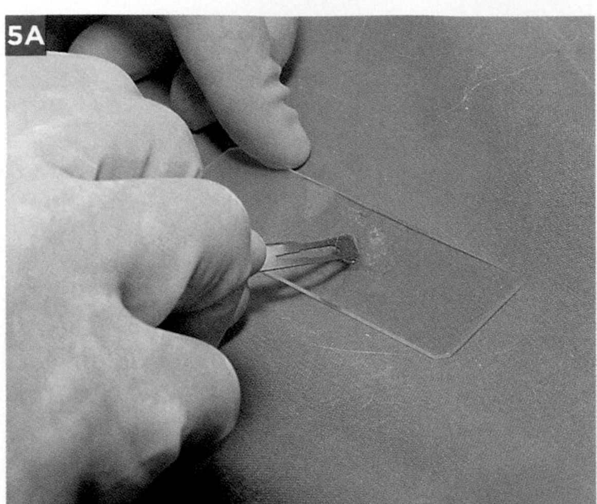

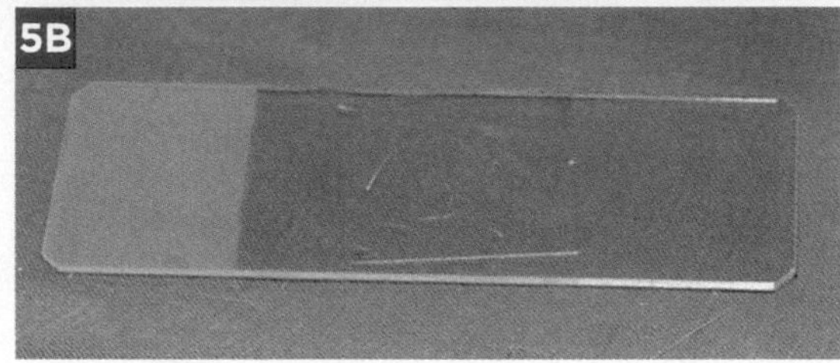

The scraped material is placed on a microscope slide in a drop of mineral oil and a coverslip applied.

RESULTS

1. Sarcoptic mange mites are difficult to find on scrapings, and at least 10 scrapings should be performed. Other methods for detection include vacuuming and occasionally skin biopsy.

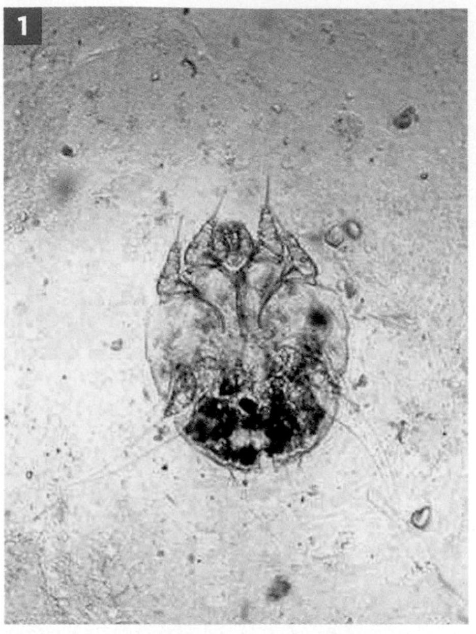

Microscopic image of sarcoptic *(Sarcoptes scabiei)* mange mite. **(Courtesy Dr. Klaas Post, University of Saskatchewan.)**

2. Demodectic mange mites are relatively easy to find, so five or six scrapings will usually be adequate. Remember to squeeze the skin first. Occasional mites may be found in normal dogs, but finding multiple mites or mites of all stages (larvae, nymphs, adults) indicates clinical demodicosis.

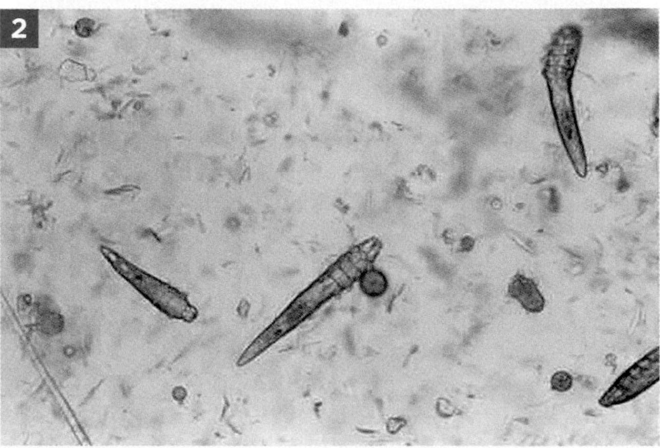

Microscopic image of demodectic *(Demodex canis)* mange mites. **(Courtesy Dr. Klaas Post, University of Saskatchewan.)**

PROCEDURE 4-2
Cellophane Tape Method

PURPOSE

To collect parasites and debris from the hair and skin surface for microscopic evaluation

INDICATIONS

1. Any animal with generalized pruritus, especially those with visible debris in the hair or on the skin surface
2. Especially useful in assessment for *Cheyletiella* mites, flea larvae, and lice
3. Can also be used to assess for cutaneous *Malassezia* (yeast) infection if the tape is stained using Diff-Quick stain before microscopic evaluation

CONTRAINDICATIONS AND CONCERNS

None

POSITIONING AND RESTRAINT

Adequate restraint to keep the animal still

EQUIPMENT

- Clean glass microscope slide
- Mineral oil
- Clear acetate cellophane tape (3M's Scotch No. 602)
- Microscope

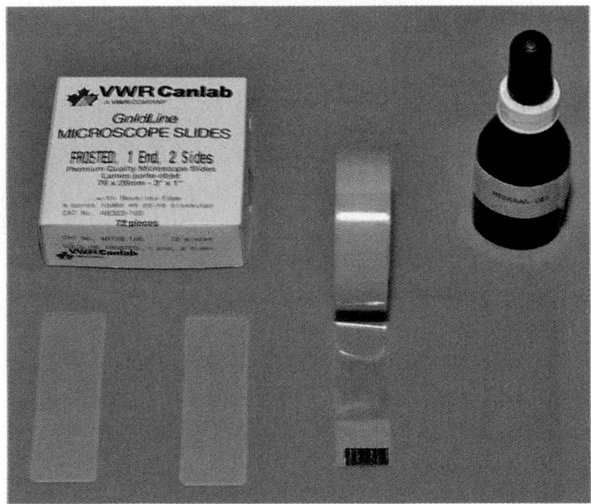

Equipment required for a cellophane tape preparation.

TECHNIQUE

1. Tear off a 1- to 2-inch piece of tape.
2. Part the hair and touch the sticky side of the tape to hair and skin, collecting flakes and debris.

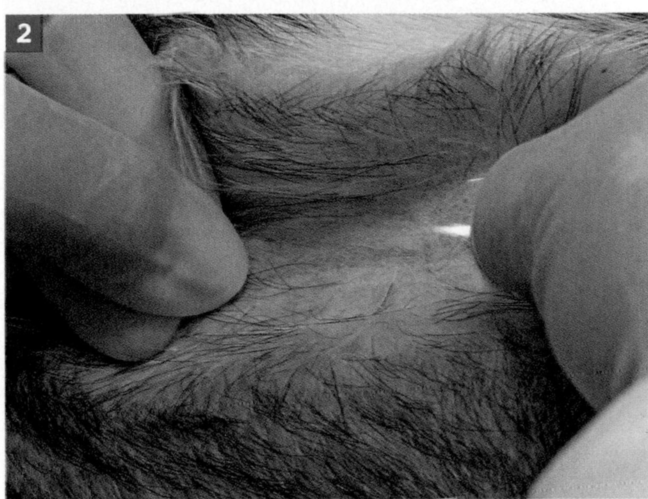

The sticky side of the tape is touched to the hair and skin in order to collect flakes and debris.

PROCEDURE 4-2 Cellophane Tape Method—cont'd

3. The tape can be applied directly, sticky side down, to a microscope slide or applied on top of a drop of mineral oil, maximizing the visibility of live *Cheyletiella* mites.

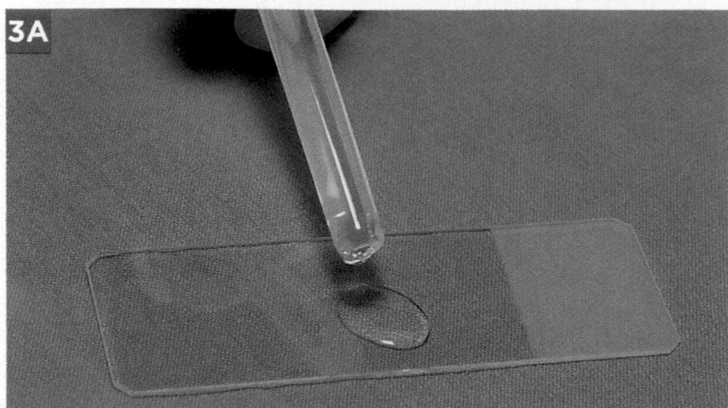

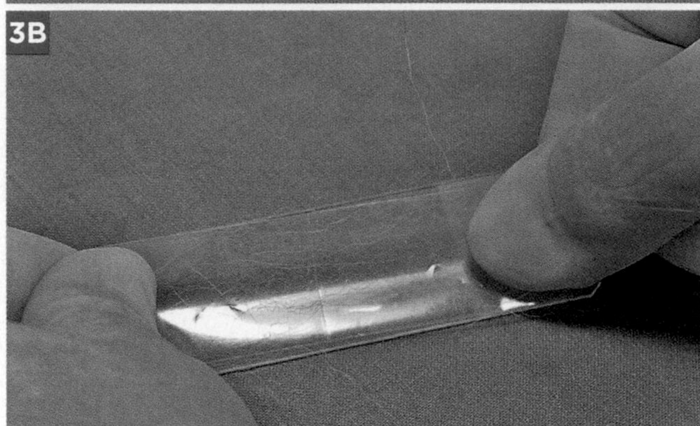

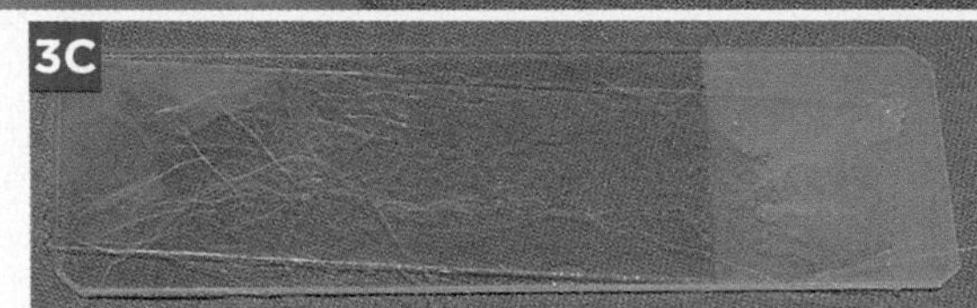

The tape is applied, sticky side down, to a microscope slide on top of a drop of mineral oil.

4. When looking for yeast, place 1 drop of the basophilic stain solution of Diff-Quick stain (the third solution) on a glass slide and press the tape, sticky side down, on the slide.
5. Examine the slide using a microscope.

RESULTS

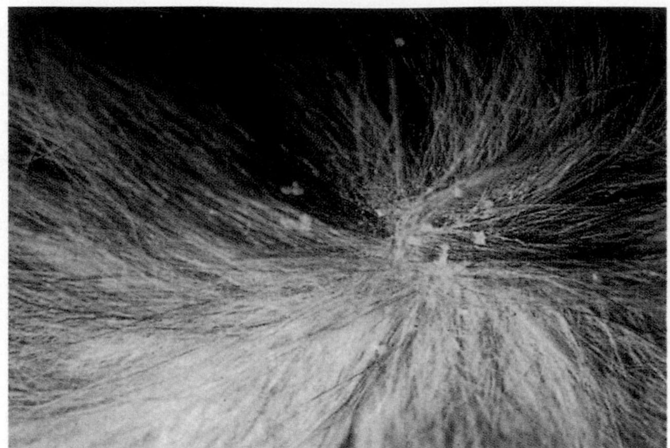

Flaking and pruritus in a young dog with *Cheyletiella* mites ("walking dandruff"). **(Courtesy Dr. Klaas Post, University of Saskatchewan.)**

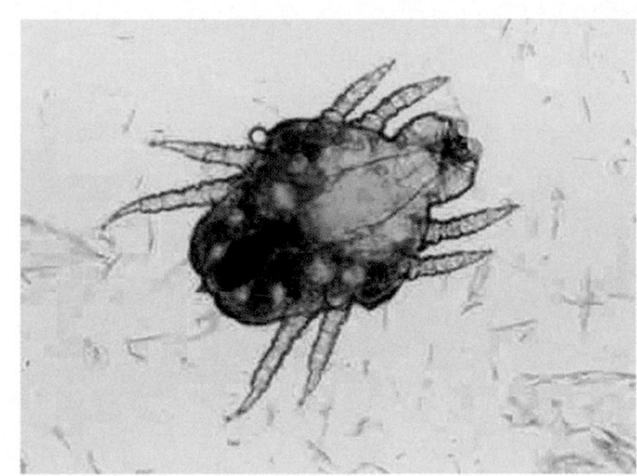

Cheyletiella yasguri mite identified microscopically using a cellophane tape preparation. **(Courtesy Dr. Klaas Post, University of Saskatchewan.)**

PROCEDURE 4-3

Vacuuming

PURPOSE

To collect parasites and debris from the hair and skin surface for microscopic evaluation

INDICATIONS

1. Any animal with generalized pruritus, especially those with visible debris in the hair or on the skin surface
2. Especially useful during assessment for *Cheyletiella* mites, sarcoptic mange mites, fleas, and lice

CONTRAINDICATIONS AND CONCERNS

None

POSITIONING AND RESTRAINT

Use adequate restraint to keep the animal still. Many animals find the noise of the vacuum disturbing, so careful restraint is required.

EQUIPMENT

- Vacuum
- Attachment
- Milk machine filter

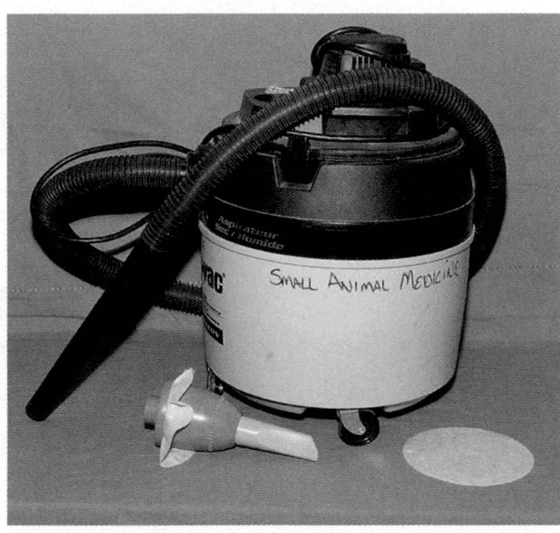

Equipment required to collect a vacuumed sample from the skin.

TECHNIQUE

1. Place filter paper in the vacuum attachment.

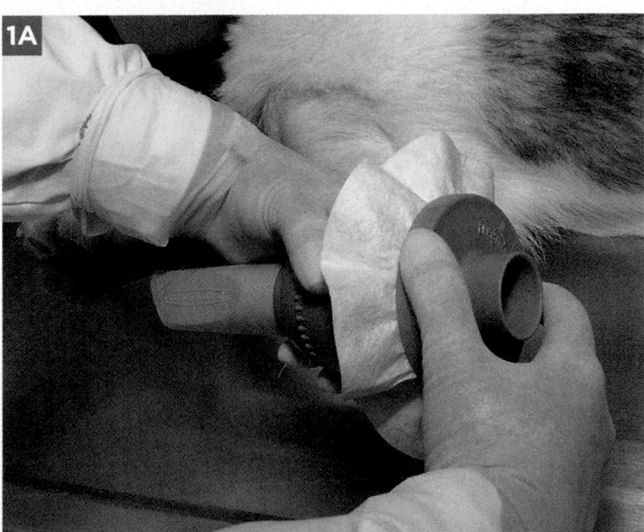

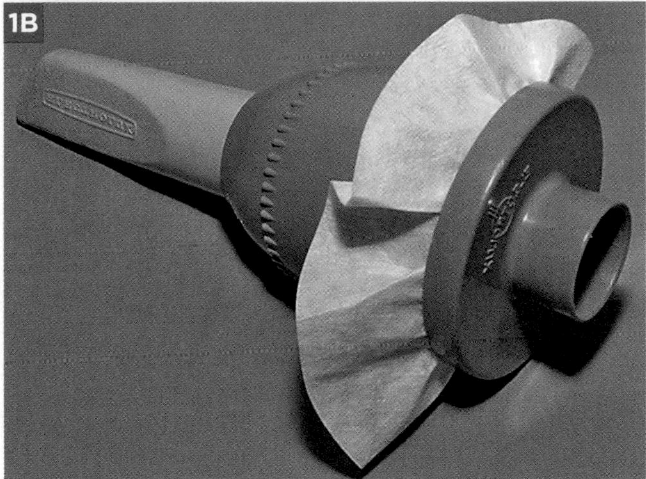

Placing filter paper in the vacuum attachment.

PROCEDURE 4-3 Vacuuming—cont'd

2. Restrain the patient.
3. Turn on the vacuum.
4. Apply suction to all areas of coat, especially regions with visible debris.

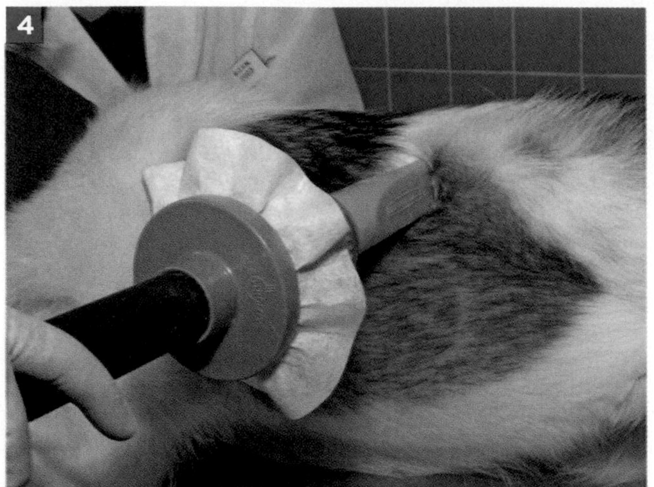

Applying suction to all areas of coat.

5. Open the attachment and examine debris collected on the filter paper.

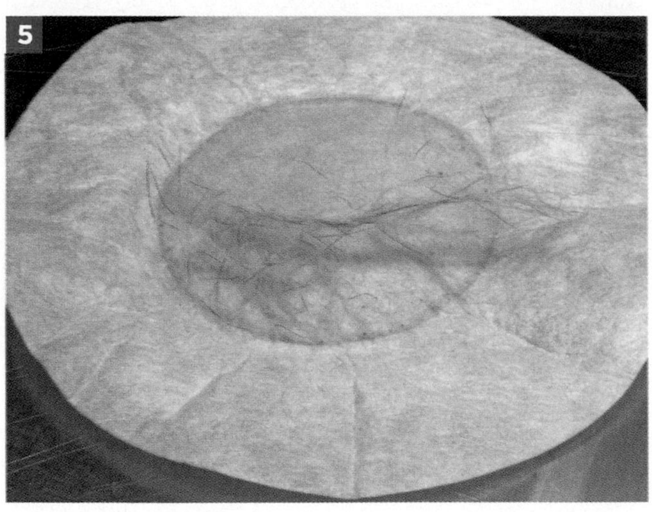

Debris collected on the filter paper during vacuuming.

RESULTS

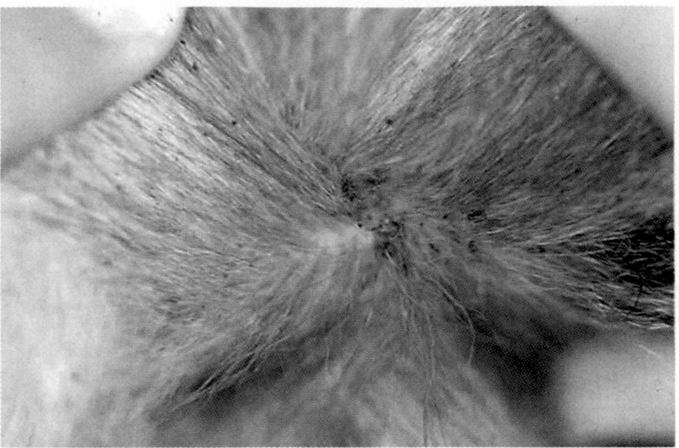

Black debris in a cat's hair, suggestive of flea feces ("flea dirt").

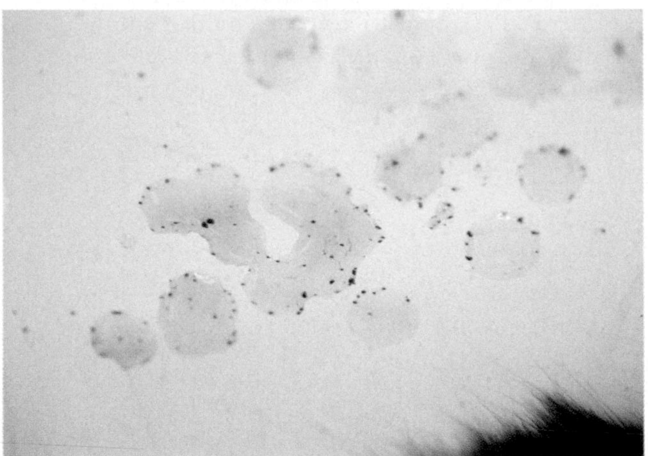

Debris collected by vacuuming is mixed with a few drops of water on a white card. Blood diffuses out of the debris, confirming that the black specks are flea dirt.

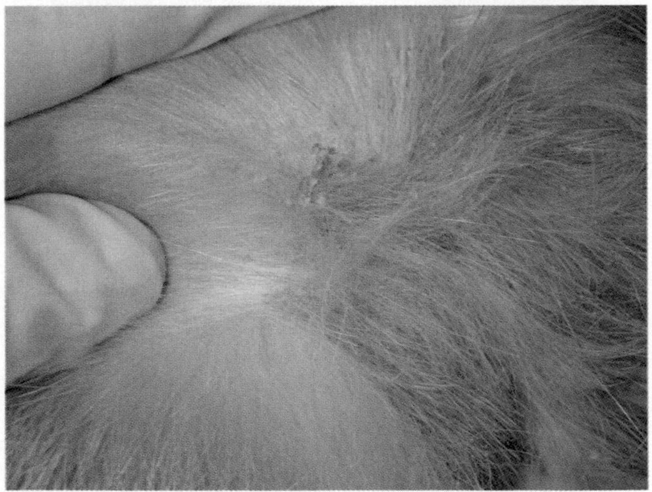

Cheyletiellosis in a rabbit. Microscopic examination of flakes obtained by vacuuming is most likely to identify *Cheyletiella parasitovorax* in this species. **(Courtesy Dr. Catherine Outerbridge, University of California–Davis.)**

PROCEDURE 4-4

Bacterial Culture of Skin Pustule

PURPOSE

To collect the contents of a pustule in order to examine the contents cytologically and to culture any causative bacteria

INDICATIONS

1. Animals with bacterial pyoderma that is recurrent or persistent in spite of antibiotic therapy
2. For the culture to be most useful, no antibiotics should have been administered during the last 48 hours.
3. Pustules on the chin of a puppy

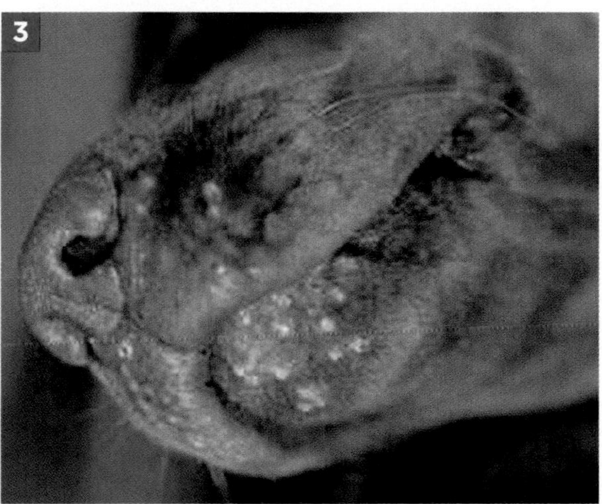

Numerous pustules on the chin of a chocolate Labrador Retriever puppy with juvenile cellulitis (puppy strangles).

CONTRAINDICATIONS AND CONCERNS

Intact pustules are fragile in dogs and cats, so should be handled with care in order to gain the benefit of collecting the contents.

POSITIONING AND RESTRAINT

Adequate restraint to keep the animal still

EQUIPMENT

- Clippers or scissors
- Alcohol
- 22-gauge needle
- Culturette swab

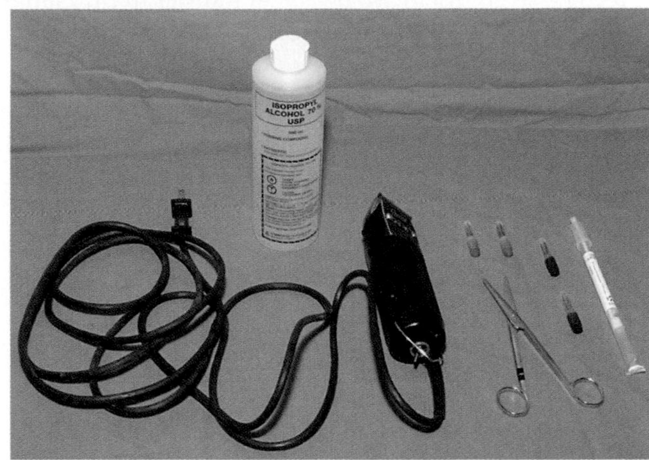

Equipment required to perform a bacterial culture from a skin pustule.

TECHNIQUE

1. Identify the pustule.

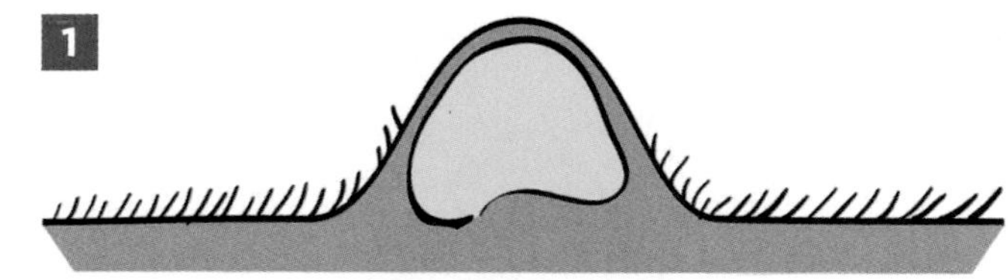

Identifying the pustule.

2. Clip long hairs around the pustule carefully, making certain to avoid touching or rupturing the pustule.

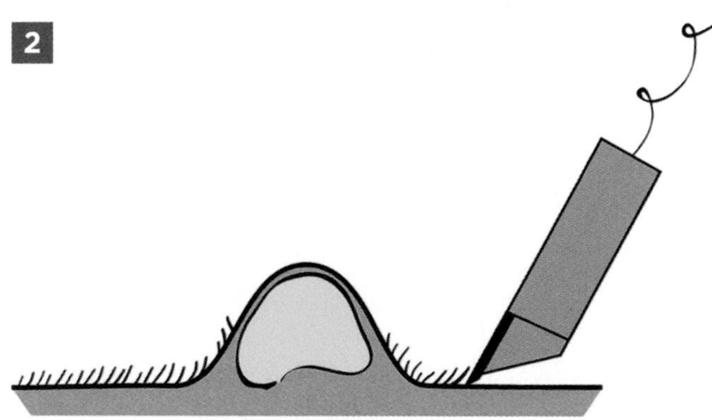

Carefully clipping the long hairs around the pustule.

PROCEDURE 4-4 Bacterial Culture of Skin Pustule—cont'd

3. Cleanse the clipped area and the surface of the pustule with 70% alcohol to remove surface contaminants. Let the region air dry to avoid alcohol transfer to the culture swab, which would inhibit bacterial growth.

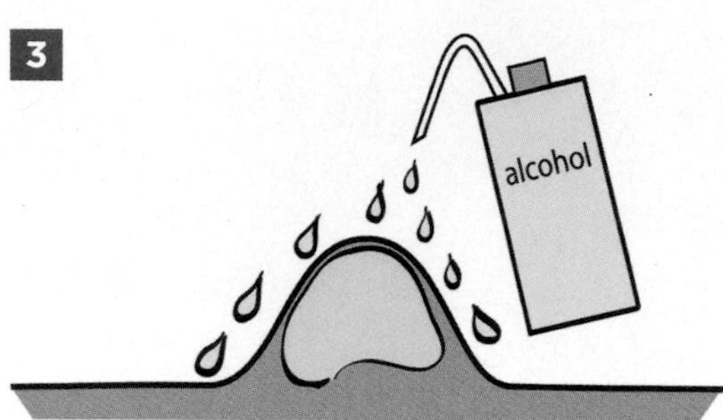

Cleansing the surface of the pustule.

4. Puncture the pustule with a sterile 22- or 25-gauge needle, then collect pus using a sterile culture swab.

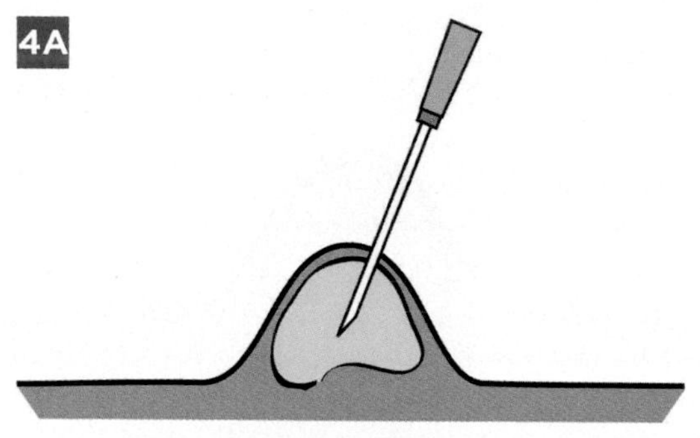

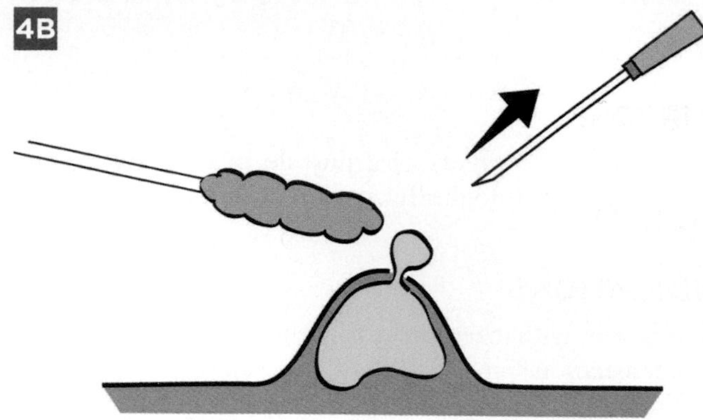

Puncturing the pustule and collecting the pus.

5. Inoculate material into suitable bacterial culture media. If sufficient material is available, collect another drop with a second swab to make a smear for cytologic evaluation.

PROCEDURE 4-5

Skin Biopsy

PURPOSE

To collect a sample of skin for histopathologic examination

INDICATIONS

1. Use in all cases in which skin neoplasia is suspected. Small lesions may be removed in their entirety, whereas larger lesions or lesions in which special surgical or adjunctive treatment is likely to be required may have incisional biopsies performed for diagnosis.
2. Dermatologic conditions that have not improved with rational therapy for the presumed diagnosis (i.e., bacterial pyoderma), so the diagnosis is uncertain
3. Dermatologic conditions suspected to be immune mediated in origin
4. Dermatologic conditions that can be definitively diagnosed only by histopathology (such as follicular dysplasia, sebaceous adenitis)
5. Once parasitic disease has been excluded, skin biopsies sometimes can help differentiate pruritus due to inhaled environmental allergens (nonspecific changes) from skin disease caused by food allergies (eosinophilic changes).

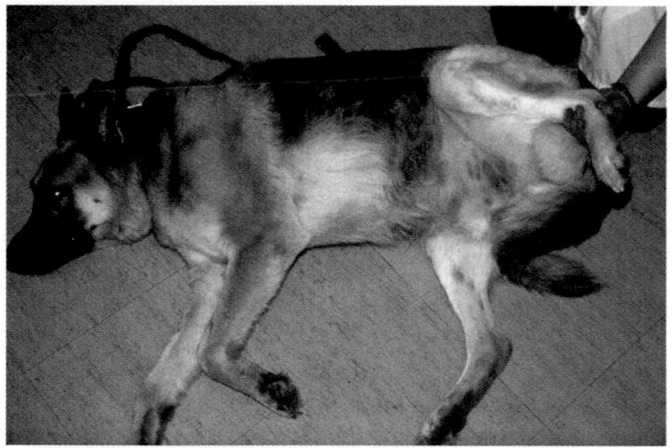

This 5-year-old Shepherd-cross had multiple painful ulcerated lesions on his ventral abdomen. Systemic lupus erythematosus was diagnosed by skin biopsy.

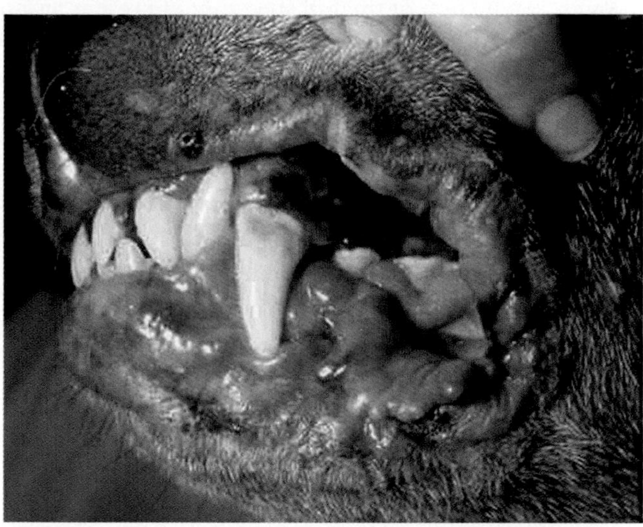

Biopsy of the reddened, hairless proliferated skin at the mucocutaneous junction in this dog yielded a diagnosis of cutaneous lymphoma.

CONTRAINDICATIONS AND CONCERNS

1. When circular punch biopsies are performed, it is important to avoid centering the biopsy on the margin of a lesion because this results in a biopsy consisting of 50% lesional skin and 50% adjacent normal skin. There is some risk that the abnormal portion of the biopsy will be lost or missed in processing.
2. Whenever possible, take multiple biopsies containing only lesional skin. New, active lesions and more chronic lesions should be sampled. As well, submit a biopsy of normal skin, but ensure that this is labeled as such for the pathologist.

POSITIONING AND RESTRAINT

1. Adequate restraint to keep the animal still
2. When local anesthesia is used, skin biopsy is not a painful procedure. Lidocaine blocking solution (2% lidocaine mixed 9:1 with 8.4% sodium bicarbonate) can be injected under the skin around the lesion to provide analgesia. The addition of bicarbonate decreases the sting of injection and speeds the local analgesic effect of the lidocaine.

PROCEDURE 4-5 Skin Biopsy—cont'd

SPECIAL ANATOMY

1. Select the appropriate biopsy site(s). The histopathologic examination of the full spectrum of present lesions gives more information than simply biopsying lesions all at one stage.
2. Avoid including a significant margin of normal skin at the edge of punch biopsy because this can cause the pathologist to miss the lesioned skin. Center the biopsy in the visible lesion.

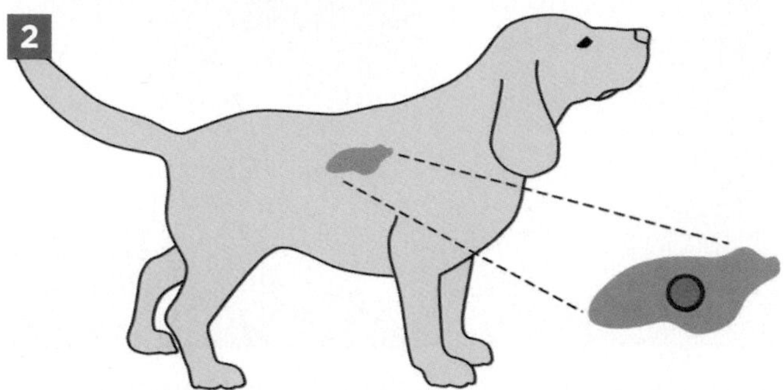

Center punch biopsies within abnormal tissue to avoid including a significant margin of normal skin at the edge of the biopsy.

3. It may be helpful to also submit a separate biopsy of normal-appearing skin, labeled as such.
4. Punch biopsies (4 to 6 mm) are adequate for many lesions. Use a small enough biopsy punch to avoid including a rim of normal tissue in the biopsy.
5. Excisional biopsies using a scalpel may be indicated to remove large lesions, to biopsy deep lesions (extending into subcutaneous tissues), and to biopsy vesicles, bullae, and pustules in which the rotary action of the punch biopsy can damage the lesion.

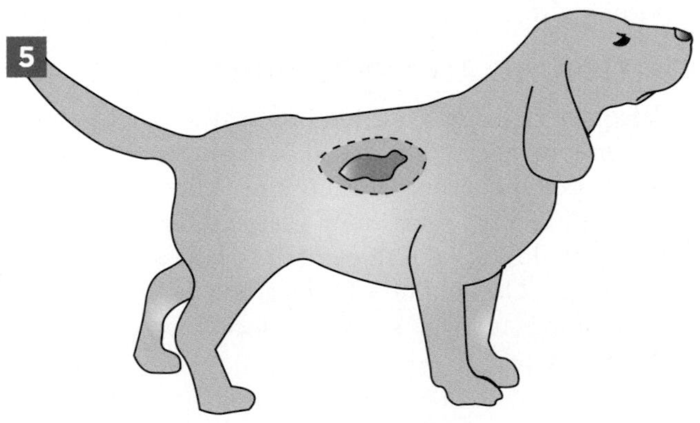

Excisional biopsy.

EQUIPMENT

- Scissors for long-haired patient
- Local anesthesia: 3-mL syringe, 25-gauge needle, lidocaine blocking solution (2% lidocaine mixed 9:1 with 8.4% sodium bicarbonate)
- Gloves
- Cutaneous 4- or 6-mm biopsy punch
- Scalpel blade
- Gauze sponges
- Fine-tooth forceps
- 25-gauge needle
- Container with 10% formalin
- Needle-holding forceps
- Nonabsorbable suture material

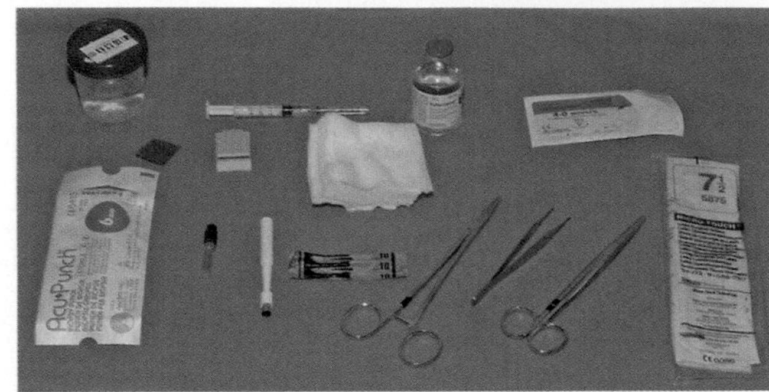

Equipment required for skin punch biopsies.

TECHNIQUE

1. Select an appropriate biopsy site. Avoid lesions caused by secondary trauma.
2. It is important to take at least four biopsies of abnormal skin and one of normal-appearing skin (labeled).
3. Clip long hair from around site with scissors, being careful to avoid traumatizing the region to be biopsied.

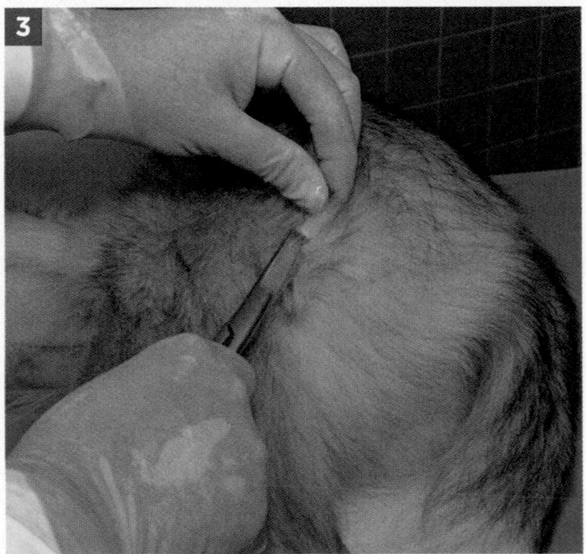

Clipping long hair from around the biopsy site with scissors.

4. Do a line block with lidocaine blocking solution around the region to be biopsied—avoid injecting lidocaine directly under the biopsy site because this can cause histopathologic changes resembling subcutaneous edema.
   A. Insert the needle, injecting lidocaine blocking solution as the needle is withdrawn, blocking the line along the needle's path.
   B. For the next line, insert the needle through the previously blocked region of skin along a line perpendicular to the first block, and inject lidocaine blocking solution as the needle is withdrawn.

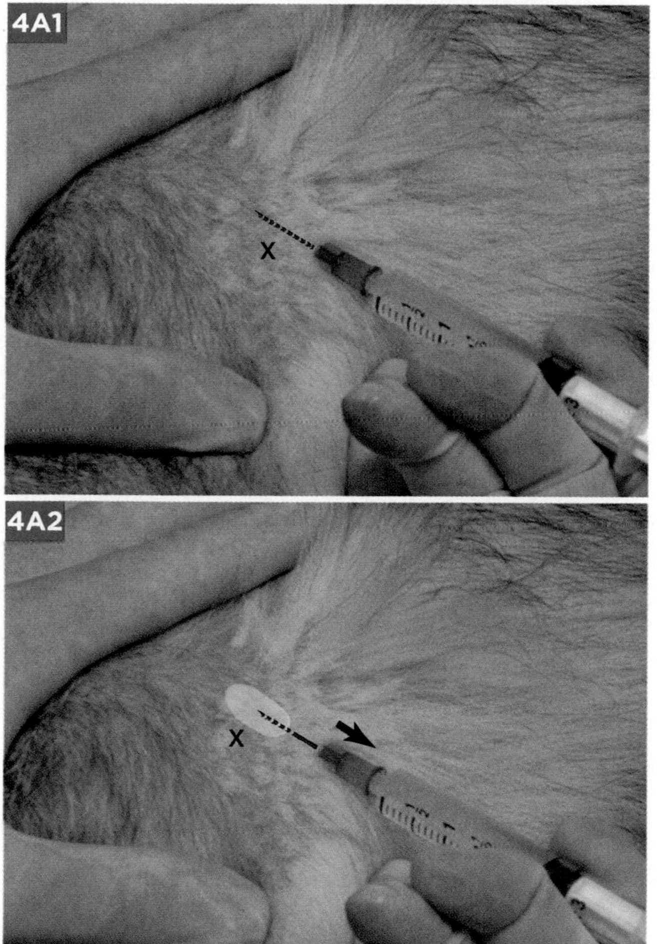

Inserting the needle and injecting lidocaine blocking solution as the needle is withdrawn.

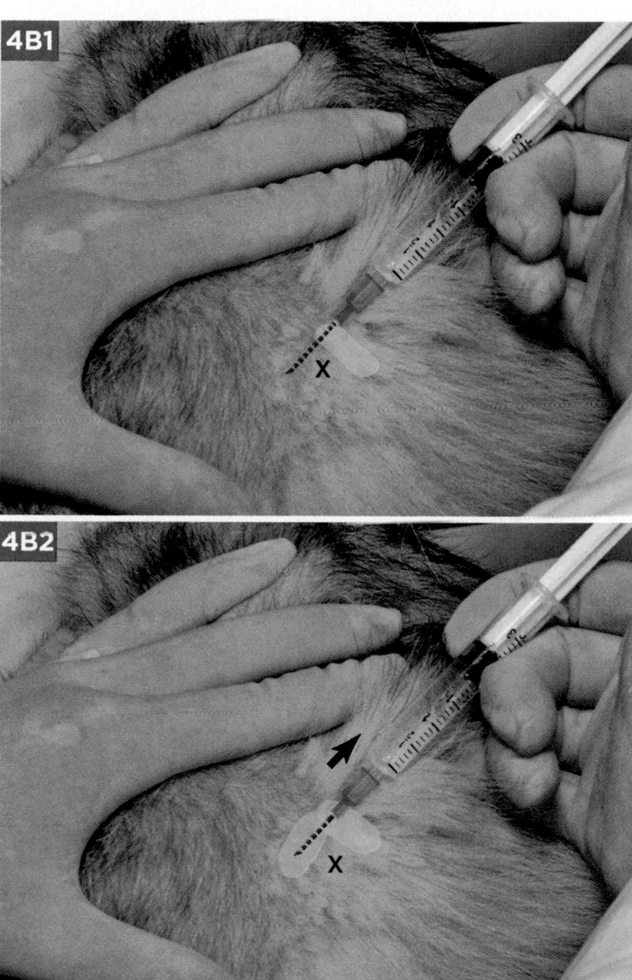

Inserting the needle through the previously blocked region of skin.

PROCEDURE 4-5 Skin Biopsy—cont'd

C. Repeat this process for each edge of the ring block, until all of the skin surrounding the area of interest has been blocked.

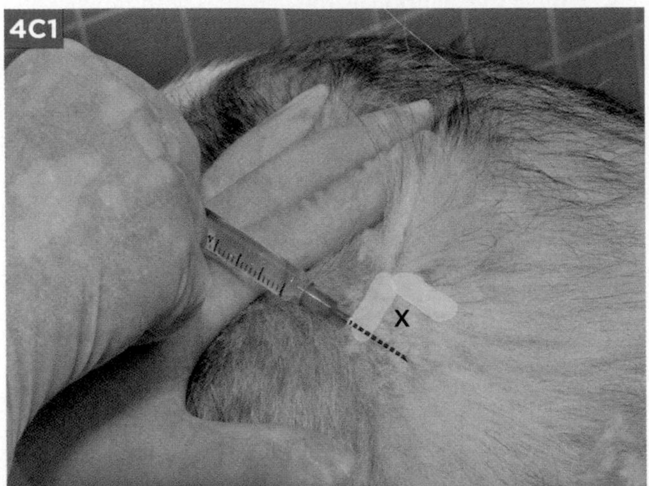

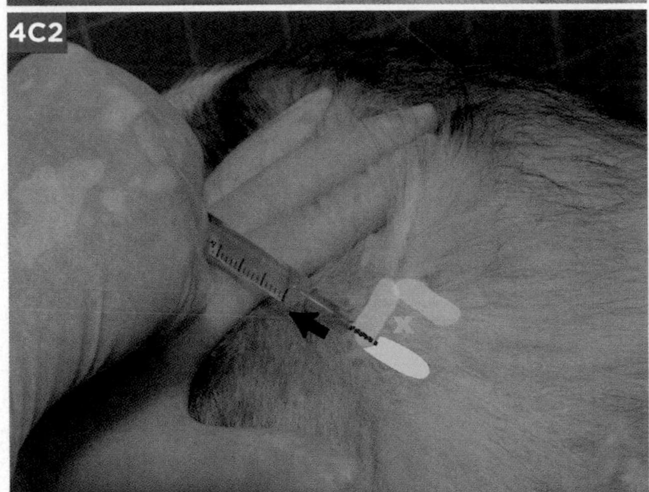

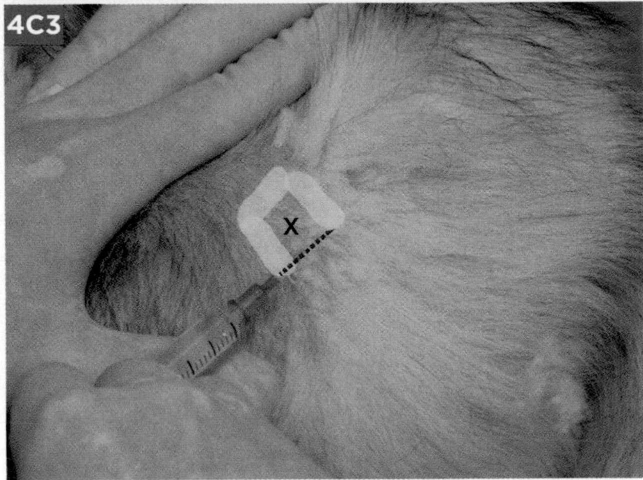

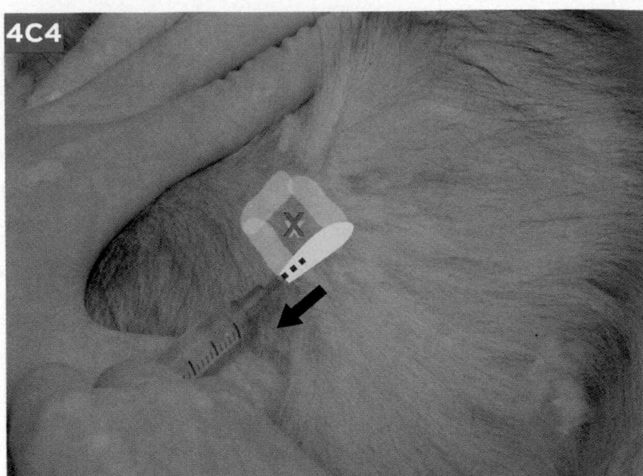

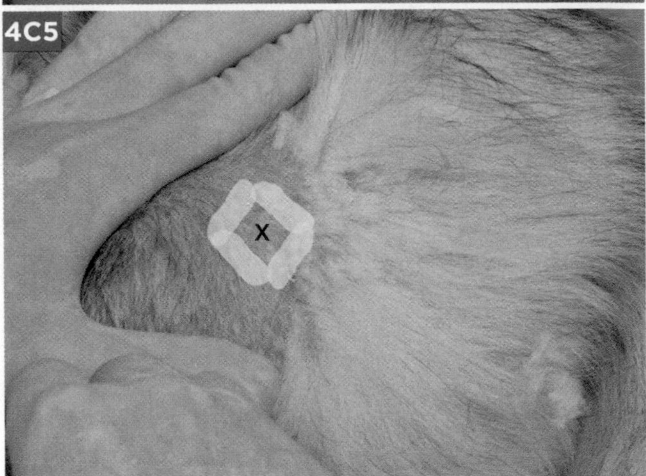

5. Wear gloves but do not prepare the skin surface in any way if the biopsies are for histopathologic evaluation.
6. Press the skin biopsy punch firmly onto the chosen site while applying a rotational motion in one direction. Continue until the full thickness of skin has been penetrated.

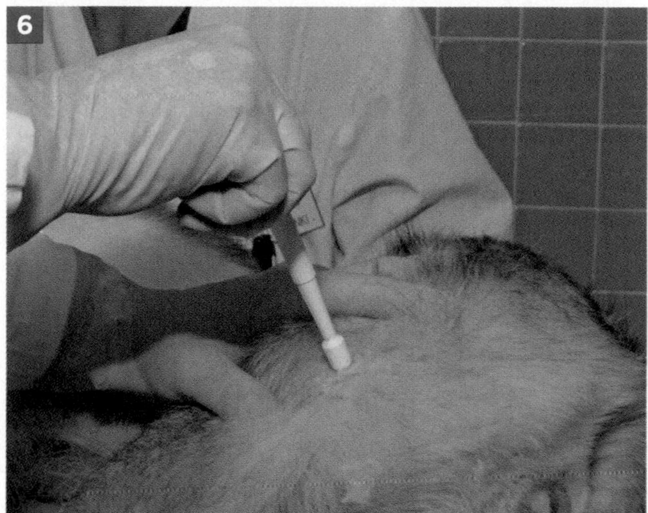

Pushing the skin biopsy punch firmly onto the chosen site while applying a rotational motion in one direction.

7. Using a forceps or needle to grasp the biopsy from underneath, cut the subcutaneous tissue if necessary with a scalpel blade.

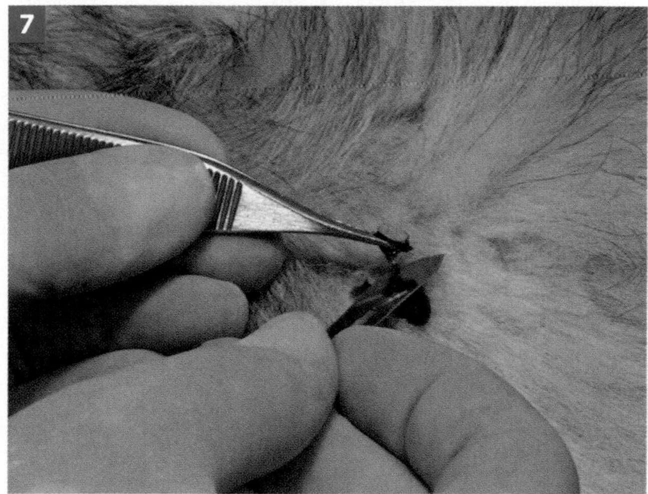

Grasping the biopsy from underneath with a forceps and cutting from the underlying subcutaneous tissue.

8. Place the biopsy in a cassette, on a piece of paper, or on a tongue depressor to maintain proper orientation (subcutaneous tissue down), and place the biopsy in formalin.

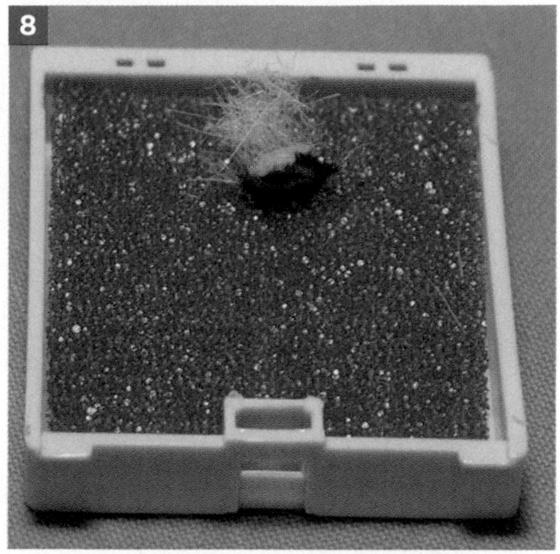

The biopsy is placed in a cassette to maintain proper orientation, then immersed in formalin.

9. Apply firm pressure to the biopsy site with gauze sponges to minimize hemorrhage.
10. Suture the biopsy site with a cruciate stitch and nonabsorbable suture material.

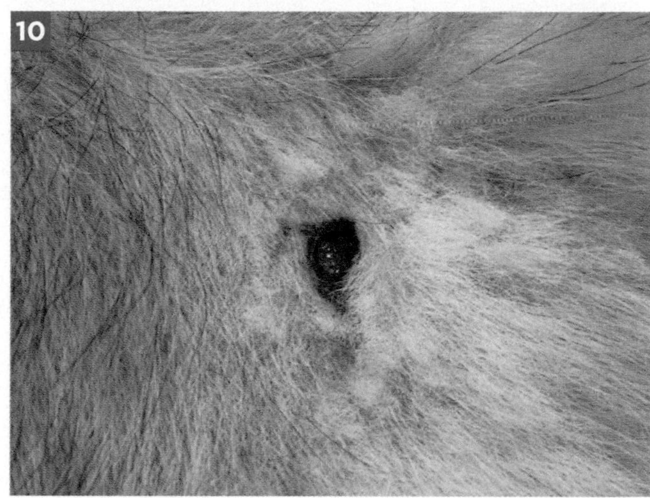

A round hole created by a punch biopsy.

PROCEDURE 4-5 Skin Biopsy—cont'd

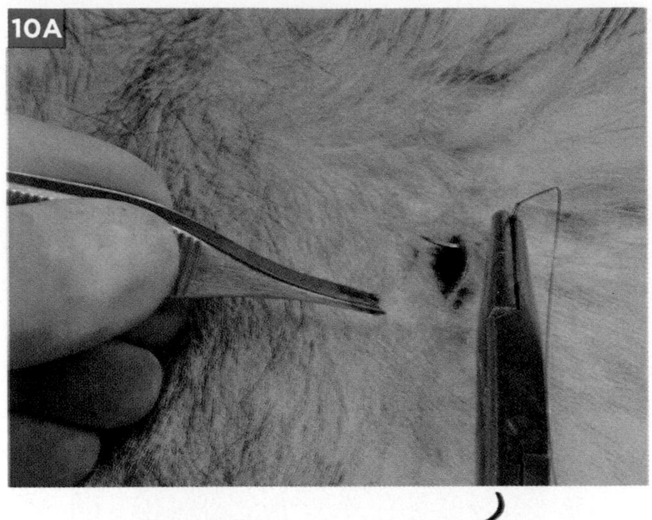

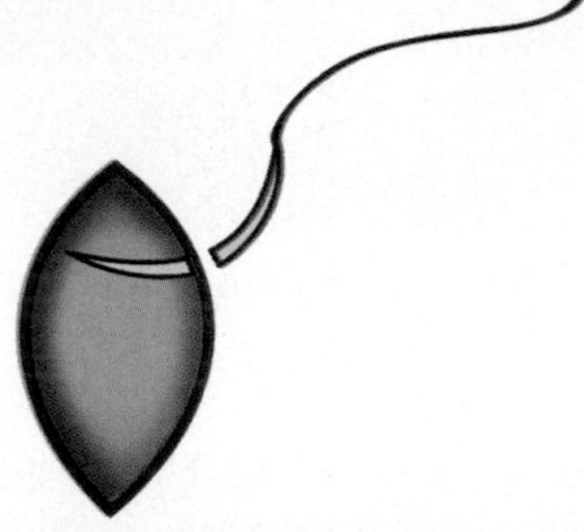

The needle is passed through the skin and tissues at one edge of the hole approximately one third of the distance from the top of the hole.

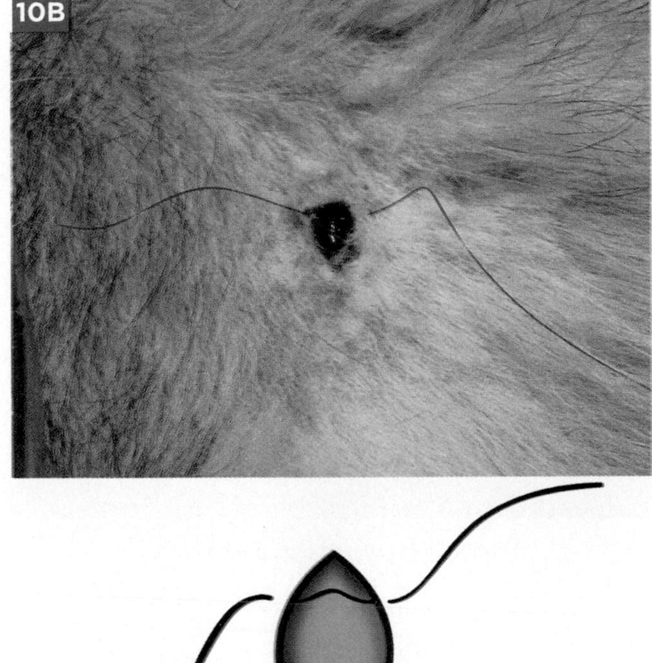

Crossing the wound, the needle is passed through the tissues and the skin at the edge of the other side of the hole, directly opposite the first needle pass, taking approximately the same-sized "bite" of tissue.

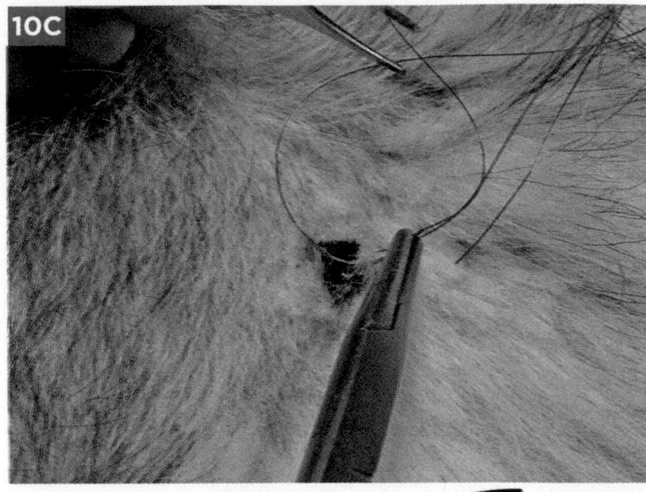

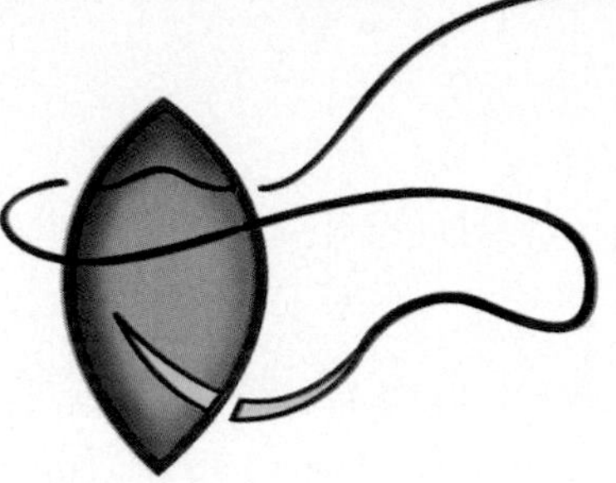

Return to the original side of the wound, and pass the needle through the skin and tissues, approximately one third of the distance from the bottom of the hole.

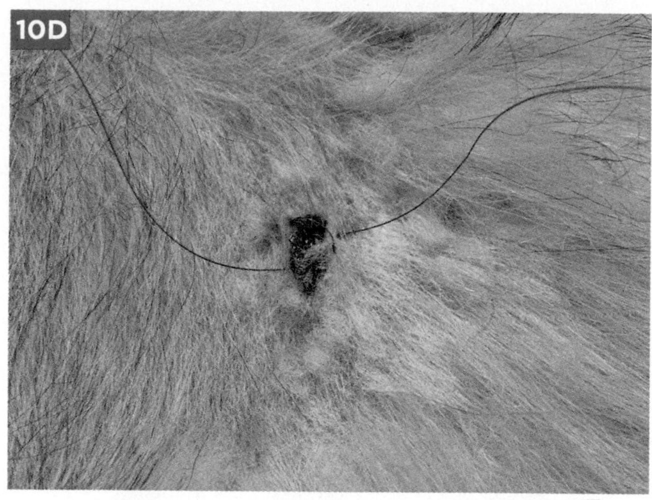

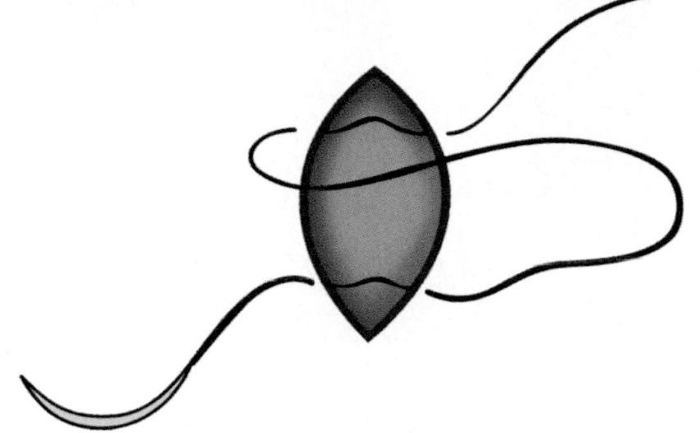

Cross the wound, and pass the needle through the tissues and the skin on the other side of the hole, again, taking approximately the same-sized bite of tissue.

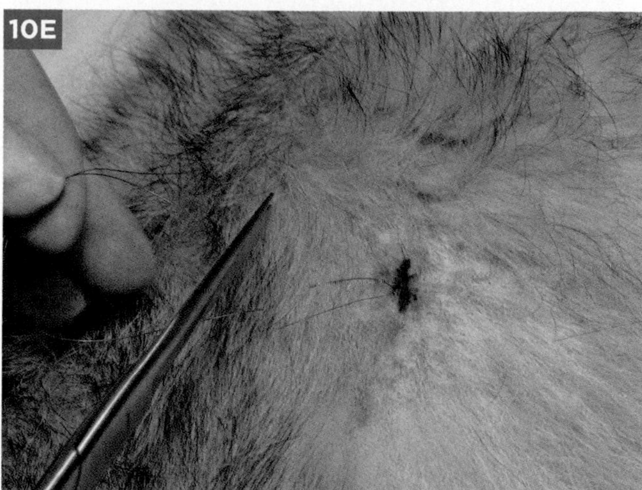

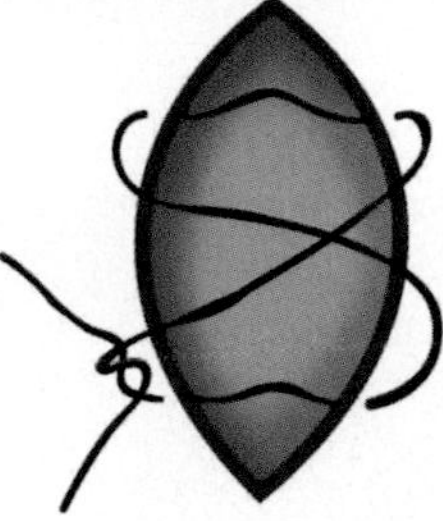

The two ends of suture are brought together and tied under minimal tension, to create the cross shape (cruciate).

Note: If a skin biopsy is being taken for culture (as may be desired in a case of bacterial pyoderma not responding appropriately to antibiotics), discontinue antibiotics for at least 48 hours before biopsy, and clip and perform a routine surgical prep of the site, followed by a water or saline rinse. Use sterile technique to collect the biopsy and submit the tissue to the laboratory for culture in a sterile red-top tube.

PROCEDURE 4-6

Wood's Lamp Examination

PURPOSE

To evaluate patients with lesions suggestive of dermatophyte (ringworm) infection

INDICATIONS

1. The evaluation of dogs and cats with dermatologic lesions that could be ringworm. The classical lesion would be well demarcated, crusted, and pruritic. Dermatophyte infection can, however, have a varied appearance, so Wood's lamp examination should be considered in any case with regional or patchy alopecia, scaling, crusting, seborrhea, pruritus, or regional folliculitis.

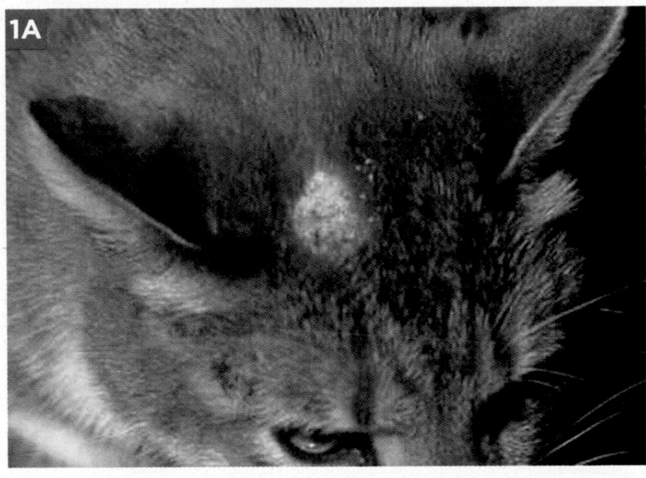

A round, crusted pruritic patch on the head of a cat with ringworm. **(Courtesy Dr. Klaas Post, University of Saskatchewan.)**

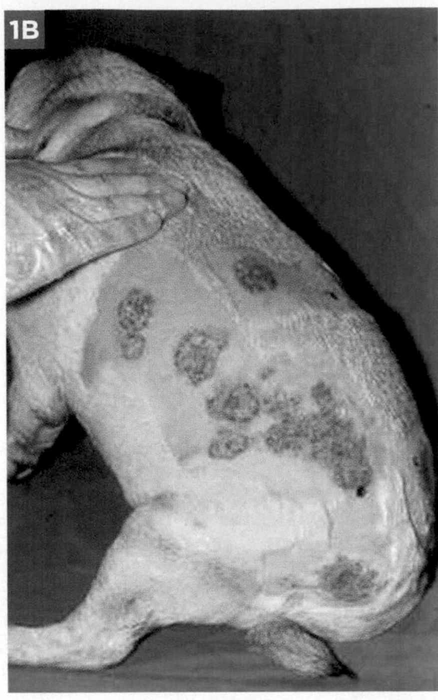

Multiple round, crusted patches in a Bulldog with *Microsporum canis* infection. **(Courtesy Dr. Klaas Post, University of Saskatchewan.)**

CONTRAINDICATIONS AND CONCERNS

1. Wear gloves because the dermatophytes infecting dogs and cats can cause lesions in humans.
2. The Wood's lamp must be turned on for 5 to 10 minutes before use because the stability of the light's wavelength and intensity is temperature dependent.
3. It is important to distinguish nonspecific fluorescence that occurs on crusts and scales from the fluorescence associated with dermatophyte infection. Scales and crusts tend to have a diffuse (not confined to hair shaft) glow that is olive-green to yellowish green. *Microsporum canis* fluorescence is confined to the individual hairs (which are often broken off) and is typically apple-green (a very bright green, like a flashlight shining through a lime lollipop).
4. The fluorescence of *M. canis* will remain even after the fungus has been killed by treatment. Over time, as the hairs grow, the dead fungus will be located near the ends of the hairs instead of near the base as expected with an active infection.

POSITIONING AND RESTRAINT

Adequate restraint to keep the animal still

EQUIPMENT

The Wood's lamp is an ultraviolet light with a lightwave filtered through a cobalt or nickel filter. Green fluorescence occurs with some dermatophytes because of the tryptophan that is produced by the fungus.

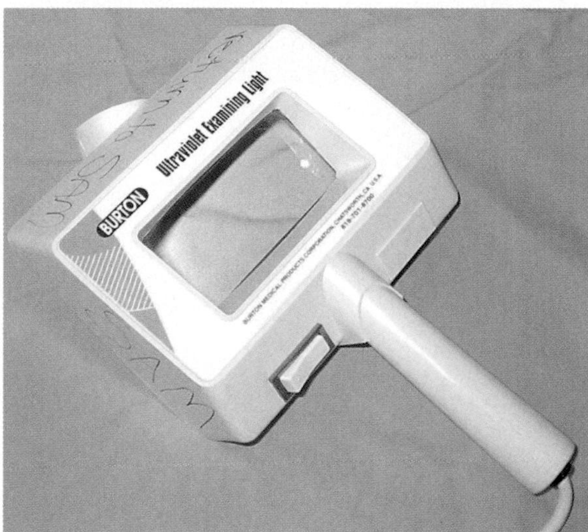

The Wood's lamp is an ultraviolet light with a lightwave filtered through a cobalt or nickel filter.

TECHNIQUE

1. Turn on the Wood's lamp at least 5 minutes before using it to examine the patient.
2. Wear gloves, and examine the patient using the Wood's lamp in a darkened room.

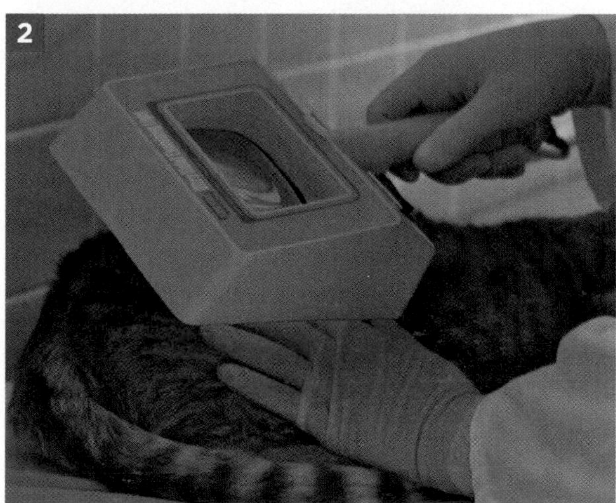

Using the Wood's lamp to examine a patient in a darkened room.

3. Look for bright green fluorescence associated with the hairs in the lesion.

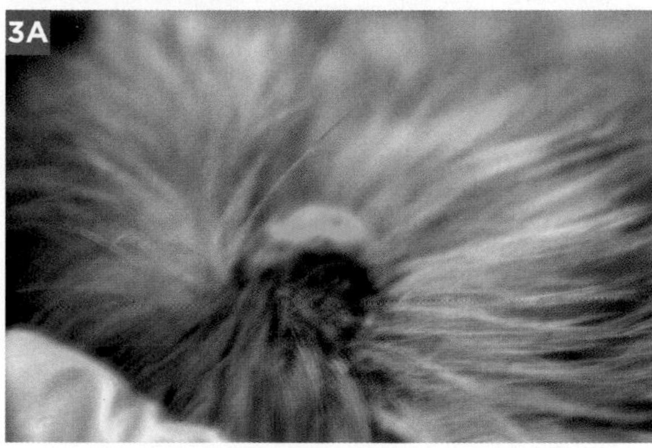

Green fluorescence of the hairs around skin lesion on a cat's neck caused by *M. canis.*

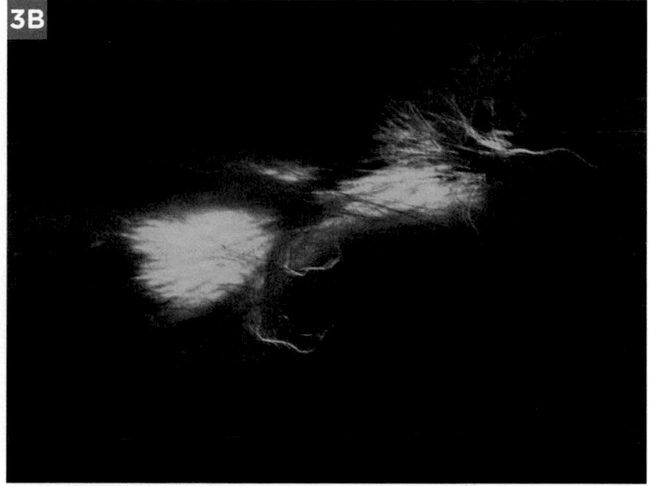

Positive Wood's lamp examination in a cat with ringworm caused by *M. canis.* **(Courtesy Dr. Catherine Outerbridge, University of California–Davis.)**

RESULTS

Only *M. canis* shows positive results, and only approximately 50% of *M. canis* infections are positive. Suspicious lesions (and all Wood's lamp–positive lesions) should have hairs, crusts, and swabs cultured to confirm the presence of a dermatophyte. *M. canis* is responsible for most dermatophyte infections in cats (>98%) and dogs (50% to 70%). Less commonly diagnosed pathogenic dermatophytes include the nonfluorescing *Trichophyton mentagrophytes* and *Microsporum gypseum*.

Ear Examination

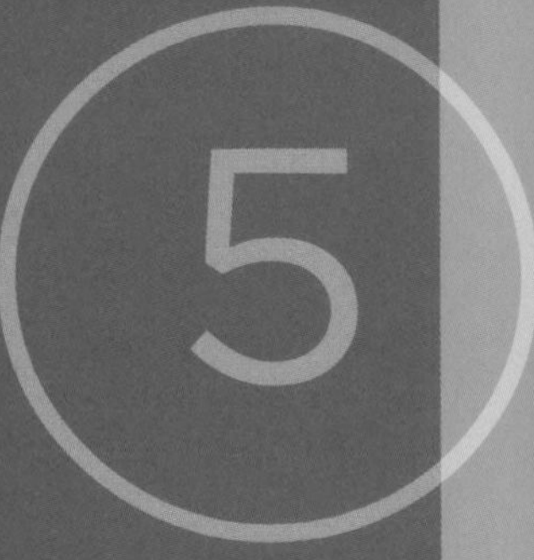

PROCEDURE 5-1

Ear Examination

PURPOSE

To examine and evaluate the external ear canal

INDICATIONS

1. Whenever possible, an external ear examination should be performed as part of a routine physical examination.
2. A complete external ear exam is especially important in animals exhibiting head shaking, ear scratching, ear odor or discharge, hair loss around the ears, deafness, head tilt, or incoordination.

CONTRAINDICATIONS AND WARNINGS

1. Few dogs or cats with inflammatory disease of the external ear canal will allow thorough examination of the ear canals without heavy sedation or general anesthesia.
2. Examination of the external ear canal in a struggling patient could lead to injury to the tympanic membrane.
3. When an external ear canal is filled with exudate or debris, the ear canal should be cleaned and lavaged with warm saline or another nondetergent, nonalcoholic flushing solution before thorough examination. This usually requires sedation or anesthesia.

POSITIONING AND RESTRAINT

1. The animal should be positioned standing, sitting, or in sternal or lateral recumbency.
2. The holder should firmly grasp the closed muzzle of the patient with one hand while restraining the body of the patient with the other hand.
3. Sedation or general anesthesia should be administered if necessary.

SPECIAL ANATOMY

1. The pinna, or auricle, is the external flap of the ear.
2. The external ear canal is composed of a long vertical ear canal that at its end bends approximately 75 degrees to form the shorter horizontal ear canal. The ear canal is lined with a stratified squamous epithelium containing sebaceous and ceruminous glands that normally secrete earwax (cerumen). The horizontal and vertical canals are largely surrounded by cartilage. However, adjacent to the tympanic membrane, the horizontal canal is supported by bone.

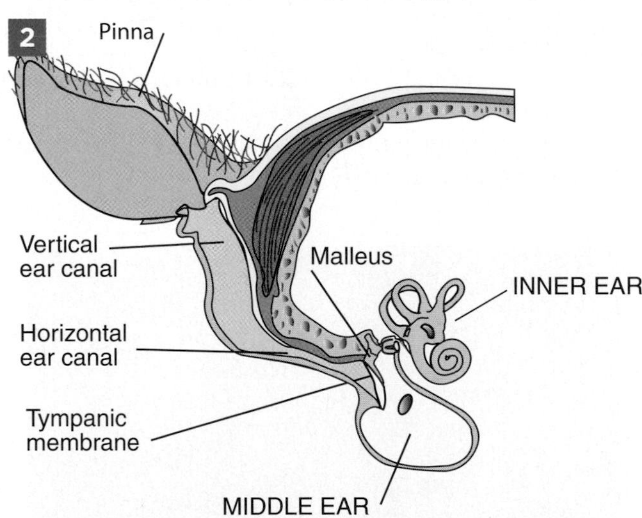

Anatomy of the external ear canal

3. The eardrum, or tympanic membrane, is a thin semitransparent sheet that forms the barrier between the external ear canal and the middle ear and transmits sound waves from the external ear onto the auditory ossicles of the middle ear.
4. The tympanic membrane is surrounded by and suspended within the tympanic ring. The large, thin, transparent to translucent portion of the tympanic membrane is under considerable tension and is called the pars tensa. The

smaller triangular dorsal to anterodorsal portion of the tympanic membrane is an opaque pink or white membrane containing a network of small vessels. This is the pars flaccida. In an inflamed ear, this "vascular strip" can become edematous and resemble a mass. The pars flaccida contains blood vessels that are important to the health and repair of the germinal epithelium of the eardrum.

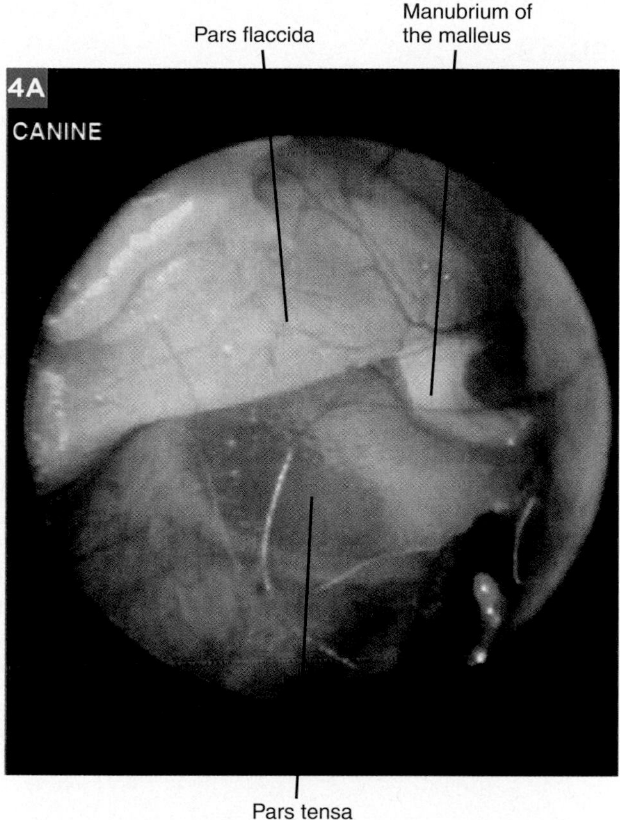

Anatomy of a normal canine right tympanic membrane. The dog's nose is to the right. **(Courtesy Dr. Louis Gotthelf, Montgomery, Alabama.)**

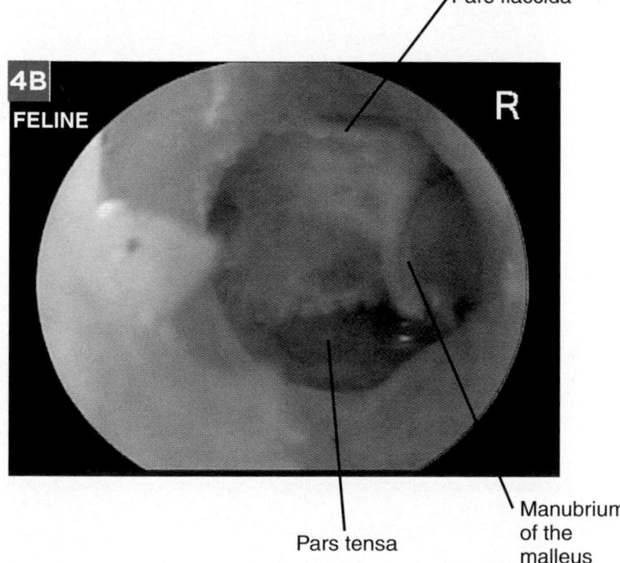

Anatomy of a normal feline right tympanic membrane. The cat's nose is to the right. **(Courtesy Dr. Louis Gotthelf, Montgomery, Alabama.)**

5. The manubrium (footplate) of the malleus ossicle is attached to the fibrous layer of the tympanum, pulling it inward and resulting in a mildly concave outer contour of the normal eardrum. Striations may be seen in the pars tensa extending from the attached manubrium to the periphery. The malleus is oriented dorsoventrally, with its free (ventral) end forming a gentle curve or hook—the open end of the resulting reverse C shape is pointed toward the animal's nose.

EQUIPMENT

- Otoscope and appropriately sized otoscope cone
- A video otoscope with flush, suction, and biopsy capabilities can be a very useful tool for otoscopic examination.

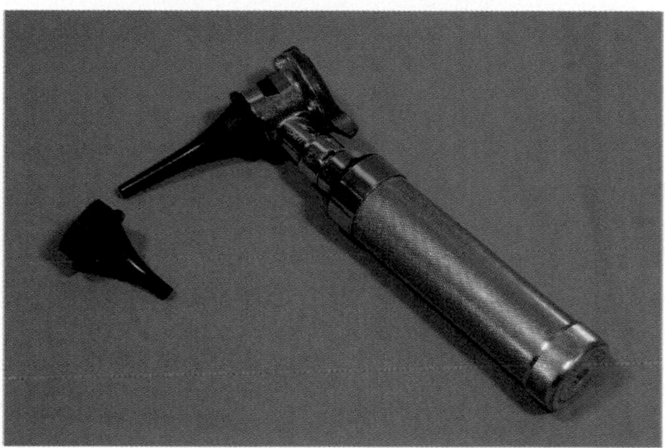

Equipment required for external ear examination.

PROCEDURE

1. Examine the pinna for any evidence of inflammation or exudate before performing otoscopic examination of the ear.

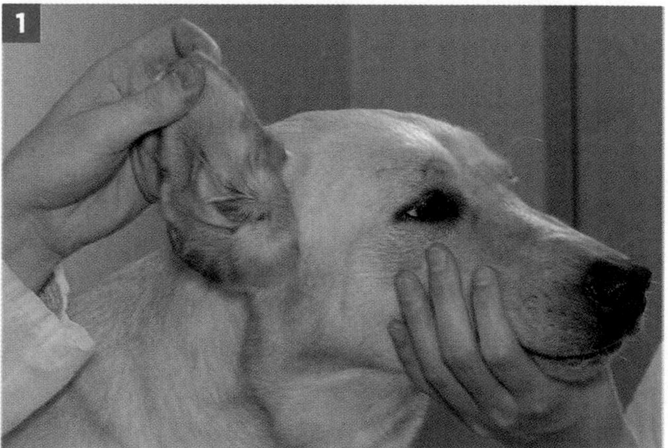

Examining the pinna for any evidence of inflammation or exudate.

PROCEDURE 5-1 Ear Examination—cont'd

2. With the animal standing, the examiner should insert the otoscope into the vertical canal of the external ear while pulling up on the pinna.

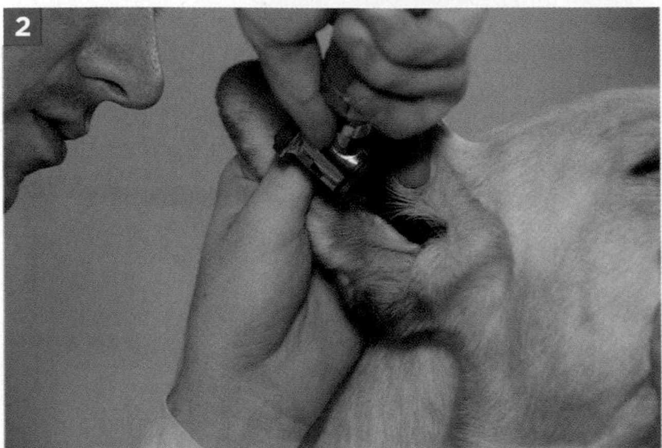

Inserting the otoscope into the vertical canal of the external ear while pulling up on the pinna.

3. Once the tip of the otoscope is at the junction between the vertical and horizontal canals, the otoscope cone can be slowly returned to a horizontal orientation so that the horizontal canal and the tympanic membrane can be visualized. This examination is not possible if the patient is uncooperative or in pain.

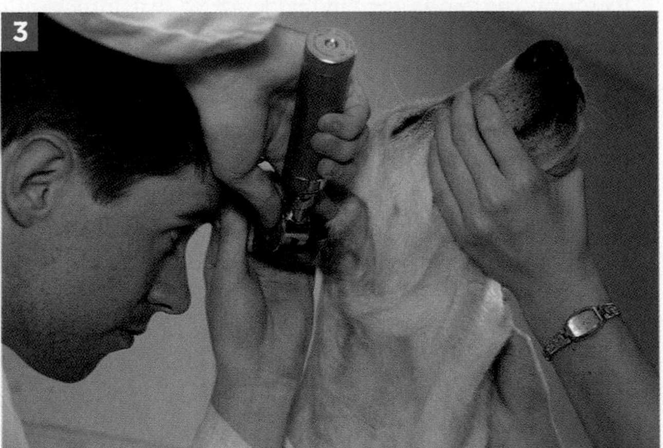

Visualizing the horizontal canal and the tympanic membrane.

4. With the animal sedated or anesthetized and in lateral recumbency, a more thorough otic examination can be performed. The pinna can be lifted (pulled laterally) to straighten out the curved ear canal, making insertion of the otoscope easier.

RESULTS

1. The ear canals can be evaluated for patency or stenosis, proliferation, ulceration, exudates, foreign bodies, parasites, tumors, and excessive wax or hair accumulation. Suspicious lesions can be biopsied.
2. Whenever there is otic exudate, a cytologic preparation should be made. A disinfected otoscope cone should be placed into the vertical ear canal with its tip near the junction with the horizontal canal. A cotton-tipped swab is inserted through the otoscope cone and extended beyond the cone to collect a sample. The swab is then withdrawn.
   - **A.** To look for mites, the ear swab is rolled in a drop of mineral oil on a microscope slide, a coverslip is applied, and the slide is examined under low power (40× to 100×).
   - **B.** To look for cellular debris, bacteria, and yeast the swab is rolled on a clean, dry microscope slide. The slide is heat-fixed and stained, and then covered with a coverslip for evaluation. The slide should be examined under low power (40× to 100×) for an overall view of cellular debris and under high power (440× to 1000×) for bacteria and yeast.

Ocular Techniques

6

PROCEDURE 6-1
Schirmer Tear Test

PURPOSE

To measure the aqueous component of basal and reflex tear production

INDICATIONS

1. Any animal with a red eye
2. Any animal with a mucoid or purulent ocular discharge
3. Any animal with pigmentary keratitis
4. Monitoring treatment of any animal with known keratoconjunctivitis sicca (dry eye)
5. Monitoring dogs being treated with medications that may decrease tear production (sulfonamides, etodolac, others)

COMPLICATIONS

1. It is important to perform a Schirmer tear test (STT) before any other ocular procedures are performed in order to obtain accurate results.
2. Avoid any excessive manipulation of the eyelids and the administration of topical anesthetic or systemic medications before STT measurement.

SPECIAL ANATOMY

The precorneal tear film is essential for maintaining corneal health. It consists of three layers (Table 6-1). Tears comprise the middle aqueous layer and are produced by the lacrimal gland and the gland of the third eyelid. Tears provide oxygen and nutrients to the cornea, flush away particulate debris, maintain hydration of the cornea and conjunctiva, and inhibit bacterial growth. Tears are continuously produced at a basal rate, and production is stimulated by corneal irritation.

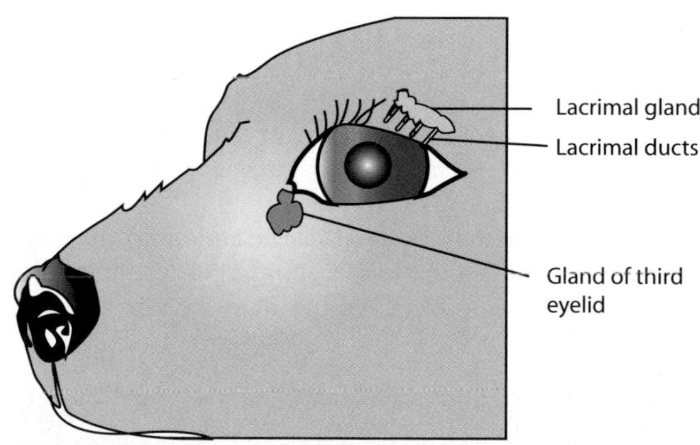

Tears are produced by the lacrimal gland and the gland of the third eyelid.

TABLE 6-1

The Three Layers of the Precorneal Tear Film

LAYER	COMPONENT	ORIGIN
Inner layer	Mucin	Conjunctival goblet cells
Middle layer	Aqueous	Lacrimal gland, third eyelid gland
Outer layer	Lipid	Meibomian (tarsal) glands

PROCEDURE 6-1 Schirmer Tear Test—cont'd

EQUIPMENT

- Schirmer tear test strips

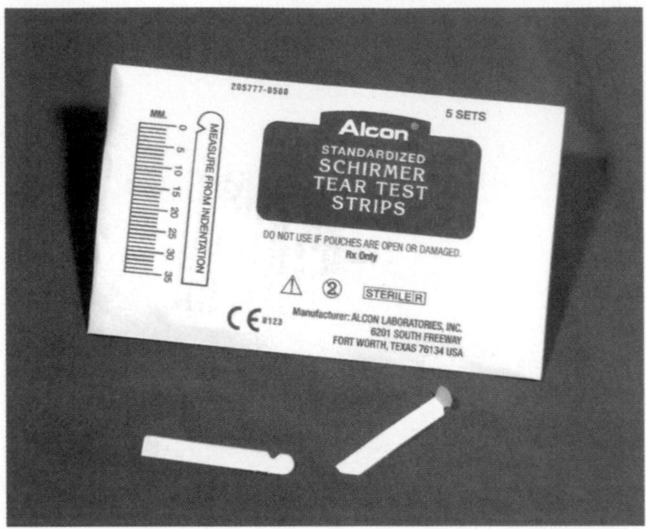

Equipment needed to measure tear production.

TECHNIQUE

1. Fold the notched (rounded) end of the sterile filter paper strip within the sterile package, thus keeping this end of the strip sterile.
2. Remove the strip from the package, and insert the folded end between the lower eyelid and the cornea, at the junction of the middle and lateral third of the lower eyelid.

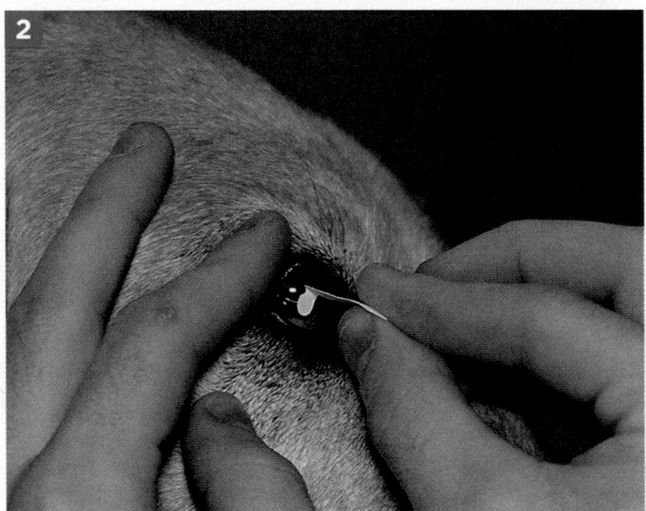

Inserting the strip between the lower eyelid and the cornea, at the junction of the middle and lateral third of the lower eyelid.

3. The rate of basal and reflex tear production is measured as the animal tears in response to the sensation of the strip contacting the cornea.

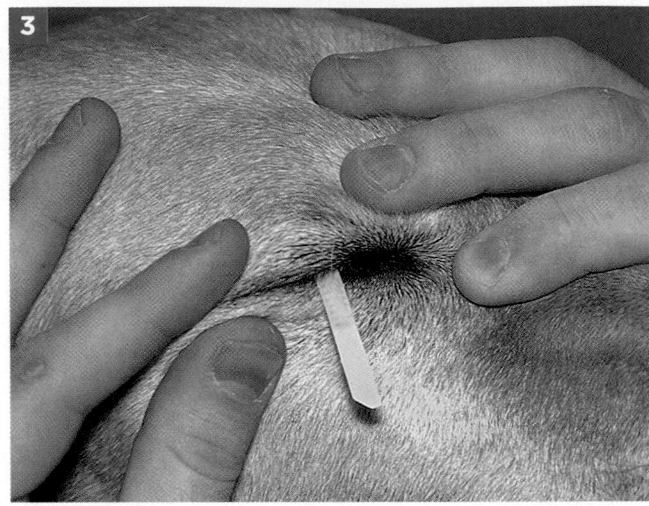

The animal tears in response to the sensation of the strip contacting the cornea.

4. Allow the strip to stay in place for exactly 1 minute. The eye may be closed or open.

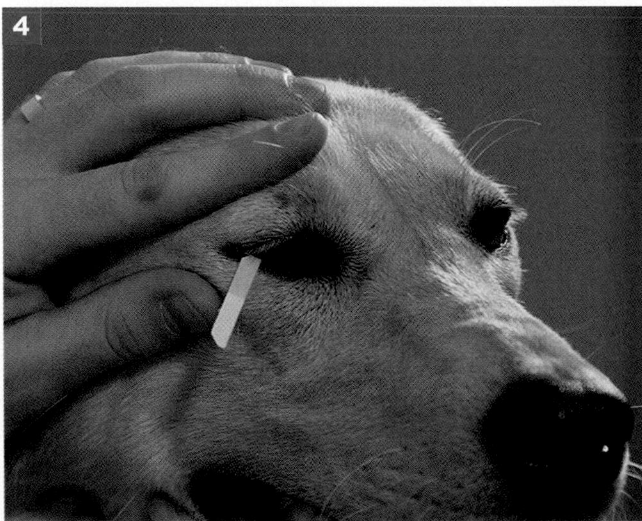

The strip in place.

5. Remove the strip and measure the wet portion of the strip from the notch to the wet/dry interface against the millimeter scale on the package.

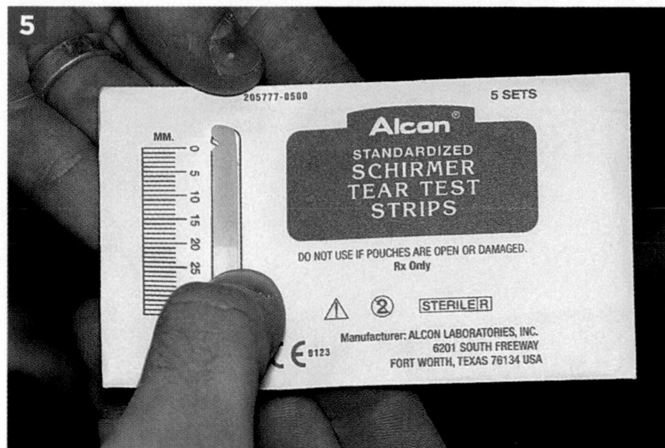

Measuring the wet portion of the strip from the notch to the wet-dry interface.

6. Normal values for dogs are 15 mm or greater, whereas normal values in cats can be lower (5 mm/min).

7. Repeat the procedure in the opposite eye.

PROCEDURE 6-2

Conjunctival Culture

PURPOSE

To identify infectious pathogens of the conjunctiva

INDICATION

Severe chronic conjunctivitis that has not improved with empirical antibiotic therapy

EQUIPMENT

- Sterile swabs for bacterial and fungal culture
- Transport medium

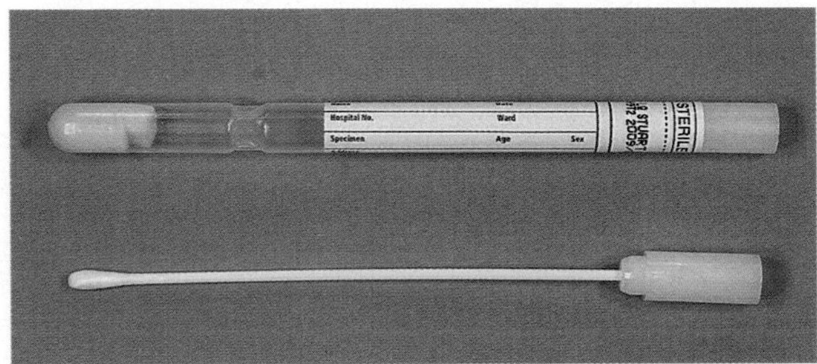

Equipment needed for conjunctival culture.

CONTRAINDICATIONS AND WARNINGS

Primary bacterial pathogens rarely cause persistent conjunctivitis in dogs and cats. When presumed bacterial conjunctivitis does not respond to empirical topical antibiotic treatment, it is important to carefully evaluate the eyelids, the nasolacrimal system, the cornea, and the systemic health of the animal before concluding that incorrect antibiotic choice is the reason for the problem. Ideally, topical and systemic antibiotic treatments should be discontinued for 5 days before obtaining a conjunctival culture.

TECHNIQUE

1. Moisten the end of a sterile cotton-tipped swab with sterile saline.

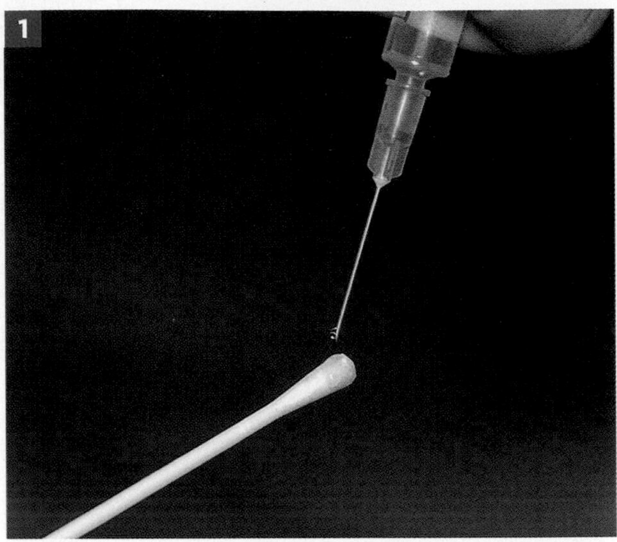

The end of a sterile cotton tipped swab is moistened with sterile saline.

2. Evert the lower lid by pulling downward on the skin just below the eyelid margins with the index finger.
3. Gently swab the conjunctival sac, avoiding the eyelid margins.

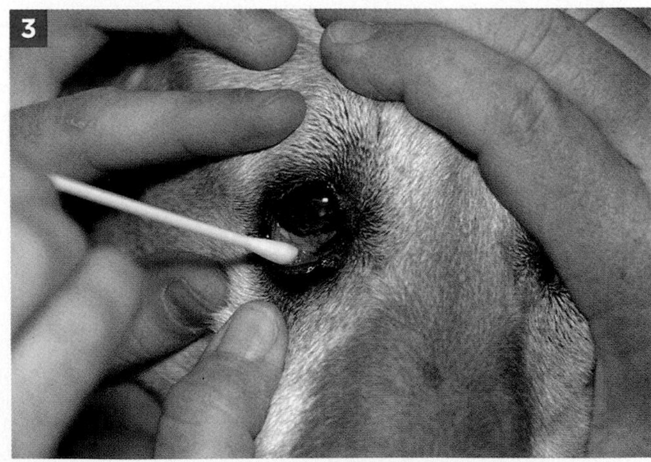

Swabbing the conjunctival sac, avoiding the eyelid margins.

4. Replace the swab in transport tube or inoculate media immediately.

PROCEDURE 6-3

Fluorescein Staining

PURPOSE

To detect and characterize corneal ulcers, as well as to assess the patency of the nasolacrimal ducts

INDICATIONS

1. Animals with a painful or red eye
2. Animals with a visible irregularity or clouding of the cornea
3. Animals with a chronic watery ocular discharge
4. Animals with a mucoid or purulent ocular discharge

SPECIAL ANATOMY

Fluorescein, which is water soluble, distributes within the preocular tear film, resulting in a faint yellow-orange appearance. The corneal epithelium is lipid selective and resists penetration by this water-soluble stain. In the presence of an epithelial defect (ulcer), fluorescein dye rapidly diffuses into the corneal stroma and is retained there even after rinsing. A region of fluorescein retention by the corneal stroma therefore indicates an epithelial defect such as an ulcer or erosion.

Drainage of tears from the eye takes place through the superior and inferior lacrimal puncta, oval openings located on the inner conjunctival surface of the upper and lower lids adjacent to the medial canthus. These puncta are sometimes surrounded by a rim of pigment. Tears drain through the nasolacrimal puncta into the nasolacrimal duct, which travels down the nose, exiting within the anterior nose adjacent to the attached margin of the alar fold. When fluorescein stain is instilled into the eye, stained tears should drain through the puncta into the nasolacrimal duct, resulting in the appearance of dye in the nostril on the same side. Failure to drain could indicate obstruction to the nasolacrimal duct within the nose due to compression by a mass or (more commonly) obstruction of the nasolacrimal puncta by cellular debris or swelling.

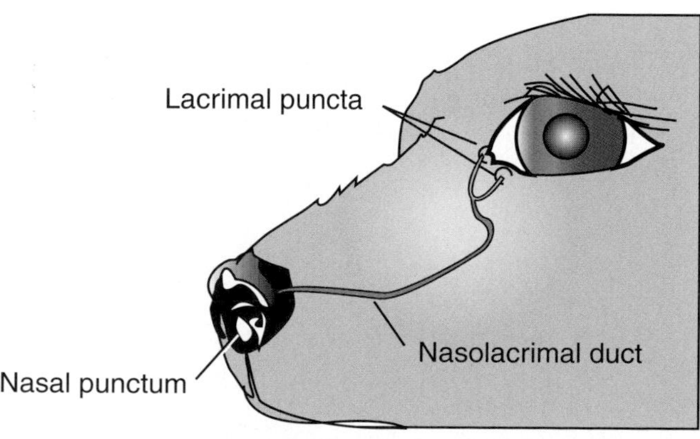

Anatomy of the nasolacrimal system.

EQUIPMENT

- Fluoroscein test strips
- Eyewash
- Gauze sponges
- Light source

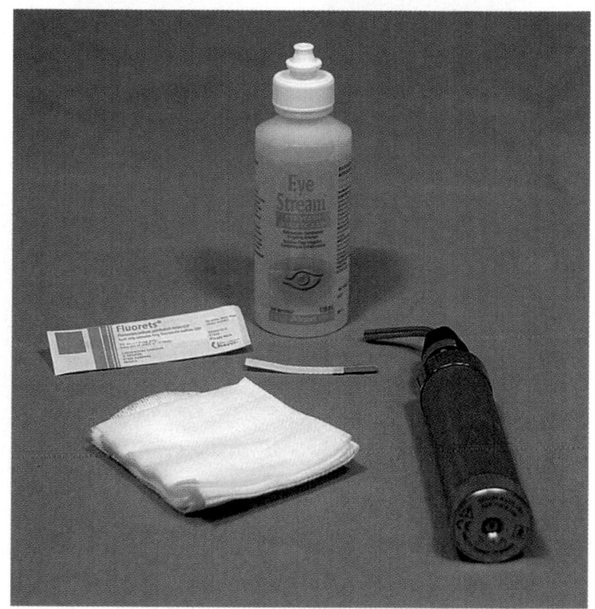

Equipment required to perform fluoroscein staining.

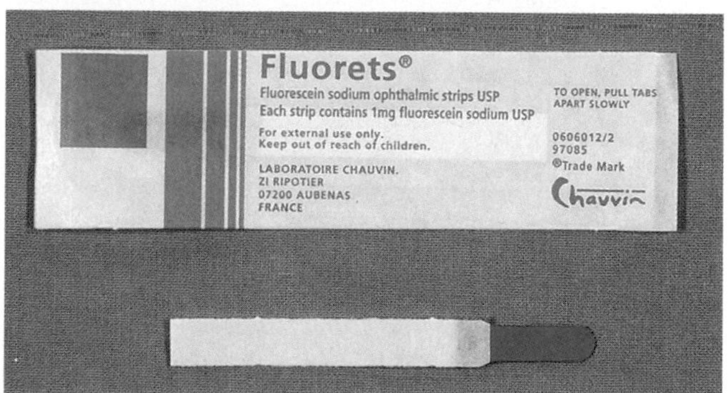

Fluoroscein test strips.

PROCEDURE 6-3 Fluorescein Staining—cont'd

TECHNIQUE

1. Moisten the end of a strip of fluorescein with a few drops of sterile eyewash.

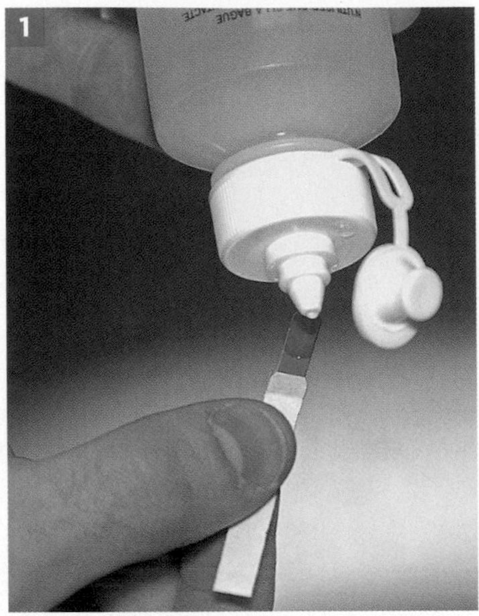

Moistening the end of a strip of fluorescein with a few drops of sterile eyewash.

2. Elevate the upper eyelid and touch the moistened tip of the fluorescein strip against the bulbar conjunctiva for 2 seconds.

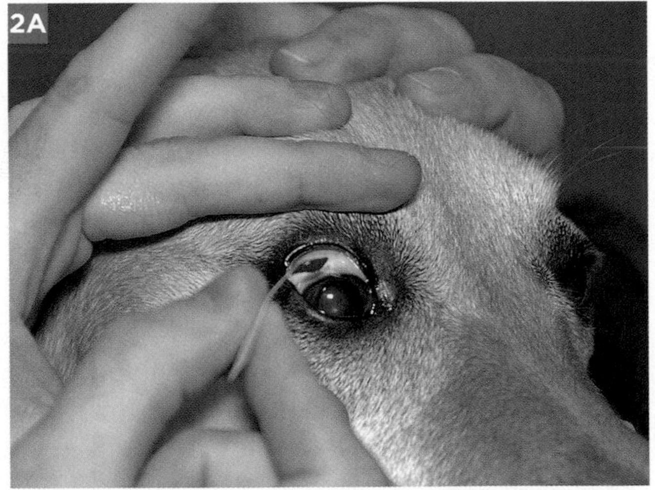

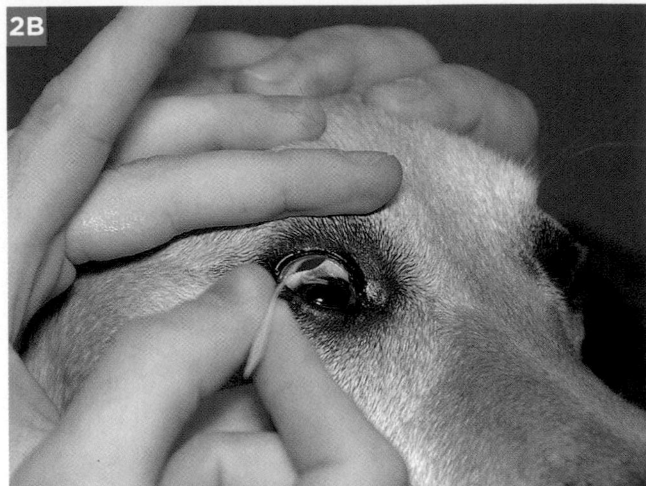

Elevating the upper eyelid and touching the moistened tip of the fluorescein strip against the bulbar conjunctiva.

3. Remove the strip and allow the patient to blink to distribute the stain.

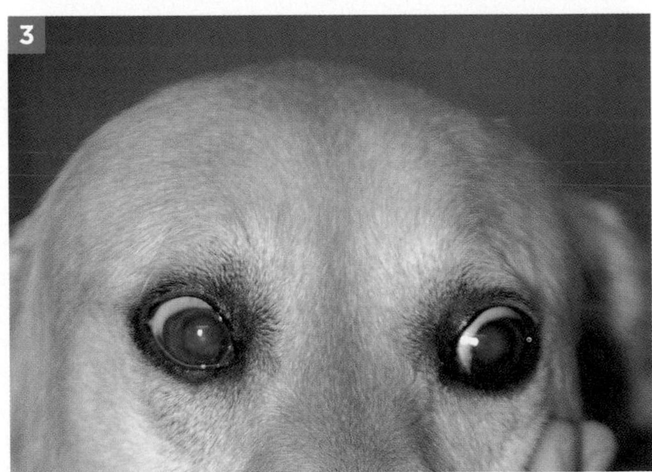

The stain is distributed throughout the tear film as the dog blinks.

4. Liberally rinse the eye with ophthalmic irrigating solution, which will remove the unbound excess stain and enhance the visibility of stain retained within a corneal defect.

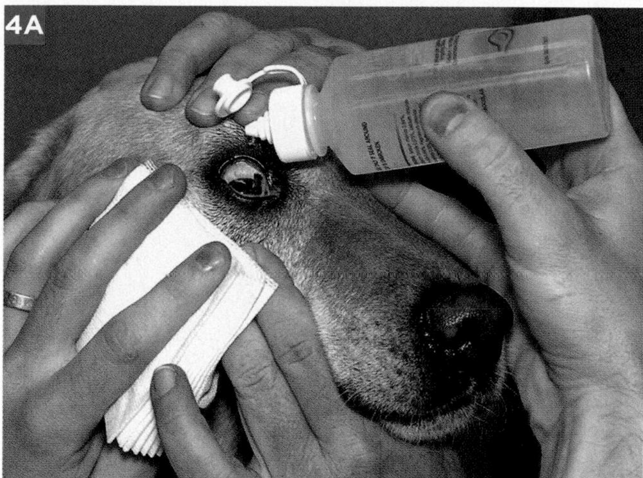

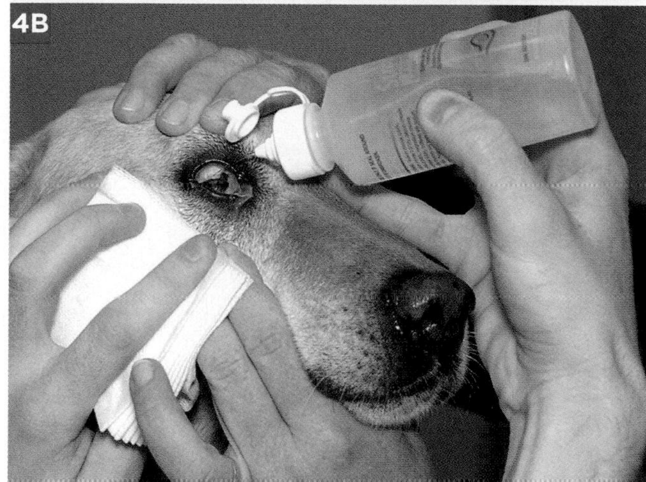

Rinsing the eye with ophthalmic irrigating solution to remove unbound stain.

5. Examine the cornea in a partially darkened room with a white light and also with an ultraviolet light source or a cobalt blue filter on the tip of a handheld transilluminator to excite the fluorescein molecules, making them glow green.

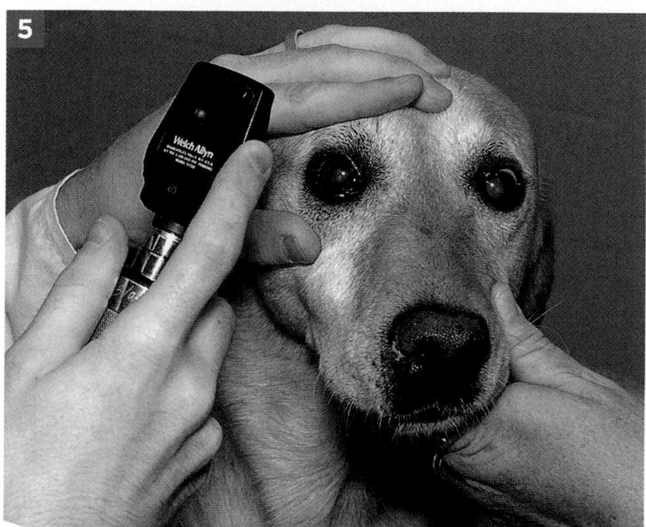

Examining the cornea for fluorescein retention.

6. Stain uptake on the cornea indicates a disruption in the epithelium, suggesting a corneal ulcer or erosion.

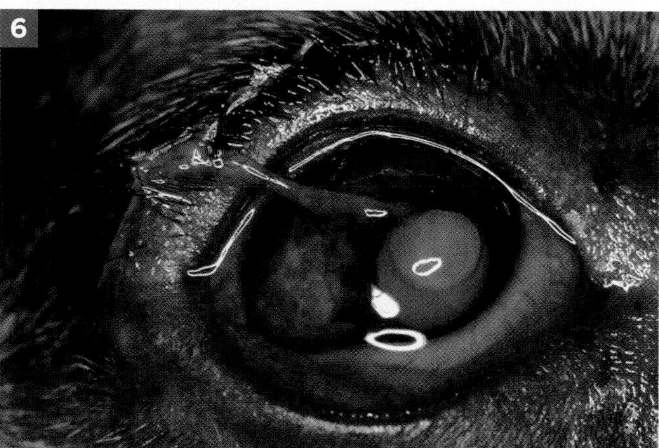

Stain uptake on the cornea indicates a disruption in the epithelium caused by a corneal ulcer. **(Courtesy Dr. Bruce Grahn, University of Saskatchewan.)**

7. Observe external nares for the appearance of green dye, indicating patency of the nasolacrimal puncta and duct.

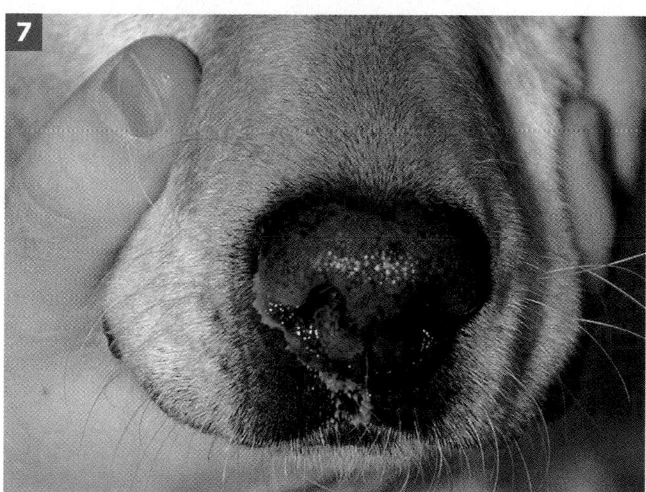

The appearance of green dye at the external nares indicates that the nasolacrimal punctum and duct are patent.

PROCEDURE 6-4

Flushing the Nasolacrimal Ducts

PURPOSE

To relieve minor obstructions of the nasolacrimal duct

INDICATIONS

Any animal with a watery or mucoid ocular discharge that does not have a patent nasolacrimal duct as assessed with the fluorescein dye test

SPECIAL ANATOMY

Drainage of tears from the eye through the superior and inferior puncta into the nasolacrimal duct and into the nose can be obstructed by cellular debris or mucus or by mass lesions compressing the nasolacrimal duct during its passage through the nasal cavity. Scarring and blockage of the puncta can occur, especially secondary to herpes keratoconjunctivitis in kittens and cats. Imperforate puncta and punctal aplasia also can occur as congenital abnormalities.

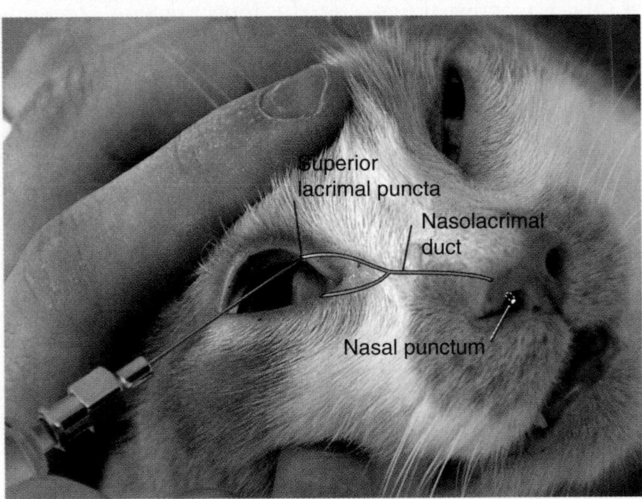

Anatomy of tear drainage through the nasolacrimal duct.

EQUIPMENT

- Gauze sponges
- Topical ophthalmic anesthetic
- Sterile 23- to 27-gauge nasolacrimal cannula
- 3-mL syringe containing sterile saline or eyewash

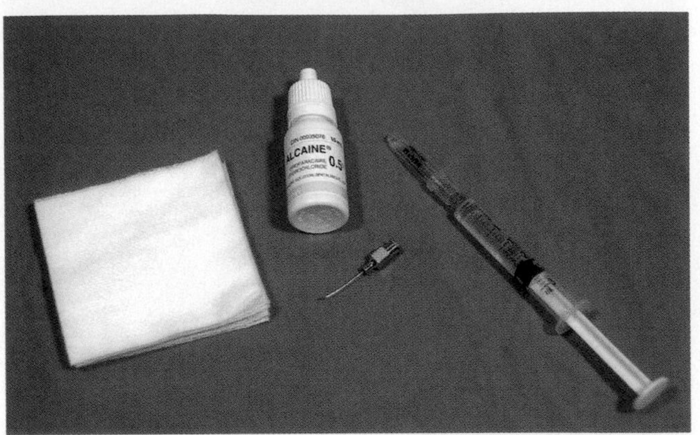

Equipment required to flush the nasolacrimal duct.

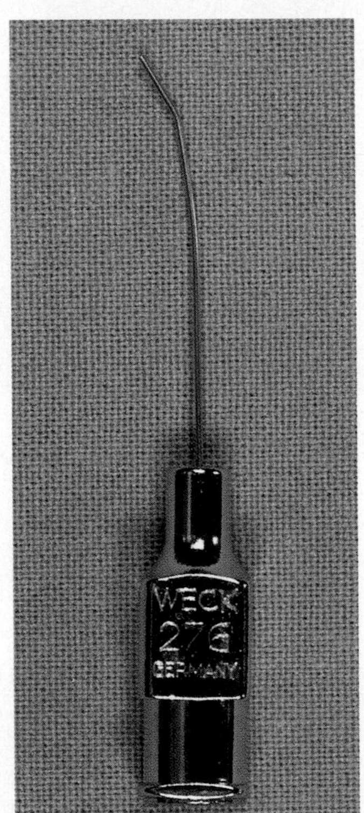

Nasolacrimal cannula.

TECHNIQUE

1. Sedation may be required, depending on the temperament of the animal.
2. Wipe out any excess discharge.
3. Instill 2 drops of topical ophthalmic anesthetic, wait 30 seconds, then apply 2 more drops.

4. While the head is restrained to prevent movement, apply tension to the upper eyelid and roll it out to expose the superior punctum.

5. Using a commercial lacrimal cannula or a small IV catheter (needle removed), slide the cannula along the inner lid margin toward the medial canthus until the punctum is located.

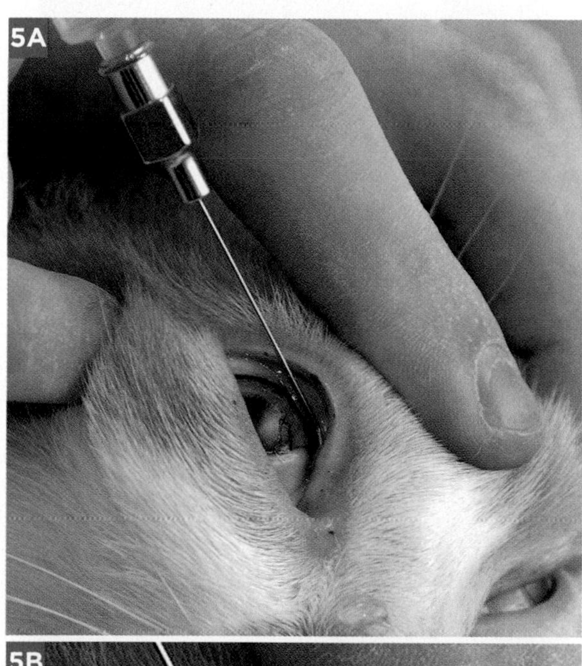

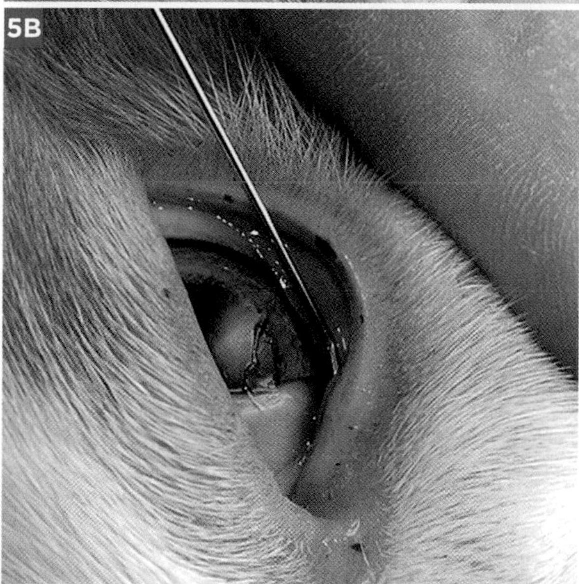

The tip of the cannula is directed along the inner lid margin toward the medial canthus until the superior punctum is located.

6. Once the cannula is well seated, flush 2 to 3 mL of sterile saline through the punctum, and observe fluid emerging from the inferior punctum.

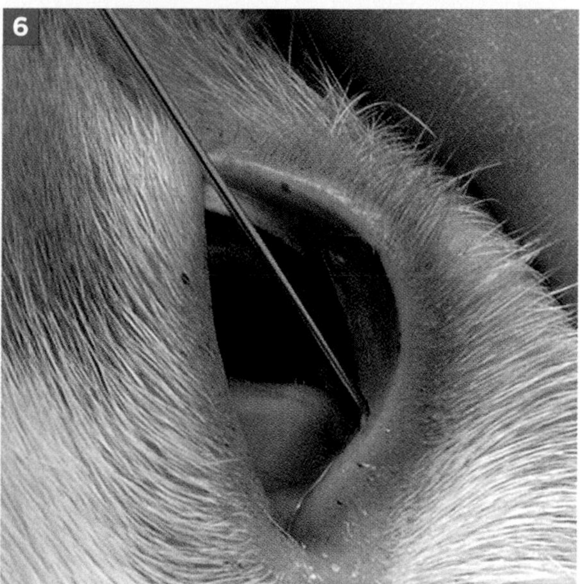

Flush saline through the punctum.

7. If saline does not flow, the lower punctum should be cannulated and flushed as well.

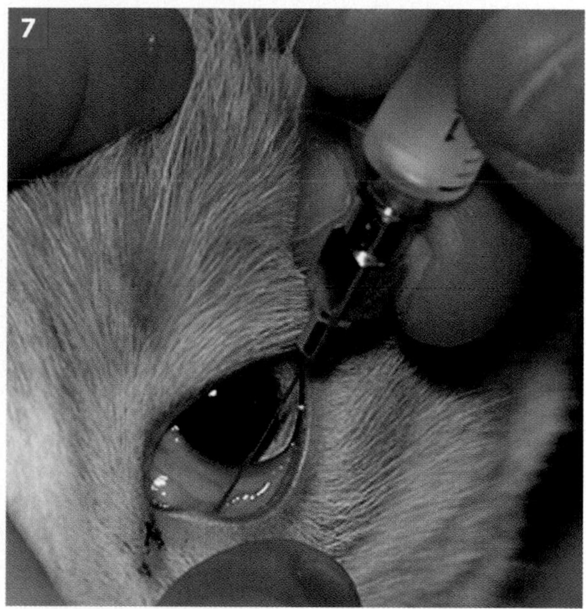

The nasolacrimal punctum on the lower lid also can be flushed.

8. While flushing the upper punctum it should be possible to occlude the lower punctum and observe fluid coming from the nostril.

PROCEDURE 6-5

Applying Topical Medications in the Eye

PURPOSE

To place ointment or drops in the eye

INDICATIONS

Medicating the eye

TECHNIQUE

1. Use warm water on a tissue or a gauze sponge to cleanse the region around the eye and to remove any discharge.
2. If there is abundant debris, use an ophthalmic irrigating solution to wash away the debris and discharge, and then blot with a tissue or gauze sponge to remove excess fluid.
3. Tilt the animal's head back and use fingers to lift the upper eyelid.
4. Instill 1 or 2 drops of solution or a small ribbon (¼ inch) of ointment on the sclera at approximately the 12 o'clock position.

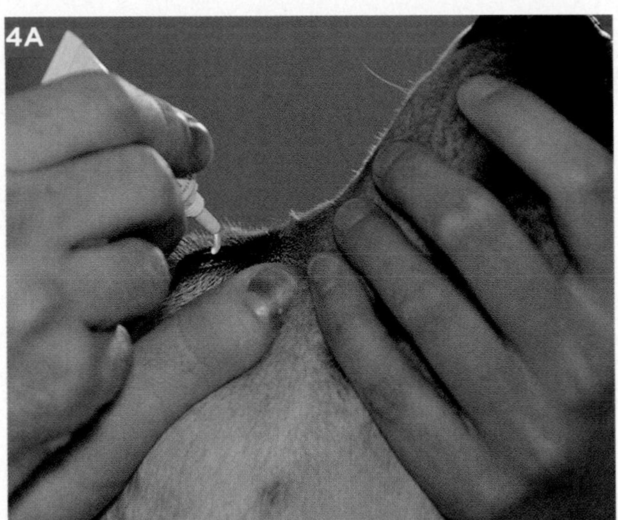

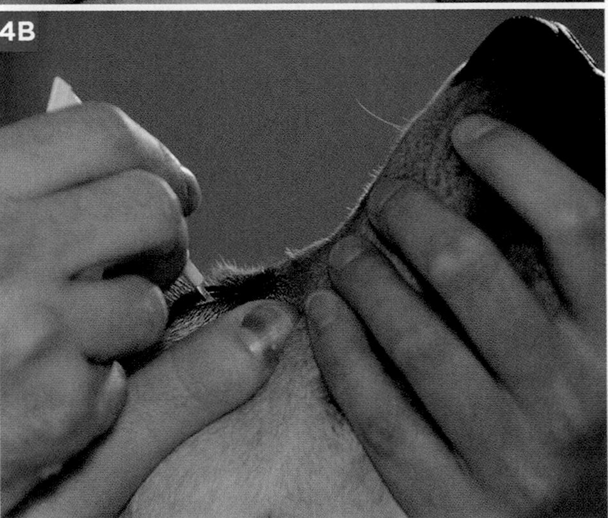

The head is tilted back and a small ribbon of ointment is deposited on the sclera at approximately 12 o'clock on the globe.

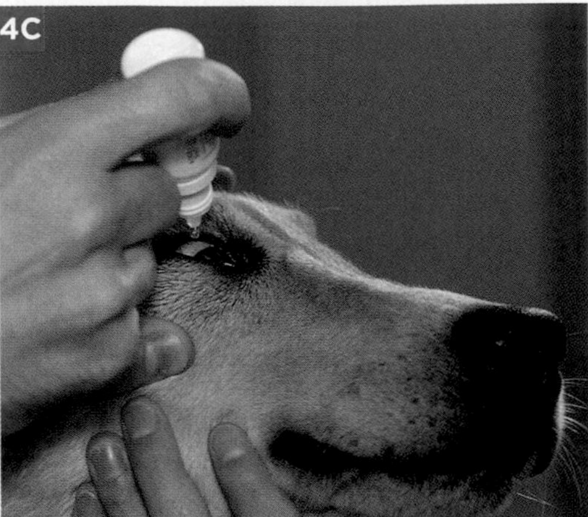

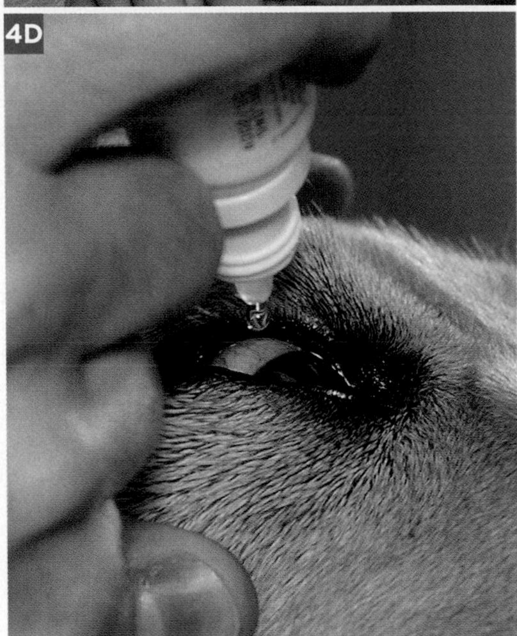

A drop of solution is instilled in the eye. Instill 1 or 2 drops of solution.

PROCEDURE 6-6
Conjunctival Scrapings

PURPOSE

To obtain cells from the conjunctival surface for evaluation

INDICATIONS

1. Animals with chronic conjunctivitis and ocular discharge
2. Dogs with suspect canine distemper infection
3. Cats with suspected chlamydial conjunctivitis
4. Animals with conjunctival masses

EQUIPMENT

- Topical ophthalmic anesthetic
- Sterile metal ocular spatula or scalpel blade
- Glass slides

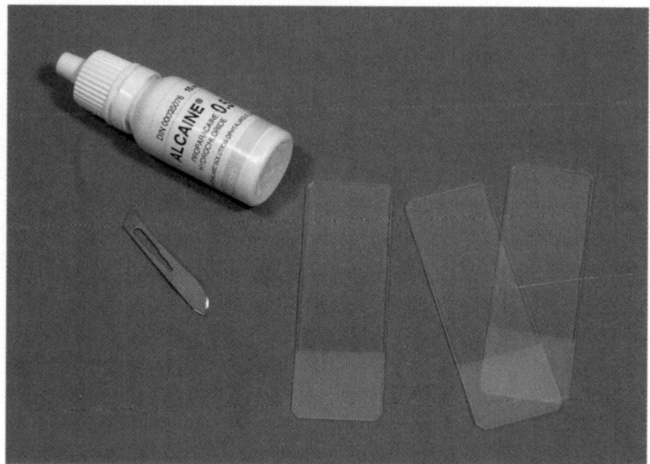

Equipment required to perform a conjunctival scraping.

TECHNIQUE

1. Wipe discharge from the eye.
2. Instill 2 drops of topical ophthalmic anesthetic, wait 30 seconds, then apply 2 more drops.

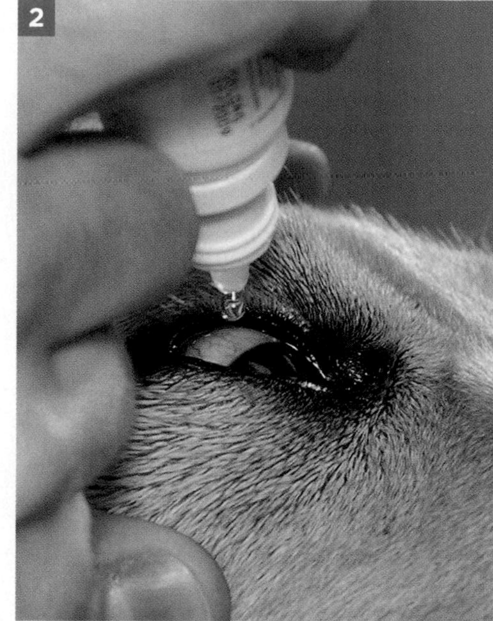

Applying topical anesthetic ophthalmic drops.

3. Use a platinum spatula designed for this purpose or the blunt snap-on end of a surgical blade.
4. Retropulse the globe to cause the third eyelid (nictitans) to protrude.

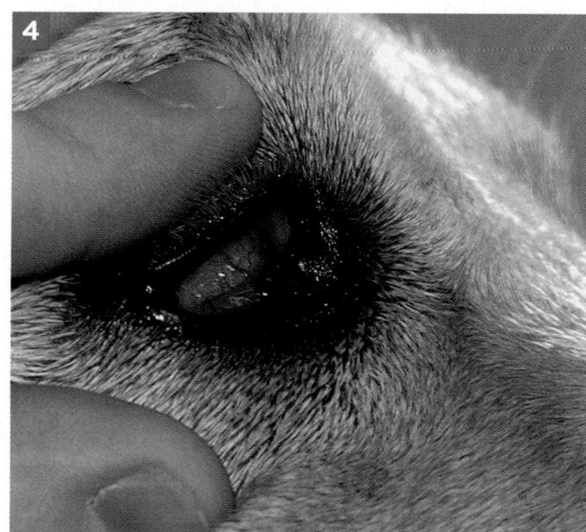

Retropulsing the globe to cause the third eyelid (nictitans) to protrude.

PROCEDURE 6-6 Conjunctival Scrapings—cont'd

5. Evert the lower eyelid by pulling down on the skin below the eyelid margin.
6. Place the spatula or blade perpendicular to the surface to be scraped, press firmly against the tissue, and scrape along the surface.

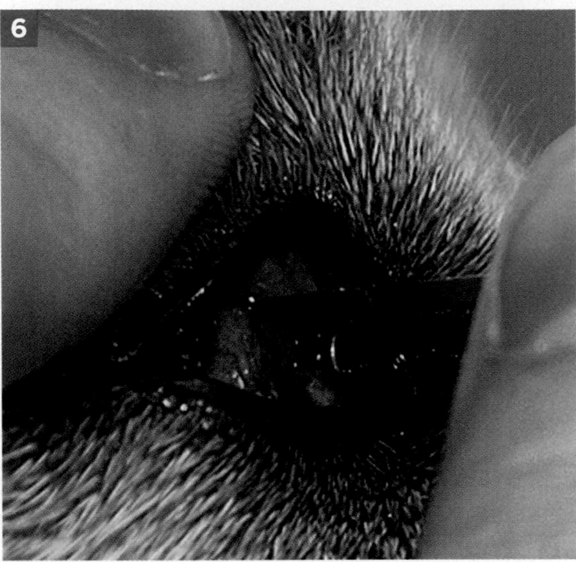

The conjunctiva is scraped while the blade is held perpendicular to the surface.

7. Gently blot the tissues obtained onto a glass slide, air dry, and stain for cytologic evaluation.
8. Alternatively, place the material obtained directly into a sterile tube or in sterile saline to submit for organism-specific polymerase chain reaction (PCR).

Respiratory System Techniques

7

PROCEDURE 7-1
Respiratory Examination and Auscultation

PURPOSE

To evaluate all aspects of the respiratory system in order to identify, localize, and characterize any abnormalities

INDICATIONS

1. A complete respiratory examination should be performed as part of a general health exam on every animal presented to the veterinarian.
2. Evaluation of a patient with symptoms of respiratory difficulty, coughing, sneezing, noisy breathing, exercise intolerance, or lethargy

CONTRAINDICATIONS AND WARNINGS

1. Animals that are stressed may be difficult to examine thoroughly, but observation of the respiratory pattern during minimal restraint often allows the examiner to localize the problem to a specific site within the respiratory system and to assess the severity of the problem.
2. Dyspneic animals may benefit from inhaling supplemental oxygen during examination. An enriched oxygen environment can be provided using blow-by oxygen, a bag, a mask, an oxygen collar, nasal oxygen, or an oxygen cage (Box 7-1, page 64).

EQUIPMENT

- Stethoscope
- A quiet room

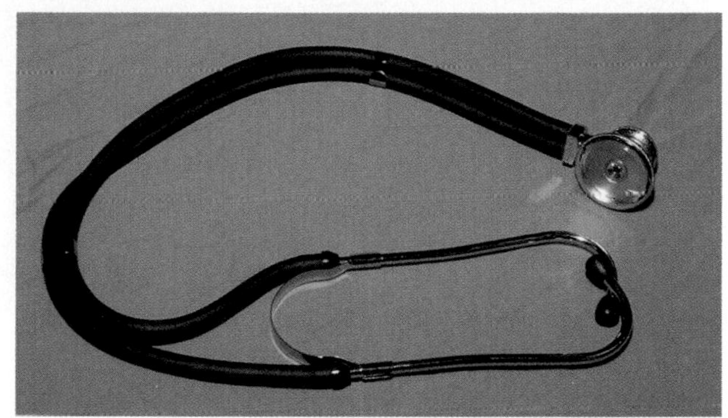

A stethoscope is the only equipment required for respiratory examination.

POSITIONING AND RESTRAINT

The animal should be standing quietly on the table or the floor during the respiratory examination.

SPECIAL ANATOMY

During auscultation it is important to examine over all regions of the lung. The lungs occupy primarily the cranial aspect of the bony thorax. Ventrally along the sternum the lung lobes extend from just cranial to the first rib to approximately the seventh rib bilaterally, whereas dorsally the caudal lung lobes extend to approximately the ninth or tenth intercostal space.

The right lung is divided into cranial, middle, accessory, and caudal lobes. The cardiac notch is a small area overlying the heart where lung tissue is not present between the heart and the body wall—this is located between the right cranial and right middle lung lobes at the ventral aspect of the fourth and fifth interspaces. The left lung is divided into cranial and caudal lobes, with a distinct separation between the cranial and caudal parts of the left cranial lung lobe.

PROCEDURE 7-1 Respiratory Examination and Auscultation—cont'd

BOX 7-1

Oxygen Therapy

Supplemental oxygen should be provided to all patients with increased respiratory rate or effort, at least until the problem can be localized and the severity of respiratory compromise can be determined. A variety of methods can be used.

Blow-by Oxygen

Tubing from an oxygen tank or an anesthetic machine is placed in front of the patient's mouth and a high flow rate (3 to 15 L/min) of oxygen is provided. This yields inspired oxygen concentration (Fio_2) of approximately 40%.

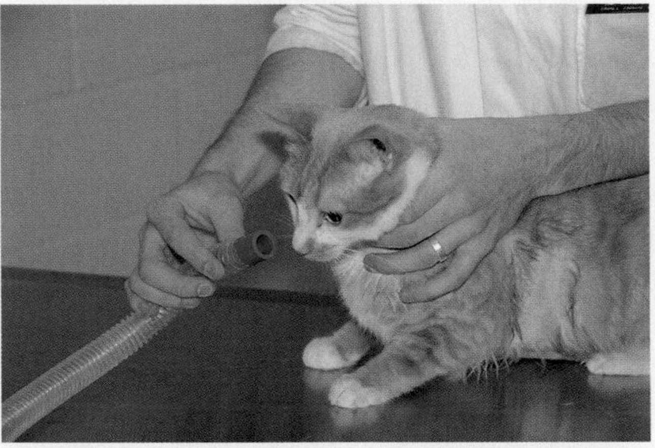

Blow-by oxygen administration.

Bag Oxygen

A small clear plastic bag can be placed over the animal's head and oxygen delivered into the bag at a rate of 1 to 5 L/minute. This delivers an Fio_2 of 70% to 80% within 1 to 2 minutes. This method allows full access to the patient for examination and treatment.

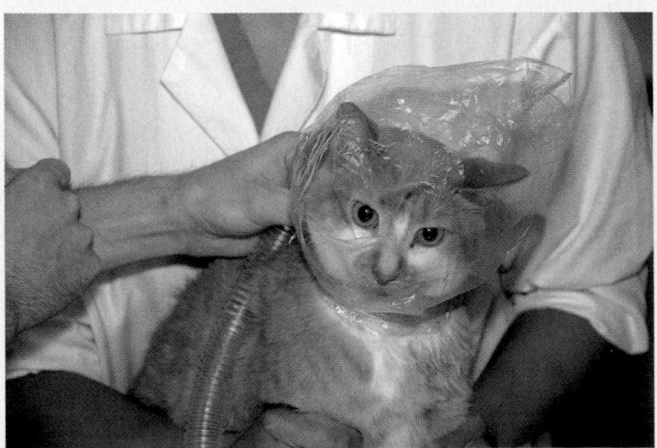

Oxygen administration into a clear bag over the animal's head is a nonstressful way to provide supplemental oxygen.

Mask Oxygen

Oxygen provided by mask provides up to 50% Fio_2, but is often not well tolerated by dyspneic patients. In order to avoid accumulation of exhaled air within the mask, high flow rates are essential (at least 100 mL/kg/min).

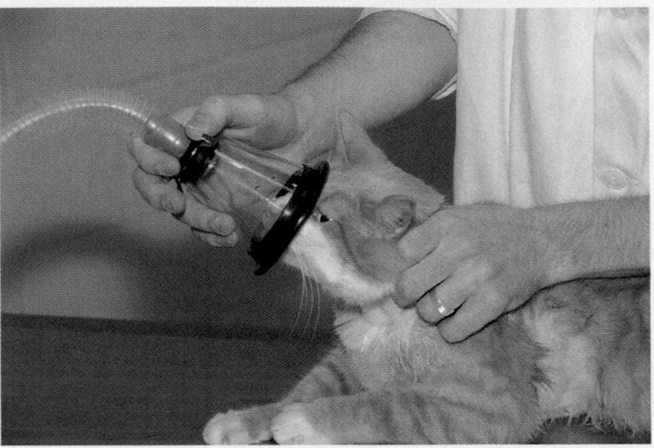

Oxygen administration by mask.

Oxygen Collar

An oversized Elizabethan collar is worn and clear plastic wrap is placed over the bottom two thirds of the collar. The supply line for oxygen is brought in under the patient's chin, with a flow of 2 to 6 L/minute. At least 60% Fio_2 can be provided with this method. No more than two thirds of the collar should be covered with the plastic wrap to prevent buildup of heat, humidity, and CO_2. This is especially effective (with or without concurrent nasal oxygen) in patients that are panting or mouth breathing.

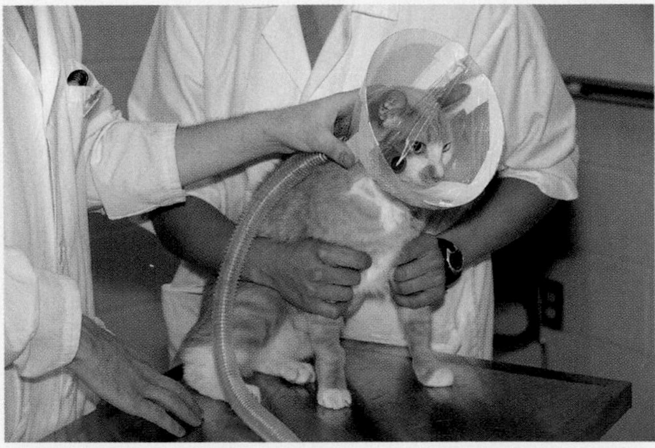

A modified Elizabethan collar can be used to provide supplemental oxygen.

BOX 7-1

Oxygen Therapy

Nasal Oxygen Catheter

A topical anesthetic is applied and the largest possible (3.5 to 8 French) soft feeding tube catheter is inserted into the ventral nasal meatus to the level of the medial canthus of the eye. The catheter is fixed in place with staples or tissue glue and oxygen is administered at 50 to 100 mL/kg/minute to achieve 40% to 80% FiO_2. This method is minimally stressful and allows easy access to the patient for examination, treatment, and monitoring.

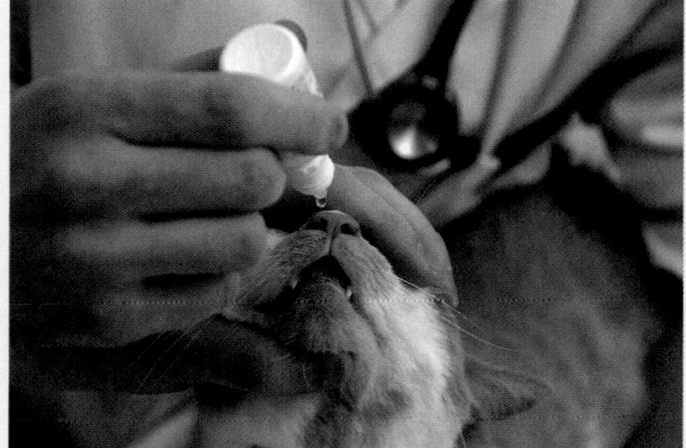

Topical anesthetic drops are placed in the nose.

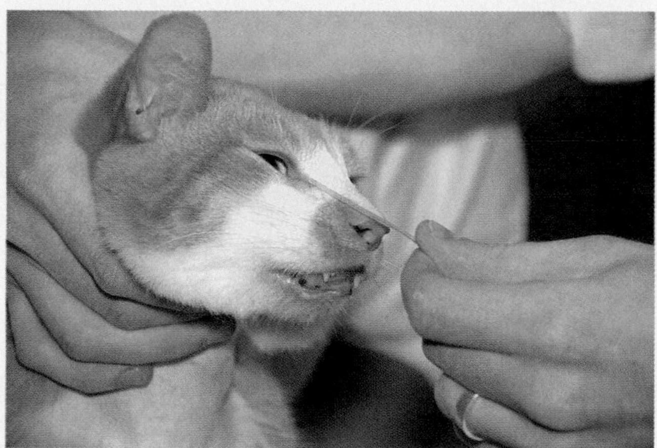

The length of the nasal catheter to be inserted is measured to the medial canthus of the eye.

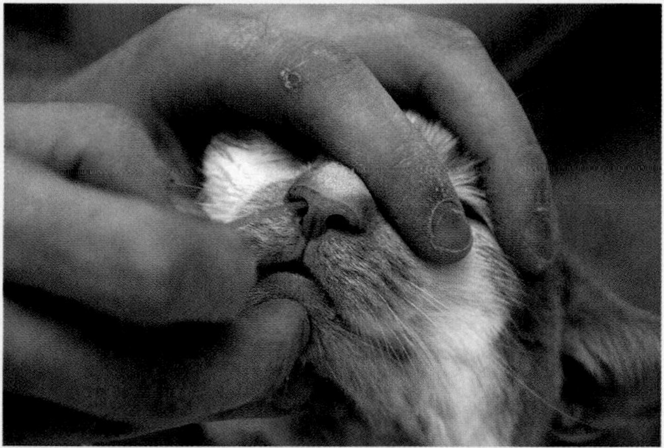

The nasal catheter is inserted into the ventral nasal meatus.

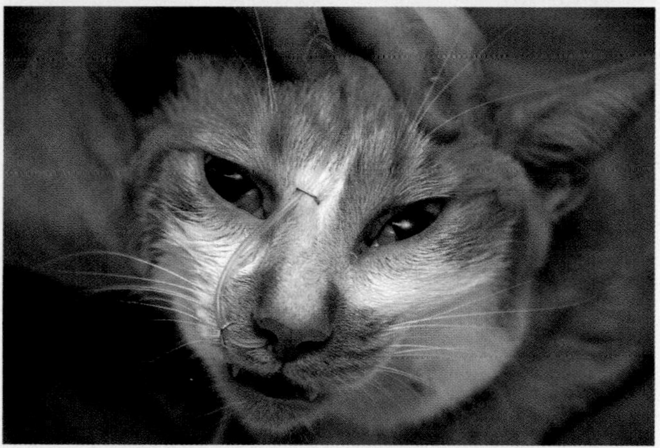

The nasal catheter is stapled or glued to the nose and head to keep it in place.

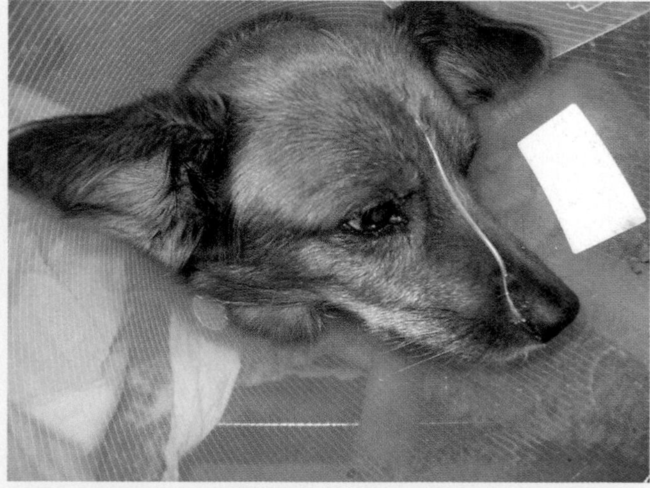

Nasal oxygen line in place in a dog with a pneumothorax and pulmonary contusions.

(Continued)

PROCEDURE 7-1 Respiratory Examination and Auscultation—cont'd

BOX 7-1

Oxygen Therapy—cont'd

Oxygen Cage

Even with very high flows of oxygen, it will take more than 20 minutes to achieve an FiO_2 greater than 50% using an oxygen cage or chamber. As well, access to the patient for hands-on examination and treatment is limited.

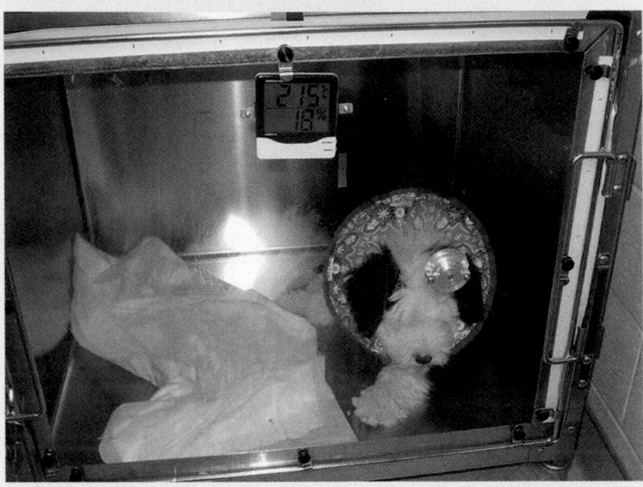

An oxygen cage can be used to provide supplemental oxygen in some stable patients.

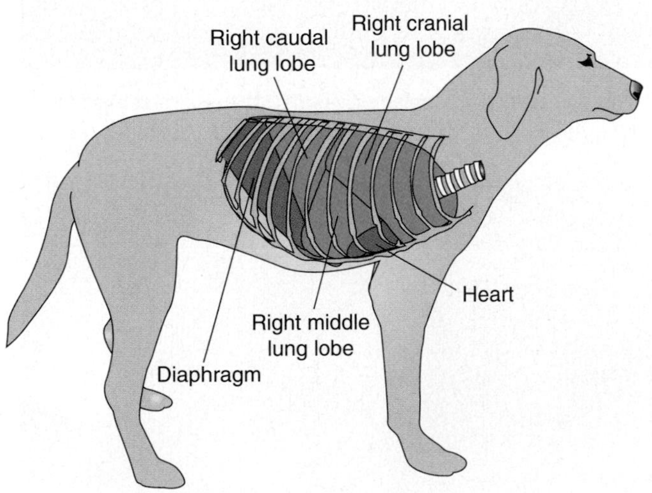

Anatomy of the right lung lobes.

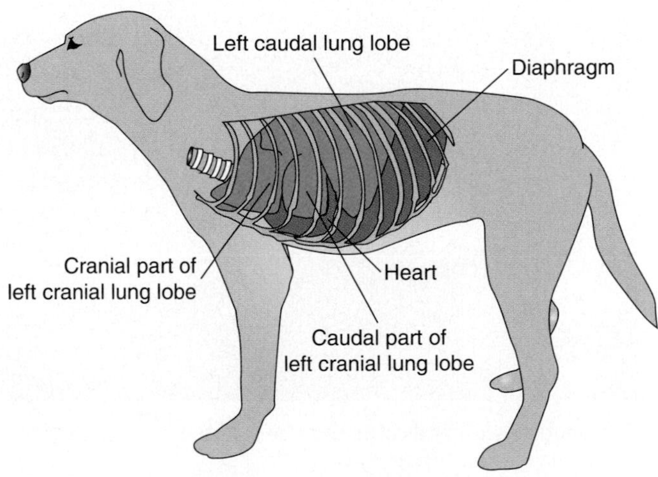

Anatomy of the left lung.

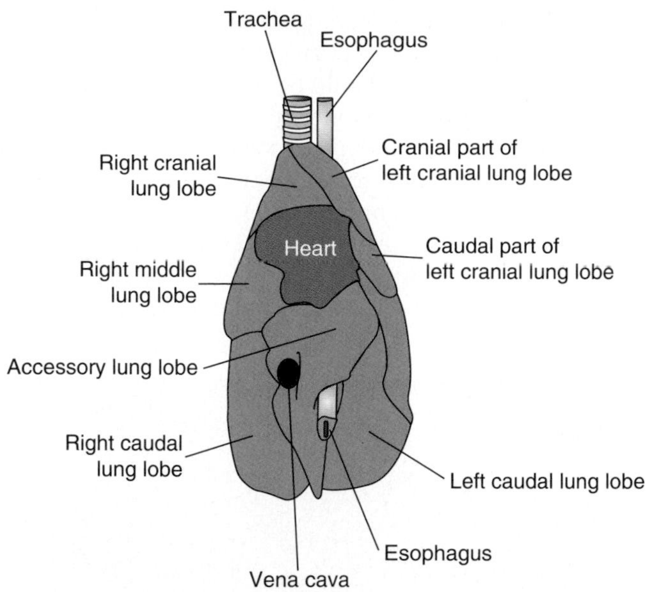

Anatomy of the lung lobes, ventrodorsal view.

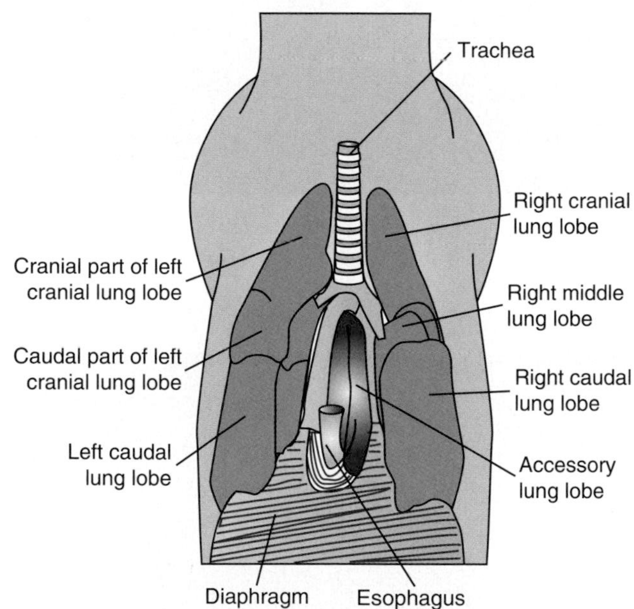

Anatomy of the lung lobes, dorsoventral view.

TECHNIQUE: RESPIRATORY EXAMINATION

1. Have the patient stand on the table or on the floor.
2. Examine the nares for any abnormal discharge.

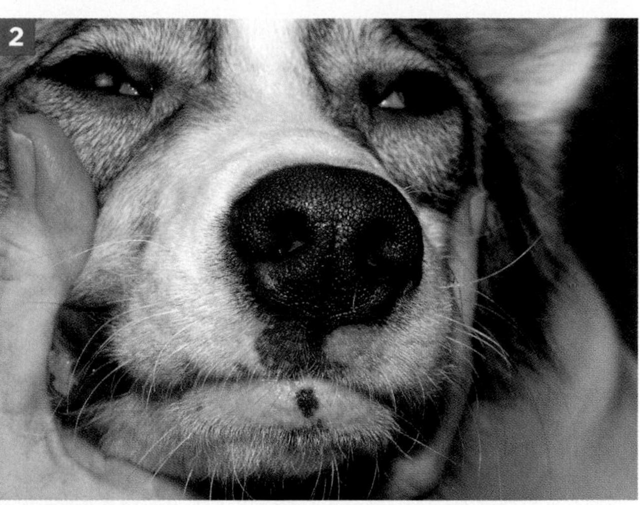

Examining the nares for any abnormal discharge.

3. Characterize any discharge as *unilateral* or *bilateral*. Very focal disease such as an inhaled foreign body, dental abscess, or oronasal fistula is most likely to cause a unilateral discharge. Progressive disorders such as fungal rhinitis and neoplasia may cause a nasal discharge that is initially unilateral but progresses to bilateral. Systemic or diffuse disorders such as allergic rhinitis and lymphoplasmacytic rhinitis typically cause bilateral discharge.

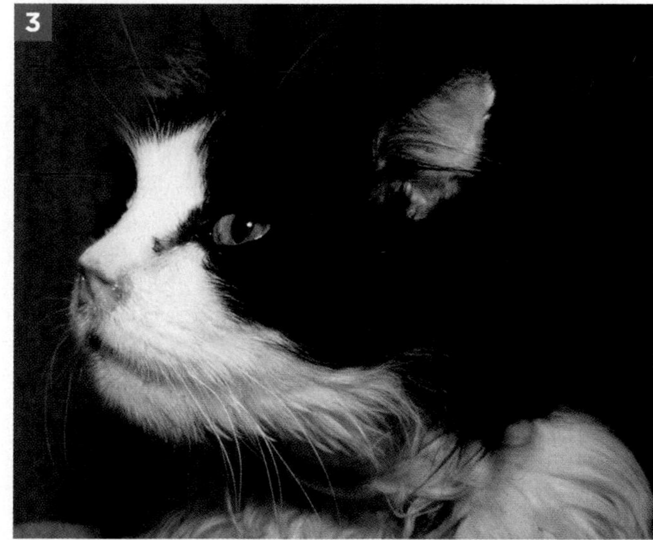

Bilateral mucopurulent nasal discharge in an old cat with nasal neoplasia.

4. Describe any discharge as watery, mucoid, purulent, or bloody.
   - **A.** A *serous* (watery) nasal discharge can be normal or can indicate a viral infection, nasal mites, or allergy. A watery discharge could also be the earliest manifestation of any of the disorders causing a purulent nasal discharge.

PROCEDURE 7-1 Respiratory Examination and Auscultation—cont'd

B. A cloudy *mucoid* discharge without an abundance of inflammatory cells can be seen in dogs with allergic rhinitis, cats with chronic viral rhinosinusitis, and dogs and cats with nasal neoplasia, particularly adenocarcinoma.

C. A *purulent* discharge is one that contains many inflammatory cells—most often neutrophils. Purulent nasal discharges are seen with most bacterial and fungal infections, foreign bodies, oronasal fistulas, tooth root abscesses, and lymphoplasmacytic rhinitis.

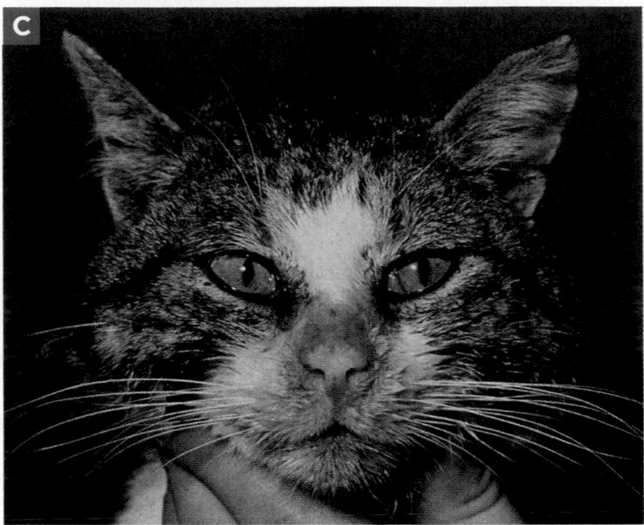

Purulent nasal discharge in a cat with chronic herpesvirus infection and secondary bacterial rhinosinusitis.

D. Bloody nasal discharge *(epistaxis)* can be caused by focal disease within the nose or by systemic disease (Box 7-2, page 69). Nasal causes of epistaxis include nasal trauma, inhaled nasal foreign bodies, neoplasia, lymphoplasmacytic rhinitis, fungal disease, and dental periapical abscessation.

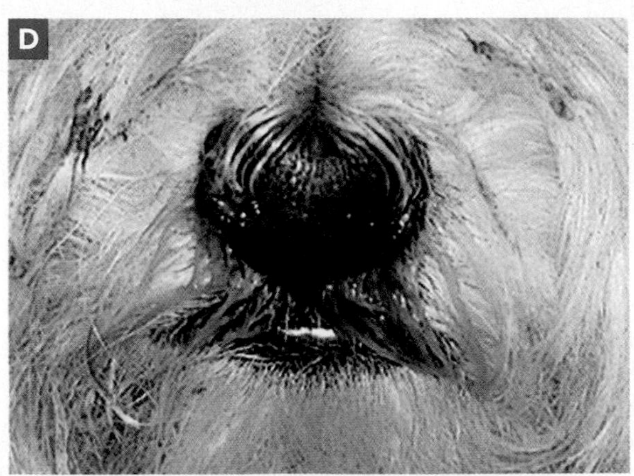

Epistaxis in a dog with nasal aspergillosis.

E. When epistaxis occurs without any prior history or physical evidence of nasal discharge or obstruction, a systemic workup should be performed (see Box 7-2). Severe thrombocytopenia (<30,000 platelets/μL) commonly results in epistaxis, as will decreased platelet function (thrombocytopathia), coagulopathies, vasculitis, and hypertension.

5. Examine the nares for erosions. Erosions around the external nares most often occur with disorders causing chronic inflammatory discharge, especially mycotic (fungal) rhinitis.

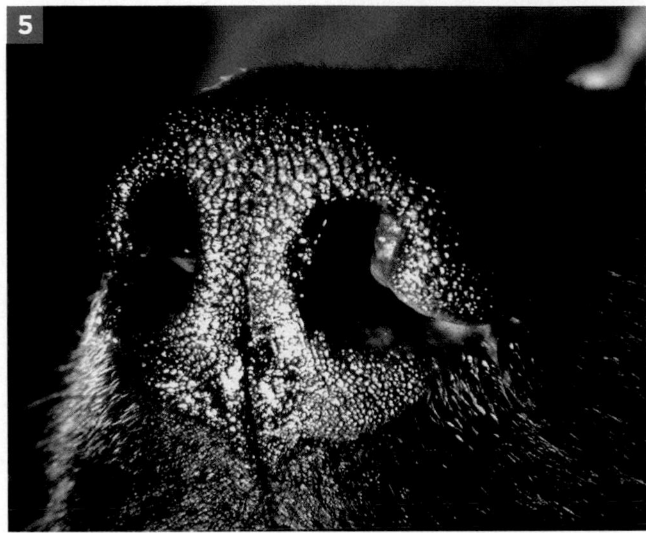

Erosions and depigmentation around the nares in a Labrador Retriever with nasal aspergillosis.

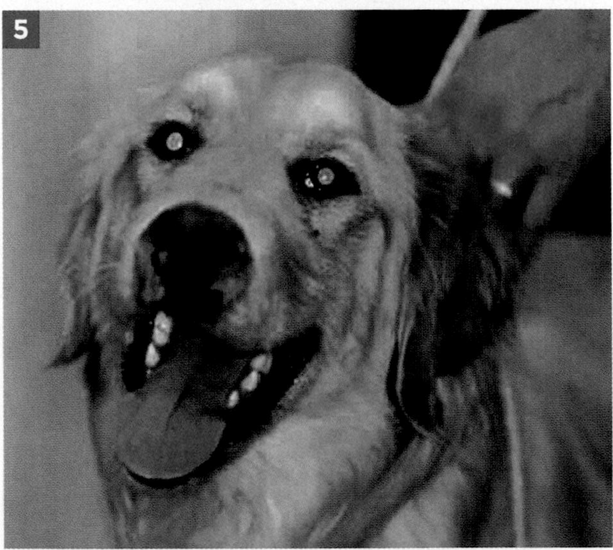

Erosion and depigmentation of the entire nasal planum in a Golden Retriever with nasal aspergillosis.

BOX 7-2

Causes of Epistaxis

Local (Nasal) Causes

- External trauma
- Neoplasia
- Inhaled foreign body
- Fungal rhinitis
- Lymphoplasmacytic rhinitis
- Tooth root abscess

Systemic Disorders

- Thrombocytopenia
- Thrombocytopathia (decreased platelet function)
    - von Willebrand's disease
    - Aspirin administration
    - Plasma cell myeloma
- Coagulopathy
- Systemic hypertension
- Vasculitis

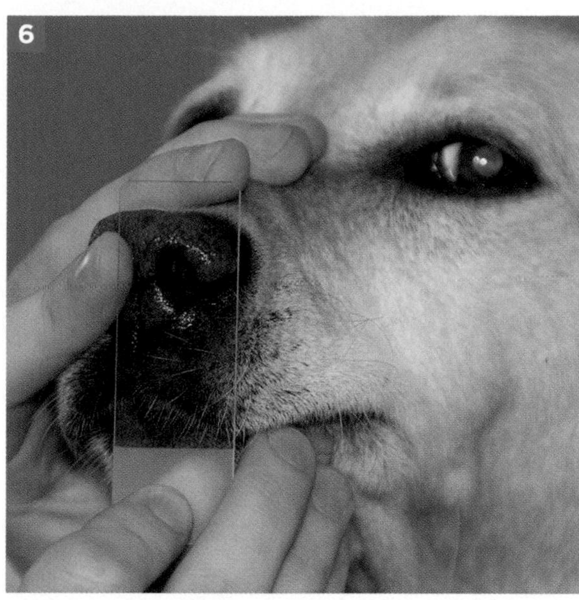

Assessing nasal airflow.

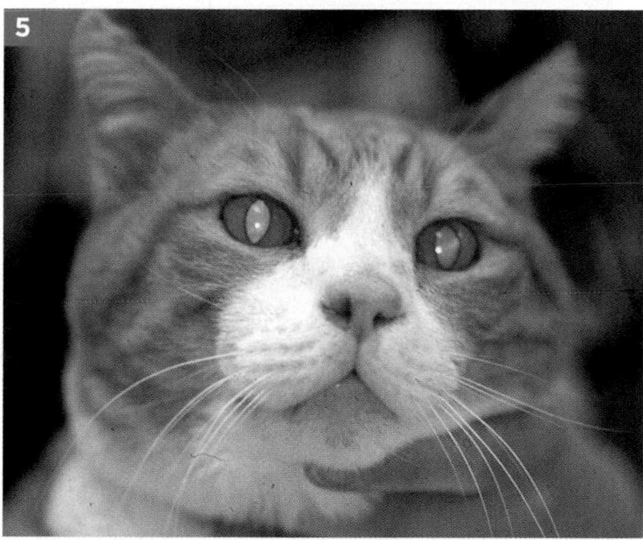

Erosion of the right nares and unilateral epistaxis in a cat with nasal *Cryptococcus* infection.

6. Assess *airflow* through each side of the nasal cavity. While occluding one nostril, determine airflow through the other nostril by palpation, by observing the movement of a wisp of cotton caused by the flow, or by observing the condensation caused on a chilled (frozen) microscope slide by the exhaled warm air. Complete obstruction to nasal airflow is most likely to occur with neoplasia.

7. Examine for *ocular discharge*. The nasolacrimal duct passes through the nasal cavity, where it can become compressed or obstructed by a mass lesion. *Epiphora* (the overflow of tears onto the face) may result. Over time this can lead to a moist dermatitis and matting of hair ventral to the eye.

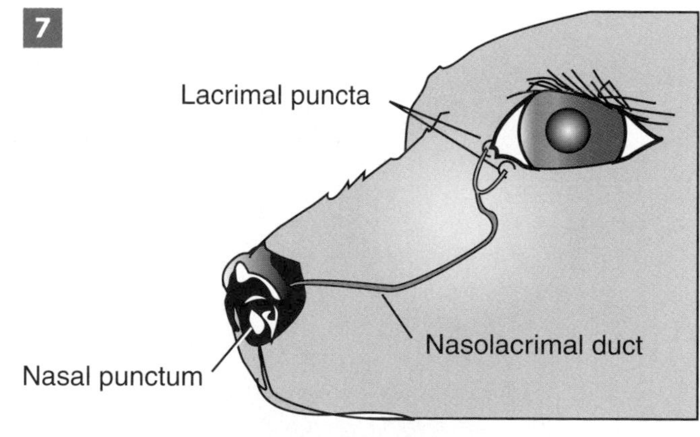

Anatomy of the nasolacrimal duct.

8. Examine for facial deformity, which is most often caused by nasal neoplasia in cats and dogs and by *Cryptococcus* spp. nasal infection in cats. Whenever nasal deformity occurs, the structural integrity of the bone has been lost, so cytologic evaluation of fine-needle aspirates taken directly from the deformed region can often be used to provide a diagnosis.

PROCEDURE 7-1 Respiratory Examination and Auscultation—cont'd

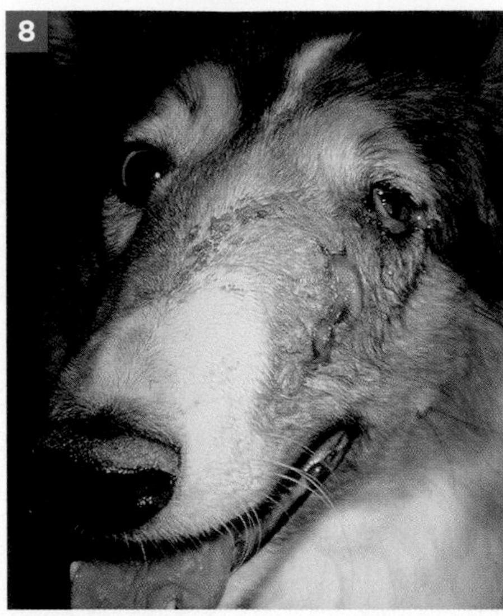

This 9-year-old collie has obvious nasal deformity and nasal bone destruction caused by a nasal adenocarcinoma.

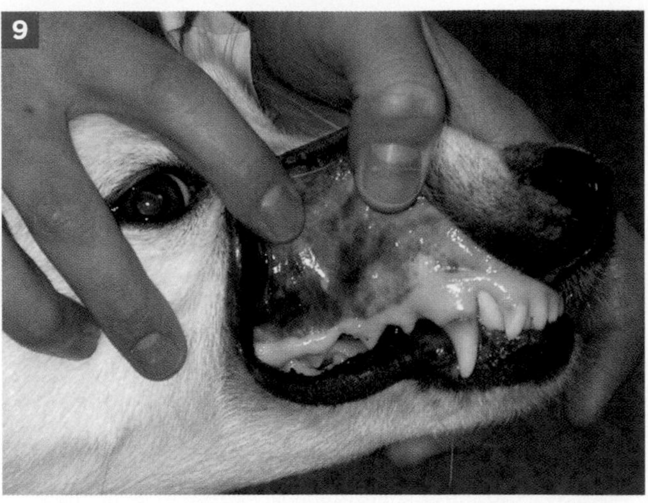

Pale tongue and oral mucous membranes in a tachypneic white German Shepherd with a bleeding intestinal neoplasm.

9. Examine *mucous membrane color*. *Pallor* (pale mucous membranes) occurs with anemia, which can cause increased respiratory rate *(tachypnea)* and exercise intolerance even in the absence of respiratory disease. *Cyanosis* (blue discoloration of the mucous membranes) is caused by an excess of unoxygenated hemoglobin in the blood (concentration >5 g/dL). Cyanosis most often occurs with severe respiratory disease or congenital heart defects.

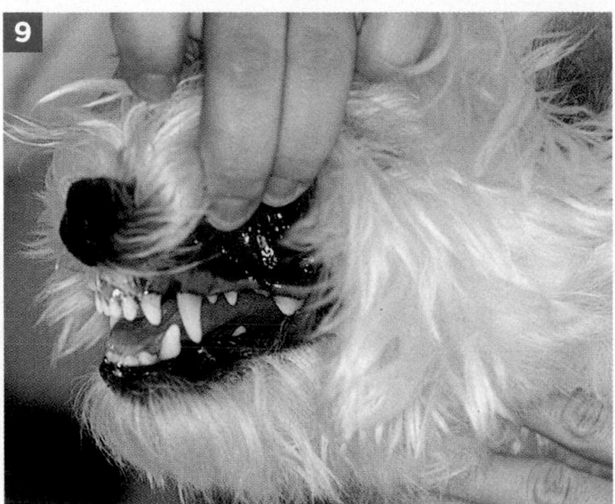

Cyanotic mucous membranes in a dyspneic West Highland White Terrier with pulmonary interstitial fibrosis.

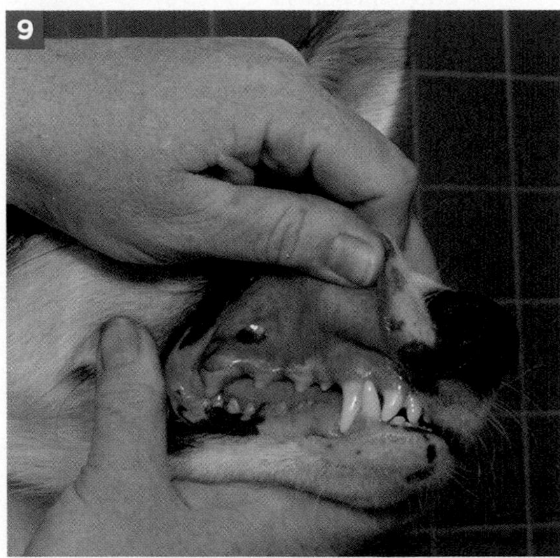

Normal pink mucous membranes.

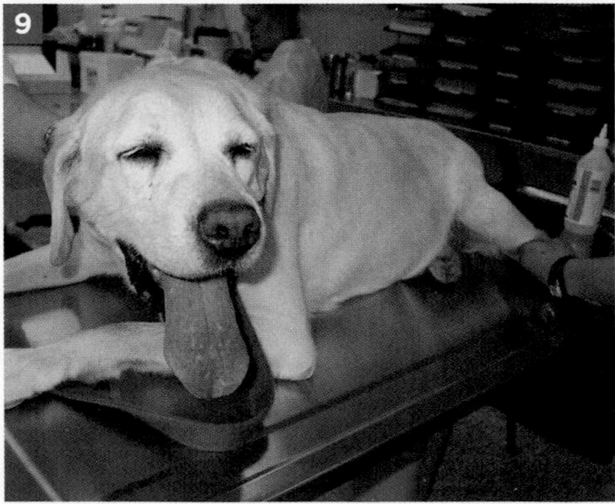

Cyanotic tongue in a 12-year-old Labrador Retriever with laryngeal paralysis.

BOX 7-3

Respiratory Patterns

Forced, Noisy, and Prolonged Inspiration

Stridor

High-pitched, musical sound with each inspiration. Most suggestive of laryngeal obstruction due to laryngeal paralysis, granulomatous laryngitis, or neoplasia.

Stertor

Loud, discontinuous snoring noises heard on inspiration. Most suggestive of pharyngeal obstruction due to elongated soft palate, pharyngeal neoplasia, or nasopharyngeal polyps.

Reverse Sneeze

Episodes of extreme inspiratory effort and noise that occur while breathing through the nose with the head and neck extended. Can be normal in some small-breed dogs. When this occurs as a new symptom, it is most suggestive of nasal disease, with the caudal flow of discharge causing nasopharyngeal spasm.

Forced and Prolonged Exhalation

Wheezing

A forced or prolonged exhalation with an expiratory or abdominal push is most typical of dogs and cats with small airway disease such as chronic bronchitis or asthma.

Rapid, Shallow Breathing

Tachypnea

Short shallow respirations are associated with stiff noncompliant lungs (as with pulmonary fibrosis) or restricted expansion of the lung due to pleural or thoracic wall diseases. This is the pattern commonly seen with thoracic effusions, pneumothorax, or diaphragmatic hernia.

Rapid, Deep Breathing

Tachypnea or Hyperpnea

Increased effort and depth of respiration are common in animals with lung parenchymal disease resulting in hypoxemia. This pattern is common in dogs and cats with pneumonia or pulmonary edema.

10. Observe the *respiratory pattern* (Box 7-3). Watch and listen to the patient while feeling the chest expand and deflate with each respiration. Assess the relative effort and time associated with each phase of respiration. If there is increased noise or effort of breathing, determine whether this is most pronounced during inspiration or expiration.

Dogs and cats normally use their diaphragm and intercostal muscles to expand their chest during inspiration, but unless their breathing is labored, chest excursions will be minimal at rest. Exhalation is normally passive as the chest muscles relax. When a patient has noisy or labored respiration, identifying the phase of respiration associated with increased noise and effort will help you localize the site of respiratory obstruction.

Increased noise and effort as the patient tries to inhale suggest obstruction of the extrathoracic airways such as the larynx, pharynx, or extrathoracic trachea. Increased noise and effort and prolonged effort during exhalation suggest collapse or obstruction of the intrathoracic airways.

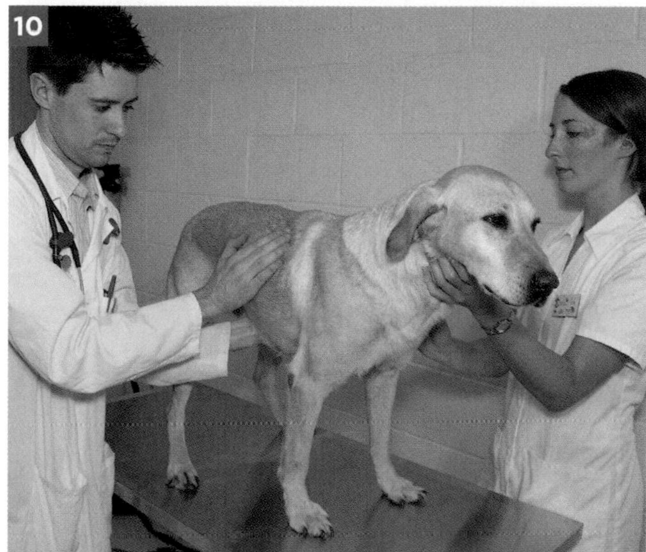

Watch and listen to the patient while feeling the chest expand and deflate with each respiration.

11. *Palpate* the larynx, cervical trachea, and external contours of the thorax for symmetry, masses, or swellings. In young cats, attempt to *compress the cranial thorax* anterior to the heart. In normal young cats this region is very pliable. In young cats with anterior mediastinal lymphoma, the chest is not compressible at this site and may actually be enlarged.

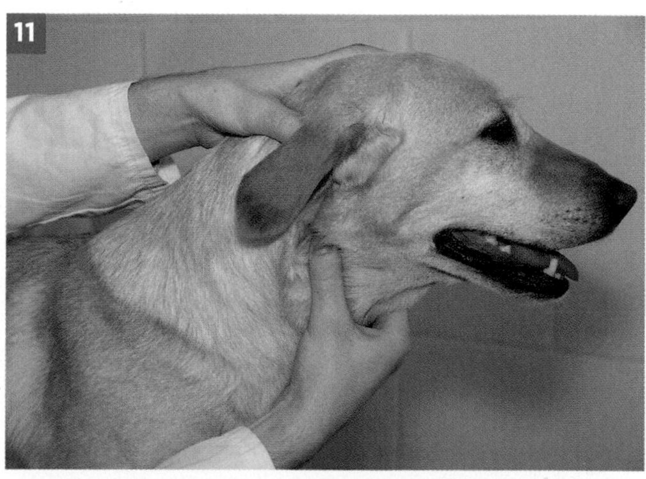

Palpating the larynx and cervical trachea.

PROCEDURE 7-1 Respiratory Examination and Auscultation—cont'd

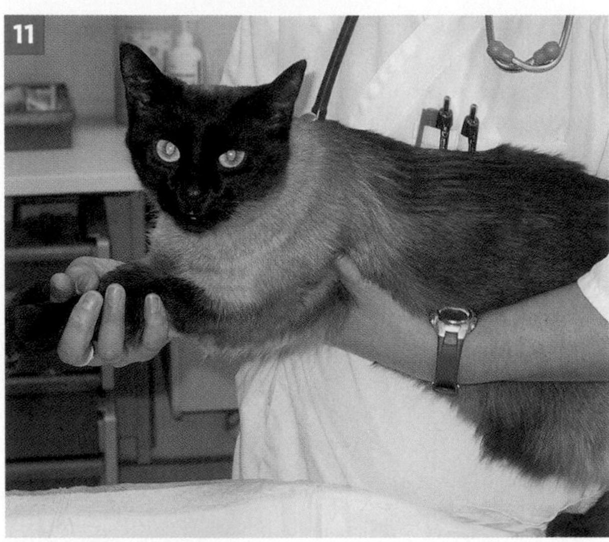

Palpating the anterior mediastinum of a cat.

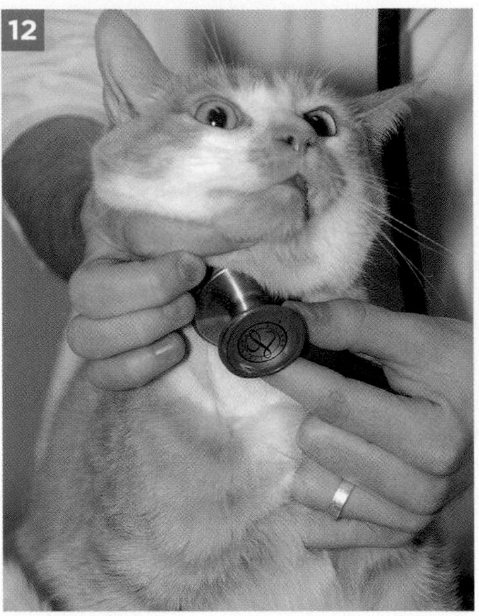

Auscultation over the larynx and trachea can help localize a site of upper airway obstruction.

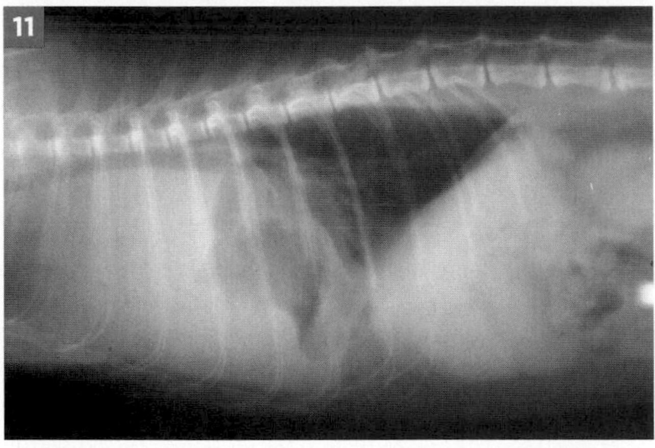

Thoracic radiographs showing a mass in the anterior mediastinum of a dyspneic cat with a noncompressible anterior thorax due to lymphoma.

12. *Auscultation of the larynx and extrathoracic trachea* should be performed by placing the diaphragm portion of the stethoscope against the skin at multiple sites from the larynx down to the thoracic inlet and auscultating during inspiration and expiration. Sounds that are referred to the lungs from the upper airways are loudest when the stethoscope is held on the skin directly over the site of restricted airflow.

13. Auscultate the lungs over all regions on the right and left side. Low-pitched breath sounds originating in the large airways normally can be heard over the lungs in dogs throughout inspiration and during the first third of exhalation. These breath sounds can be very quiet and hard to appreciate in normal cats. Breath sounds may be louder than normal (harsh) due to thin body condition, increased depth of ventilation, and when there is improved sound transmission in a region due to a consolidated lung lobe or a lung mass. Heart and lung sounds are muffled ventrally in dogs and cats with pleural effusion, and lung sounds are muffled dorsally in dogs and cats with a pneumothorax.

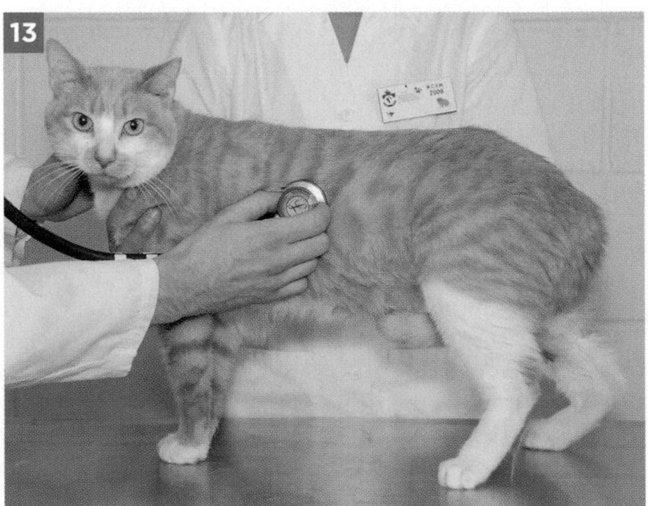

Auscultation over all lung fields is important to identify abnormalities.

14. Describe and characterize any abnormal (adventitious) lung sounds. *Crackles* are nonmusical discontinuous noises that sound like rumpling cellophane or hair rubbing between fingers. They usually indicate some fluid accumulation (edema or exudate) in the alveoli of the lung or in the airways as might be seen with pneumonia, pulmonary edema, or interstitial fibrosis. *Wheezes* are musical, continuous, high-pitched sounds that indicate airway narrowing due to bronchoconstriction, bronchial wall thickening, external airway compression, or exudate in the bronchial lumen. Wheezes are most often heard during exhalation in patients with small airway disease such as asthma or bronchitis. An *end-expiratory snap* sometimes can be heard at the end of exhalation in dogs with severe intrathoracic tracheal collapse.

15. Attempt to *induce a cough* with tracheal palpation. Normal animals will cough once or twice when their trachea is palpated. Animals with an irritated trachea may cough repeatedly. This tracheal sensitivity can be caused by tracheal, bronchial, small airway, or lung parenchymal disease. Any disorder that causes irritation or compression of the trachea or bronchi and all disorders that cause exudation of material into the airways cause cough and result in increased tracheal sensitivity. Observe carefully to determine whether the animal swallows after coughing, suggesting that the cough is productive. Productive cough can be seen with airway, lung, or cardiac disease.

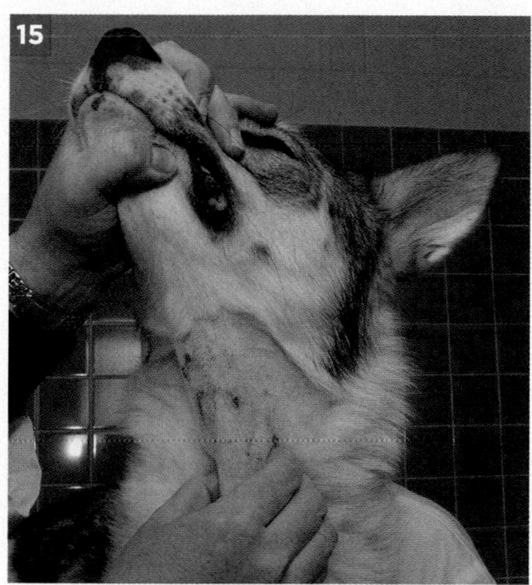

Gently squeeze the trachea in an attempt to elicit a cough.

16. Carefully evaluate the heart through auscultation, palpation of both femoral arterial pulses, and determining capillary refill time. Cardiac failure is a common cause of dyspnea and cough, so evaluation of the heart is an important part of the respiratory examination. The heart should be auscultated on both sides of the chest, listening for normal heart sounds as well as for abnormal sounds occurring during systole (ventricular contraction) or diastole (ventricular relaxation). Special attention should be paid to listening over the approximate location for the projection of sound from each heart valve in order to identify and characterize any cardiac murmurs that may be present. Heart rate is increased in most animals with respiratory distress due to cardiac failure (rate >100/min, large dogs; >160/min, small dogs; >240/min, cats). Femoral arterial pulses should be strong, regular, and correspond with each heartbeat auscultated over the thorax. Dropped beats or pulse deficits occur when a cardiac contraction is auscultated but no corresponding femoral pulse is palpated, usually suggesting a dysrhythmia.

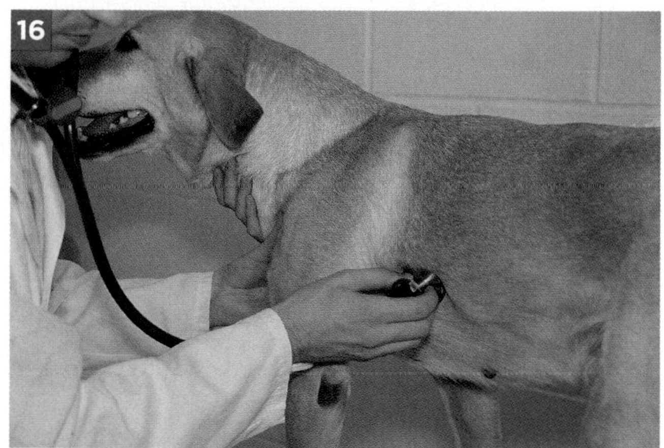

Carefully auscultate the heart on both sides of the thorax.

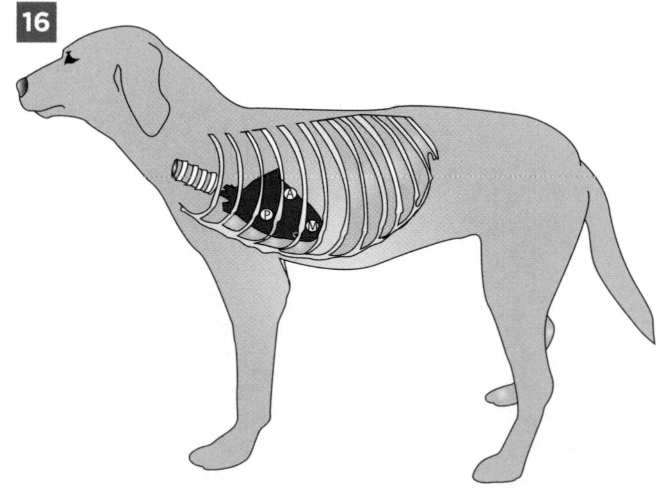

Auscultation areas on the left thorax for the pulmonic *(P)*, aortic *(A)*, and mitral *(M)* valves of the heart.

PROCEDURE 7-1 Respiratory Examination and Auscultation—cont'd

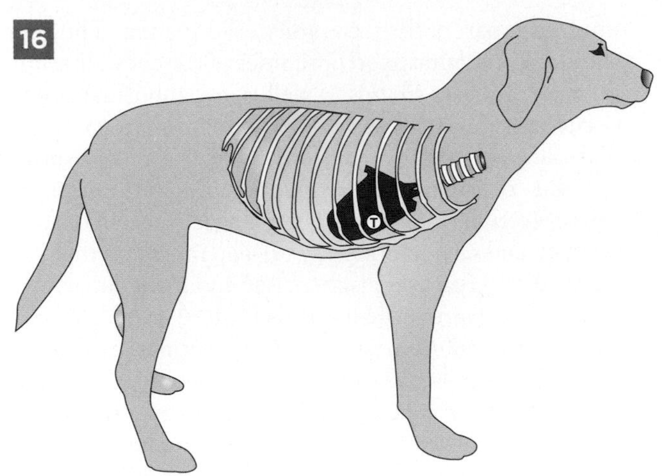

Auscultation area on the right thorax for the tricuspid (T) valve of the heart.

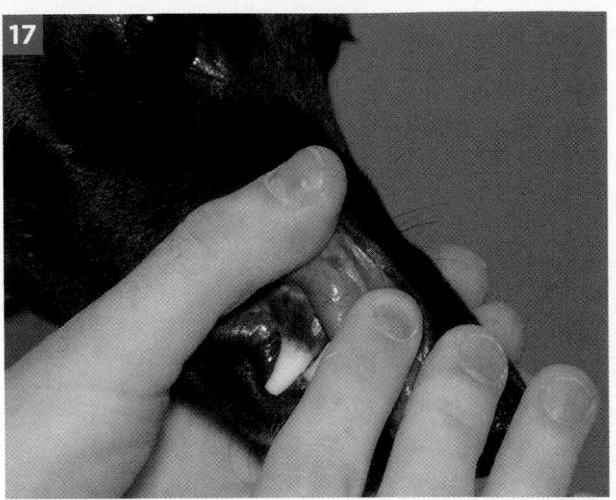

Blanch the mucous membranes with digital pressure.

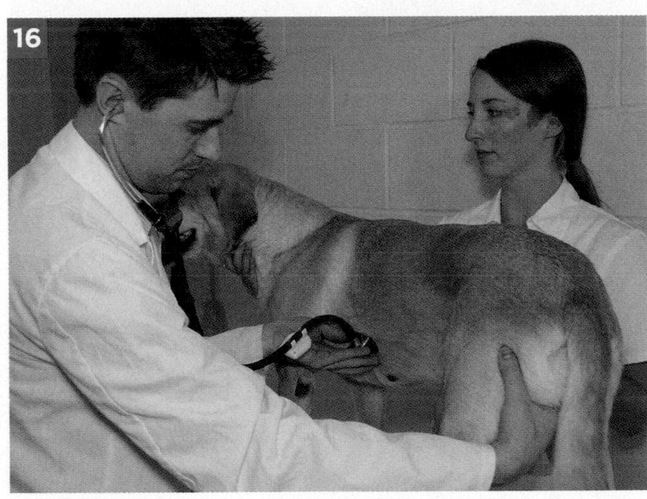

Auscultate the heart and palpate femoral pulses simultaneously to detect dysrhythmias and pulse deficits.

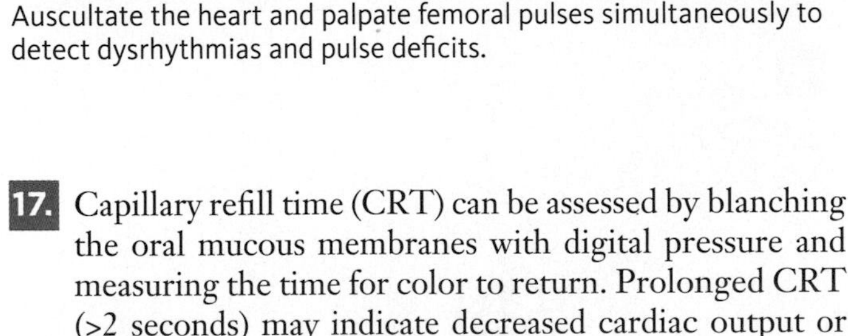

17. Capillary refill time (CRT) can be assessed by blanching the oral mucous membranes with digital pressure and measuring the time for color to return. Prolonged CRT (>2 seconds) may indicate decreased cardiac output or dehydration.

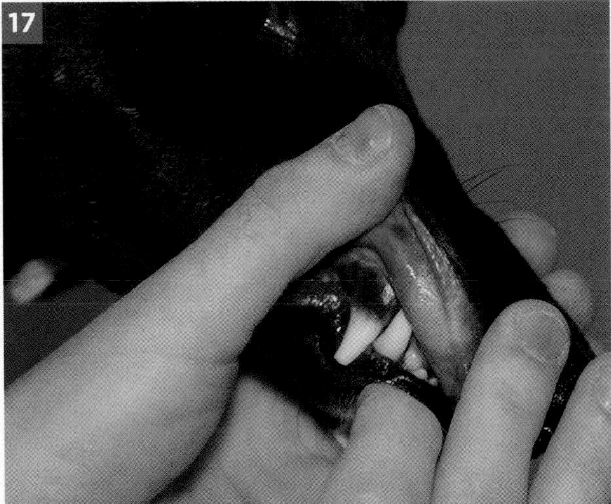

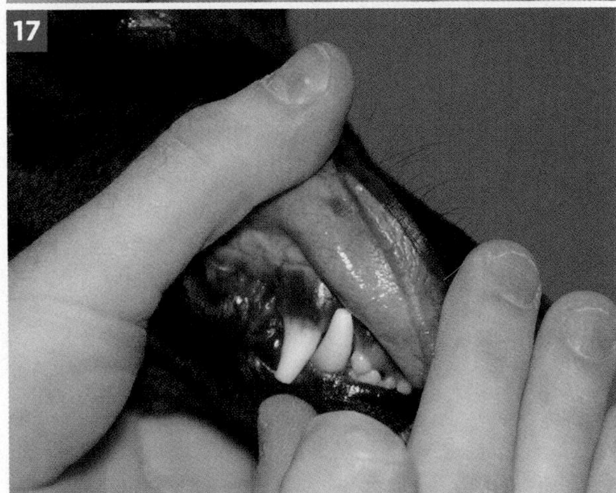

Measure the time it takes for color to return.

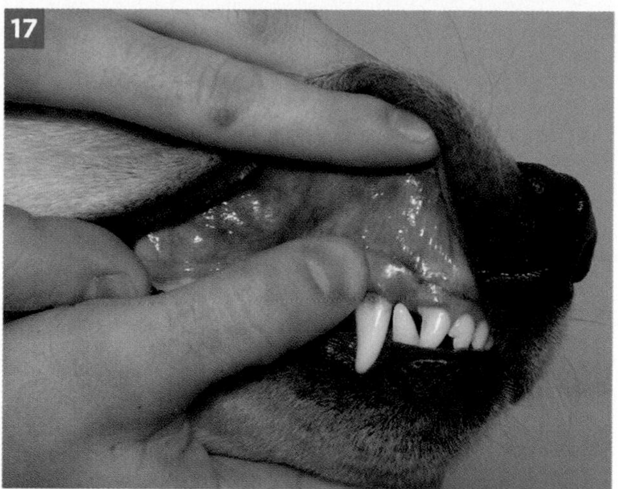

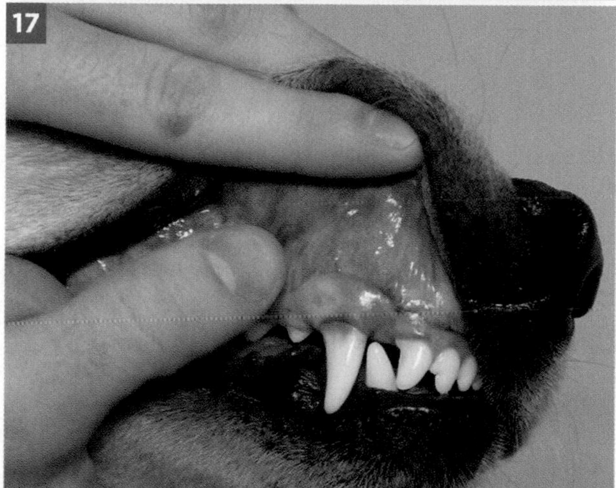

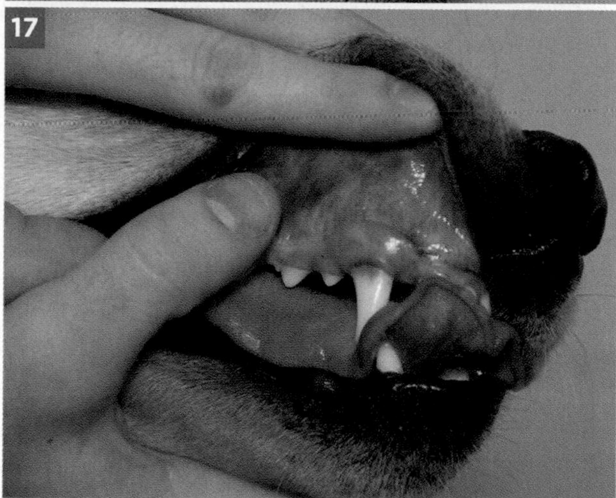

Assessing capillary refill time.

PROCEDURE 7-2

Internal Nasal Examination

PURPOSE

To examine the inside of the nasal cavity to determine the cause of localizing clinical signs

INDICATIONS

1. Evaluation of any animal with chronic nasal discharge, nasal erosions, nasal deformity, snorting, or inability to pass air through the nose
2. Any dog with an acute onset of sneezing, snorting, or pawing at the face, leading to suspicion of an inhaled foreign object

CONTRAINDICATIONS AND WARNINGS

1. Internal nasal examination (rhinoscopy) requires general anesthesia, so cannot be performed in animals that cannot be anesthetized.
2. In cats and dogs with chronic nasal discharge, a nasal swab of the exudate should be collected and evaluated cytologically before scheduling general anesthesia for internal nasal examination. Exudate immediately within the external nares is collected using a small cotton-tipped swab, rolled on a microscope slide, stained with new methylene blue, and evaluated for cryptococcal organisms. Cytology is positive in nearly 60% of animals with nasal *Cryptococcus*. Nasal swab cytology and culture are not very useful in the diagnostic approach to other nasal disorders in dogs and cats.

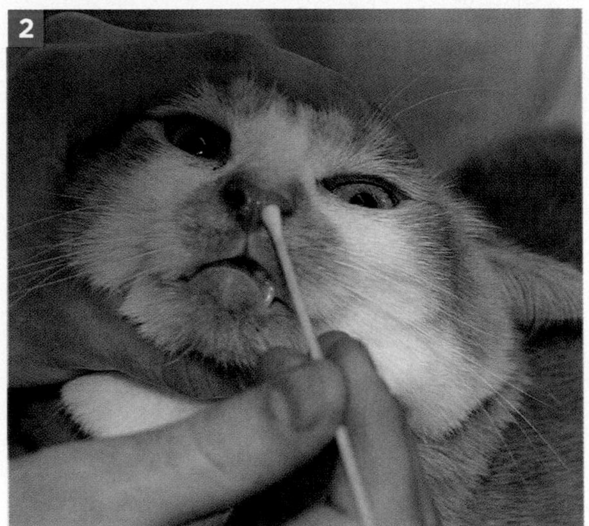

Collecting a nasal swab for cytologic evaluation.

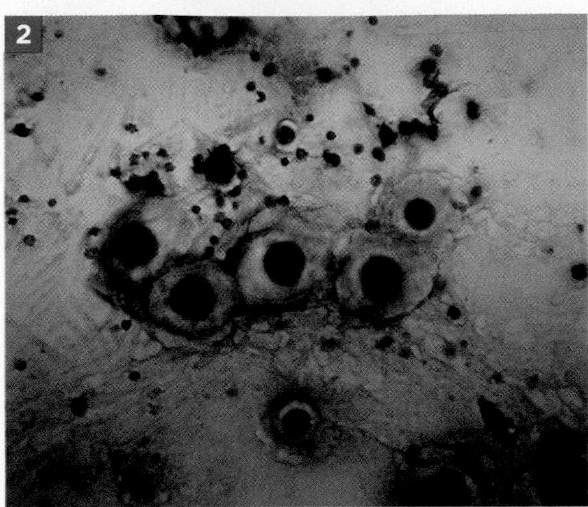

Cryptococcus neoformans identified on a nasal swab from a cat.

3. Patients with epistaxis should always be tested to eliminate extranasal reasons for hemorrhage before being anesthetized for rhinoscopy (see Box 7-2).
4. Nasal imaging such as radiographs or computed tomography (CT) should be performed before rhinoscopy in animals with chronic disease so that intranasal details are not obscured by rhinoscopy-induced hemorrhage.
5. While animals are anesthetized for internal nasal examination, thorough evaluation of the nasal cavity should be planned, including nasal flush and biopsy if a definitive diagnosis is not determined based on rhinoscopy alone.

EQUIPMENT

- An otoscope and otoscope cone can be used to examine approximately the anterior third of the nasal cavity.
- A rigid fiberoptic endoscope (2- to 3-mm diameter) or a flexible endoscope can be used to examine the anterior two thirds of the nasal cavity in large dogs.
- Lubricant

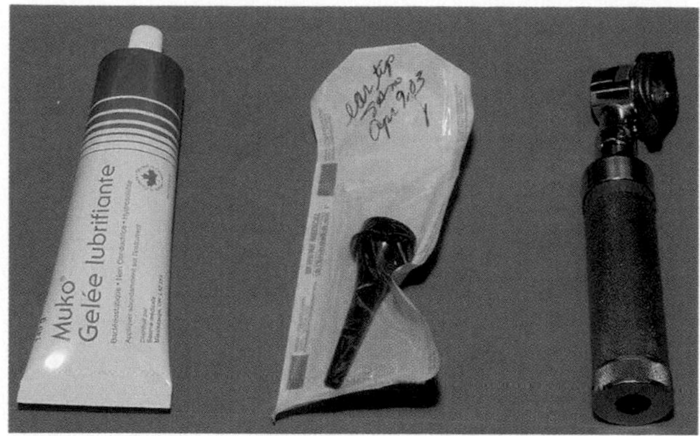

An otoscope and cone can be used for anterior nasal examination.

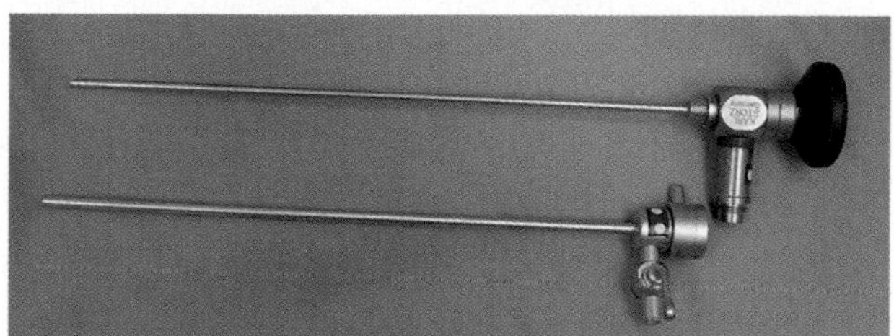
In large dogs there is better access to the middle portion of the nasal cavity using an endoscope.

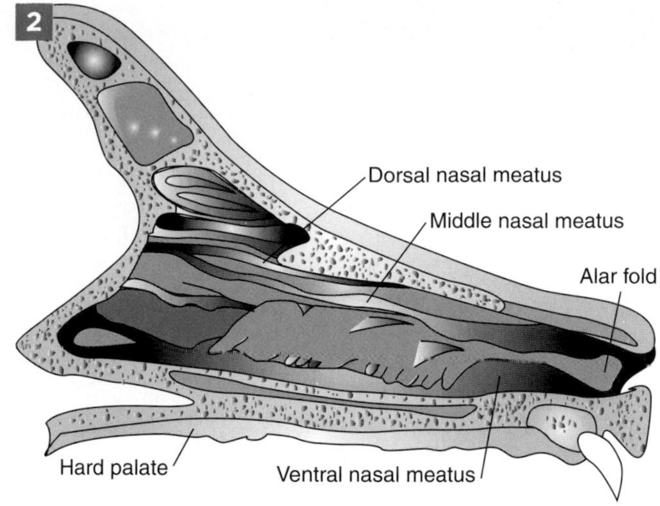

Anatomy of the nasal meatuses.

3. Anterior access to the nasal cavity with a large object like an otoscope cone or a scope is limited by the prominent alar fold ventrally and laterally. Directing the tip of the scope or cone medially and dorsally initially facilitates entry. Rhinoscopic evaluation is primarily performed within the middle meatus, although the ventral meatus also can be examined.

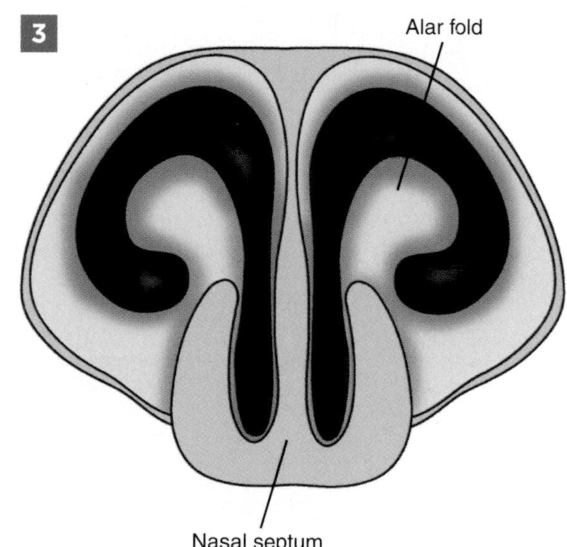

Anatomy of the alar fold.

POSITIONING AND RESTRAINT

Patient should be under general anesthesia, in sternal recumbency for this procedure

SPECIAL ANATOMY

1. The nasal cavity extends from the nostrils to the nasopharynx and is separated into two halves by the nasal septum.
2. The dorsal and ventral nasal conchae (shelves of bone covered by mucosa) project into the nasal cavity from the lateral wall, effectively dividing the nasal cavity into three passages (meatuses).
   - **A.** The dorsal nasal meatus is a narrow passage between the roof of the nasal cavity and the dorsal conchae. This meatus leads to the caudal part of the nose.
   - **B.** The middle nasal meatus lies between the dorsal and ventral conchae. This meatus also leads to the caudal part of the nose, where it splits into dorsal and ventral channels. The principal opening to the paranasal sinuses is within the middle meatus.
   - **C.** The ventral nasal meatus lies between the ventral conchae and the floor of the nasal cavity and leads directly to the nasopharynx. Most of the respiratory airflow is through this meatus.

TECHNIQUE: RHINOSCOPY

1. General anesthesia is required.
2. Unless an acutely inhaled foreign body is strongly suspected, nasal imaging (radiographs or CT) should be performed before anterior rhinoscopy. This is because rhinoscopy-induced hemorrhage can mask or mimic imaging abnormalities.

PROCEDURE 7-2 Internal Nasal Examination—cont'd

3. Before anterior rhinoscopy, the oral cavity should be examined carefully, examining and palpating the hard and soft palates for erosions, defects, and deformities.
4. Whenever possible, before anterior rhinoscopy, the caudal nasopharynx should be evaluated endoscopically (see Procedure 7-3 Pharyngeal Examination) for the presence of polyps, neoplasia, foreign bodies, and nasal mites.
5. In patients with unilateral signs of nasal disease, both sides of the nose should be evaluated. The normal side of the nose should be examined first.
6. Lubricate the otoscope cone or endoscope.

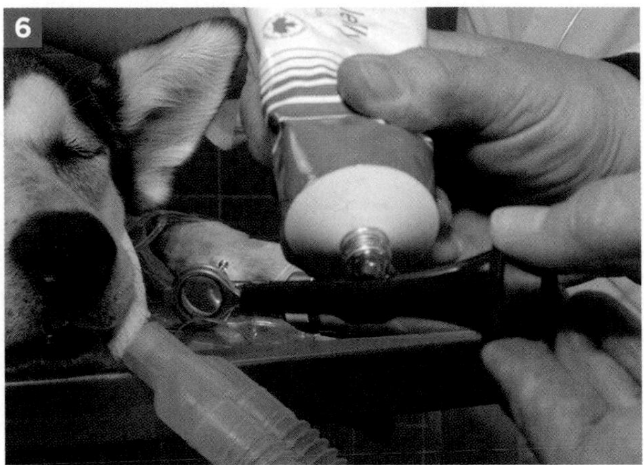

Lubricating the endoscope.

7. Insert the otoscope cone or scope into the nose, directing the tip medially and dorsally initially while applying pressure caudally.

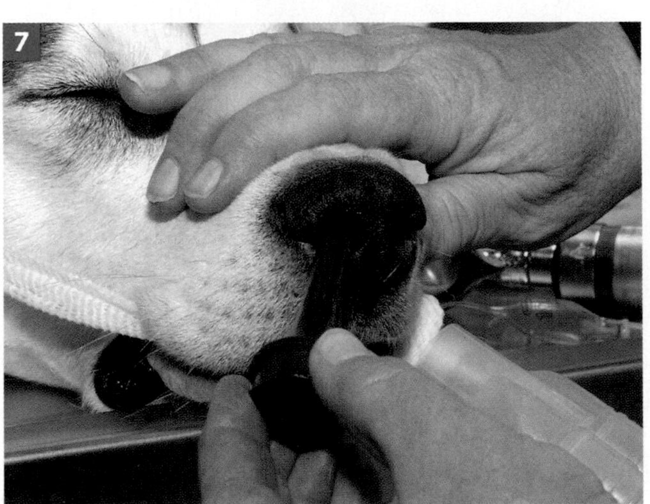

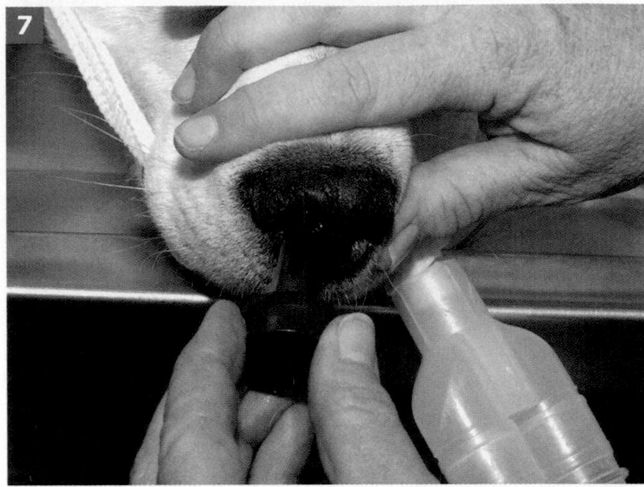

Direct the tip of the otoscope cone medially and dorsally initially while applying pressure caudally.

8. Once the otoscope cone is inserted into the nasal cavity, attach the otoscope to visualize the inside of the nasal cavity. Only the anterior one half to one third of the nose can be visualized using an otoscope cone. In large dogs there is better access to the middle portion of the nasal cavity using a rigid or flexible endoscope.

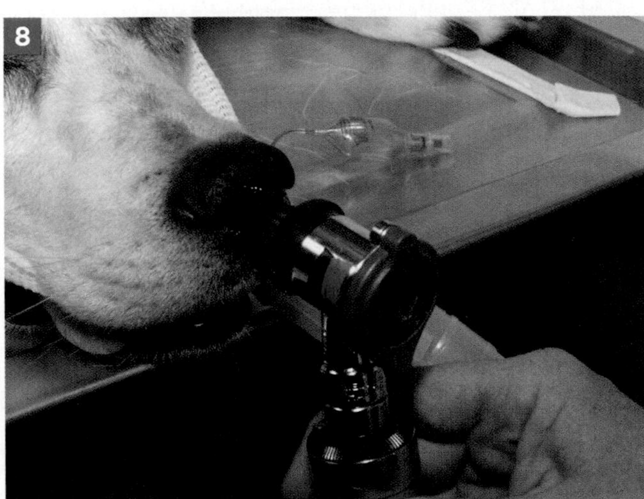

Attach the otoscope to visualize the inside of the nasal cavity.

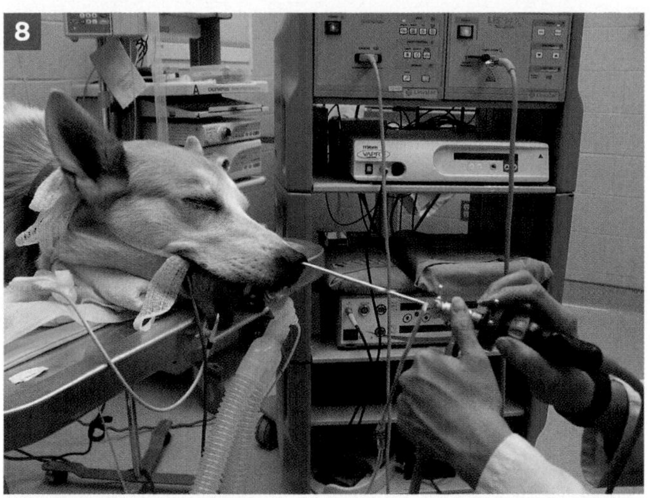

Rigid endoscopy can be used to examine most of the nasal cavity in large dogs.

9. Each nasal meatus should be systematically evaluated, beginning ventrally and working dorsally

10. The nasal mucosa is normally smooth and pink with a small amount of serous fluid. Potential abnormalities that may be visualized include inflammation of the nasal mucosa, mats of fungal hyphae, mass lesions, foreign bodies, and nasal mites.

11. When abnormalities such as masses or fungal mats are identified during rhinoscopy, samples should be collected for cytologic or histopathologic evaluation. When no abnormalities are identified during rhinoscopy, nasal flush and blind biopsies should always be performed.

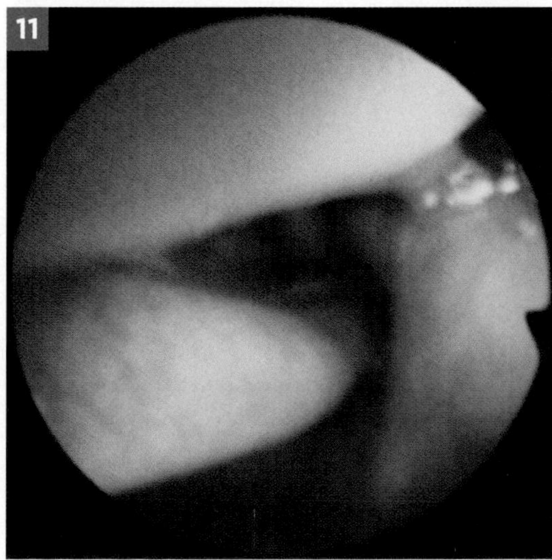

Normal anterior nasal endoscopy in a dog.

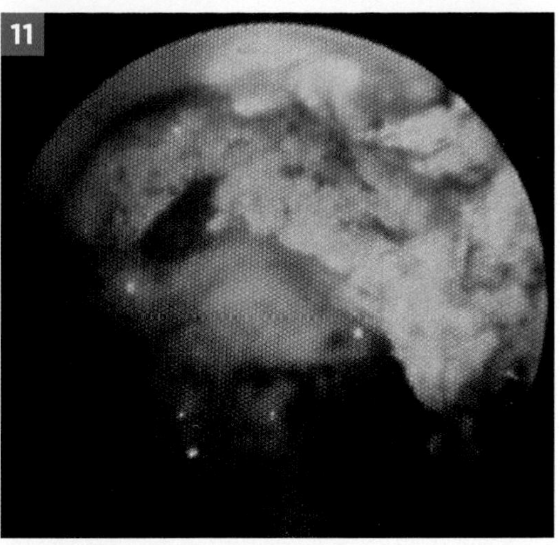

Endoscopic view of the nasal cavity in a dog with nasal aspergillosis. There is a loss of turbinate structure, the mucosa is inflamed, and fluffy gray plaques are visible. To confirm the diagnosis a small piece of the mat of fungal hyphae can be collected with a biopsy instrument, suspended in saline and submitted for cytologic evaluation. **(Courtesy Dr. Cindy Shmon, University of Saskatchewan.)**

TECHNIQUE: NASAL FLUSH

Nasal flush should always be performed if no definitive diagnosis is obtained during rhinoscopy. The patient must be under general anesthesia, and it is very important that the endotracheal tube cuff be fully inflated.

1. The caudal nasopharynx is packed with gauze sponges or gauze tape to provide a partial obstruction to the flow of saline.

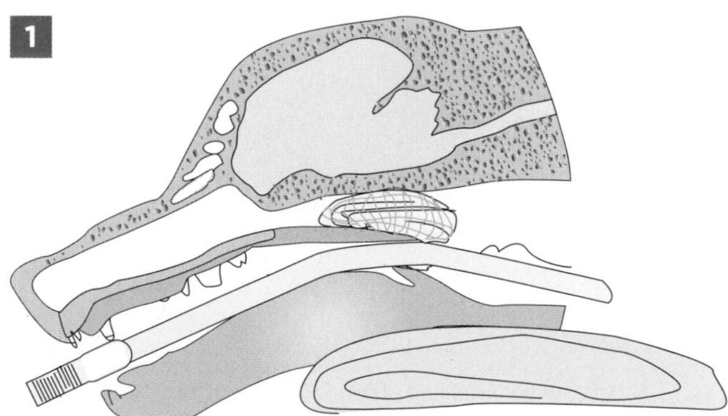

Correct positioning for nasal flush, with endotracheal tube in place and packing of the caudal nasopharynx with gauze sponges.

2. With the patient in sternal recumbency, the head is lowered off the end of the table with the nose pointed toward the floor, overlying a collection basin.

PROCEDURE 7-2 Internal Nasal Examination—cont'd

3. An ear bulb syringe is filled with approximately 30 mL of sterile saline, wedged into one nostril and squeezed so that the saline is forcibly injected into the nose. Fluid will exit the nose and the oral cavity, where it can be caught in a bowl. The flush fluid is submitted for cytologic examination together with any mucus or tissue that accumulates on the gauze sponges packing the nasopharynx. Samples obtained are often insufficient for diagnosis but occasionally nasal foreign bodies, nasal mites, and fungal hyphae can be identified using this technique.

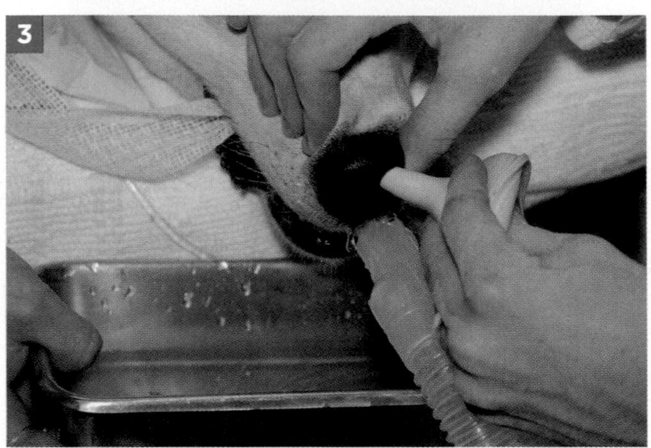

Performing a nasal flush in a dog, collecting flush fluid in a bowl.

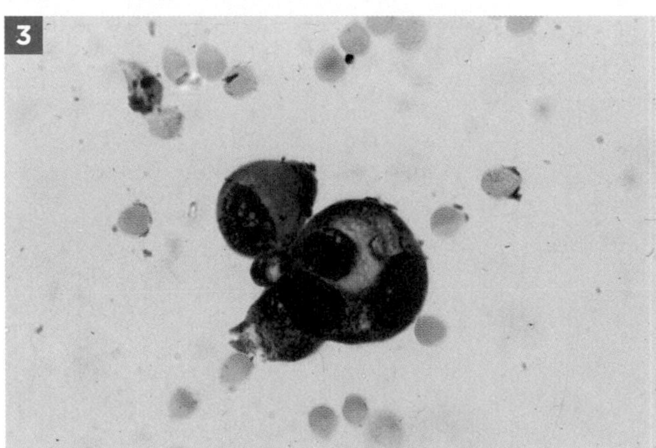

This nasal flush from a dog reveals adenocarcinoma.

TECHNIQUE: NASAL BIOPSY

Nasal biopsies should be collected for histologic examination from every patient undergoing rhinoscopy (except when rhinoscopy was performed simply to retrieve an acute nasal foreign body).

1. If a lesion was identified while scoping, small pinch biopsy forceps can be directed to the lesion using the scope. The samples obtained using these forceps are, however, quite small and are often nondiagnostic.

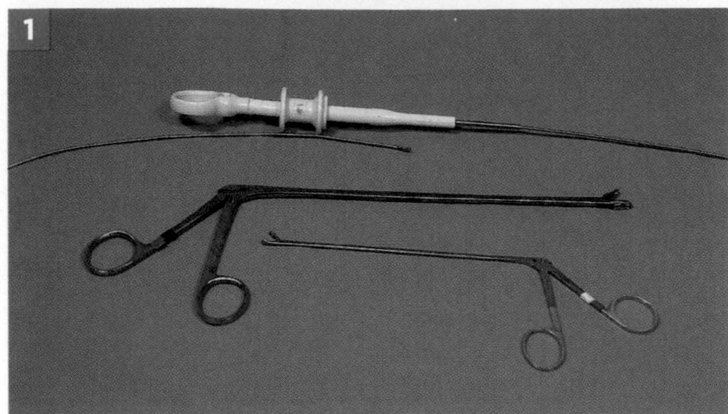

Biopsy forceps used to collect nasal biopsies in dogs and cats.

2. If no lesion was identified while scoping, but a lesion is apparent on radiographs or CT, then larger biopsy instruments such as an alligator cup biopsy forceps (minimum size 2 × 3 mm) can be directed to the region of the lesion, using maxillary teeth as landmarks to obtain biopsies.

3. If no lesion was identified during scoping or with imaging, multiple biopsies are obtained from random sites within the nasal cavity. A minimum of six tissue specimens should be collected. Avoid biopsying the floor of the nasal cavity to prevent damage to major blood vessels.

4. Biopsy forceps should never be passed into the nasal cavity deeper than the level of the medial canthus of the eye, to avoid penetrating the cribriform plate.

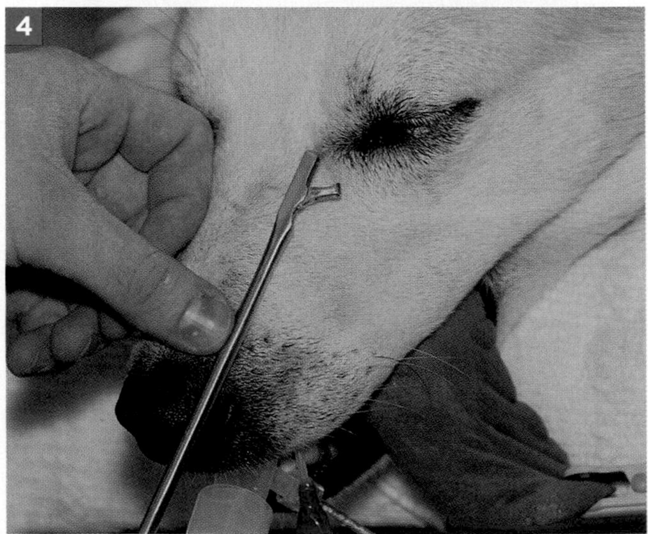

Measuring biopsy forceps to the medial canthus of the eye.

5. Biopsy forceps are passed while closed to the region to be biopsied, opened and pressed against the site, then closed tightly and withdrawn. A small-gauge needle can be used to transfer the biopsy from the forceps to a cassette for processing.

POTENTIAL COMPLICATIONS

1. Problems arising from general anesthesia
2. Excessive bleeding can occur. Hemorrhage can usually be controlled by packing the nasal cavity with cotton-tipped swabs and the nasopharynx with gauze sponges until bleeding stops.

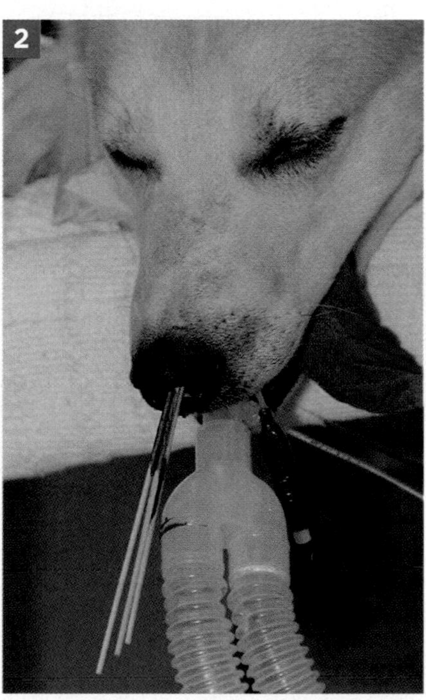

Nasal cavity is packed with cotton-tipped swabs, and nasopharynx is packed with gauze sponges to slow or prevent hemorrhage.

3. Cats with nasal obstructive disease sometimes fail to convert to mouth breathing when sedated, so may hypoventilate and could die during recovery if not monitored carefully.
4. Trauma to the brain can be avoided by never passing any object into the nasal cavity beyond the level of the medial canthus of the eye.

PROCEDURE 7-3

Pharyngeal Examination

PURPOSE

To examine the oropharynx and the nasopharynx to determine the cause of localizing clinical signs

INDICATIONS

1. Any animal with an acute onset of snorting, gagging, reverse sneezing, or repeated swallowing leading to suspicion of a pharyngeal foreign object
2. Evaluation of any animal with chronic nasal discharge, nasal erosions, nasal deformity, snorting, or inability to pass air through the nose
3. Evaluation of any patient with gagging and retching
4. Evaluation of any patient with stertorous breathing. Stertor is a loud discontinuous snoring noise heard on inspiration that is most suggestive of pharyngeal obstruction.

CONTRAINDICATIONS AND WARNINGS

1. Complete pharyngeal examination requires general anesthesia, so cannot be performed in animals that cannot be anesthetized.
2. Animals with pharyngeal obstructive disease due to a mass or redundant soft tissue are at significant risk of developing total airway obstruction and death if they are sedated and left unattended. Relaxation of redundant tissues may cause further airway obstruction during inhalation. Anesthetic induction should therefore be rapid and focused on establishing a patent airway. Personnel and equipment should be available to perform an emergency temporary tracheostomy if an endotracheal tube cannot be passed orally past an obstruction.

EQUIPMENT

- A penlight will be adequate to examine the oral cavity and oropharynx.
- A small-diameter flexible endoscope is required to adequately examine the nasopharynx (performing a caudal nasal examination).

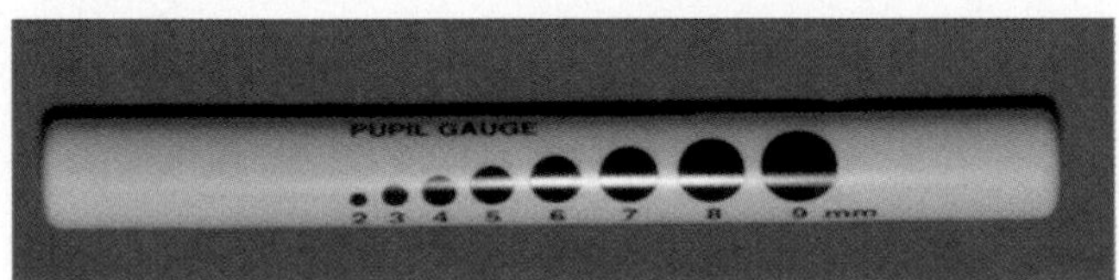

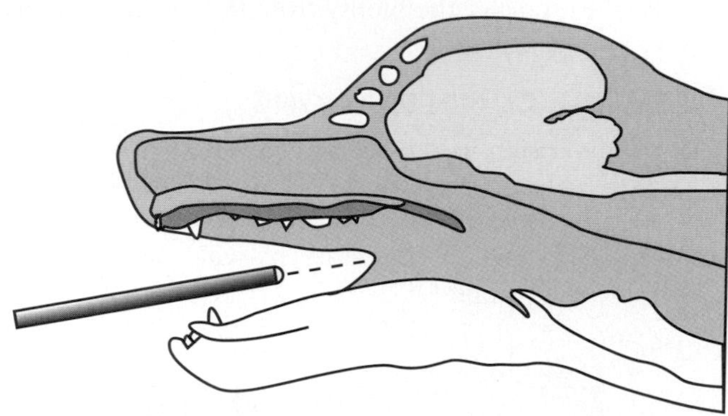

The only equipment required for complete oropharyngeal examination is a light source.

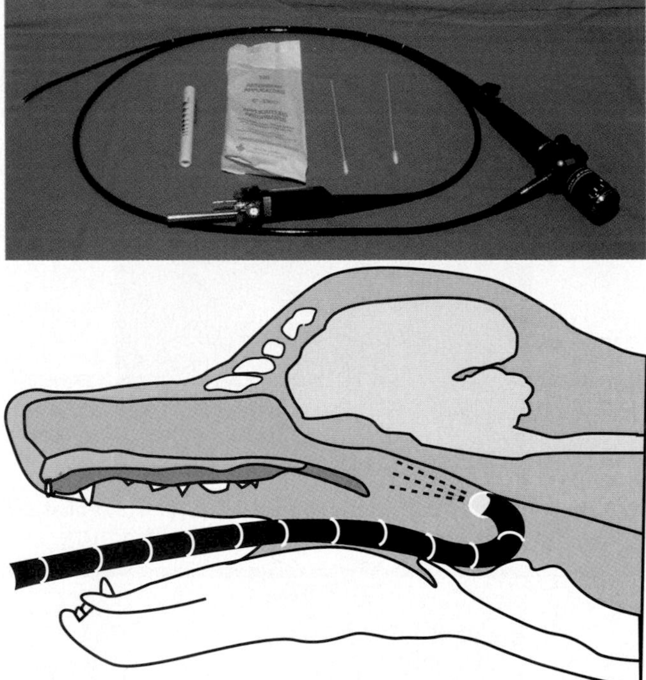

Examination of the nasopharynx requires a flexible endoscope. The endoscope tip is retroflexed and directed above the soft palate to view the nasopharynx.

POSITIONING AND RESTRAINT

The patient should be under general anesthesia, in sternal recumbency, with a mouth gag in place for this procedure.

SPECIAL ANATOMY

1. The tonsils are located in the dorsolateral pharynx, and may lie entirely within their crypts, appearing as small slits.

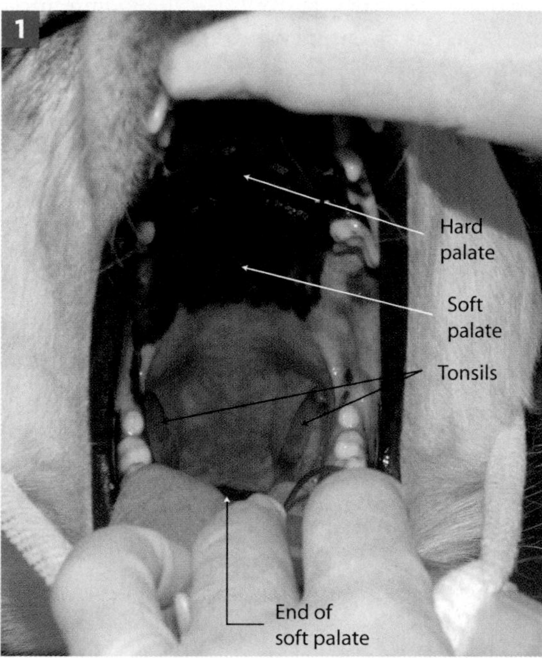

Tonsils are located in the dorsolateral pharynx.

2. The soft palate is a fleshy piece of tissue extending from the hard palate to the tip of the epiglottis, separating the oropharynx from the nasopharynx. The free edge of the soft palate just covers the tip of the epiglottis in the normal dog. It extends no farther than the caudal aspect of the tonsillar crypts.

3. The nasopharynx is the space dorsal to the soft palate.

4. The oropharynx is the region of the throat that is between the soft palate, the tongue, and the epiglottis.

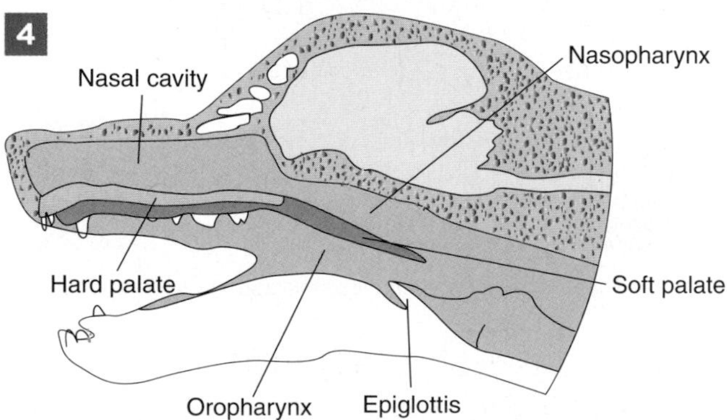

Lateral drawing of pharyngeal anatomy.

TECHNIQUE

1. General anesthesia is required. A deep plane of anesthesia is required for the nasopharyngeal examination because this technique strongly stimulates the gag reflex.

2. Inspect the tonsils, everting them from their crypts if necessary using a cotton-tipped swab. Probe the tonsillar crypts for foreign objects such as grass awns.

3. Palpate the hard and soft palate in order to detect any deformities, soft areas, or mass lesions.

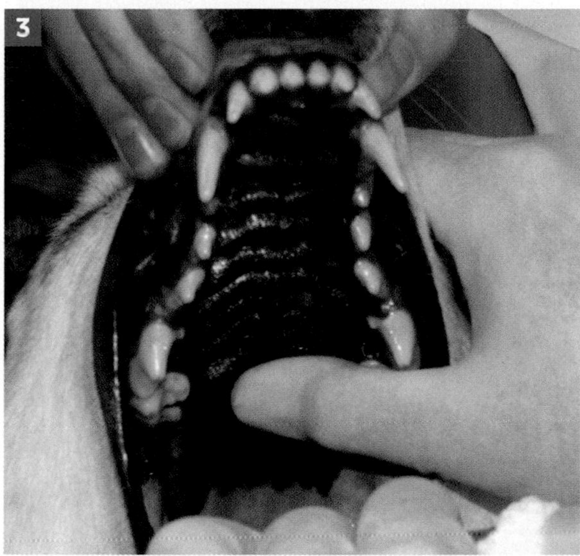

Palpating the hard palate for deformities, soft areas, or masses.

4. Assess the length and shape of the soft palate. The soft palate normally ends at the cranial edge of the epiglottis, without significant overlap. In most dogs, the soft palate extends no farther caudal than a line connecting the caudal aspect of the two tonsillar crypts. In dogs with upper airway obstruction due to an elongated soft palate, the soft palate stretches and elongates as it is sucked into the larynx and trachea, giving the caudal edge a pointed appearance.

PROCEDURE 7-3 Pharyngeal Examination—cont'd

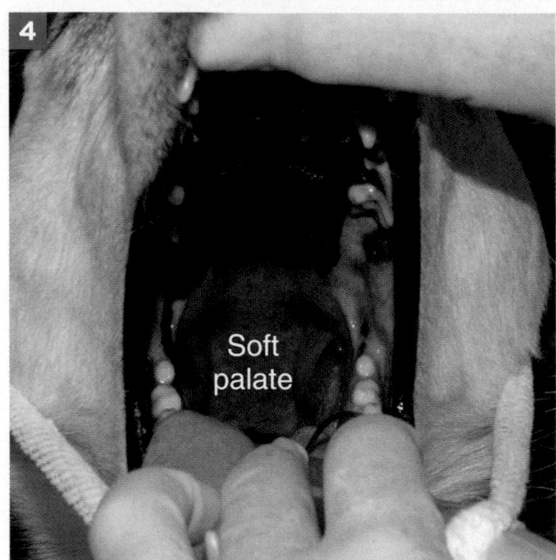

Normal soft palate length in a dog.

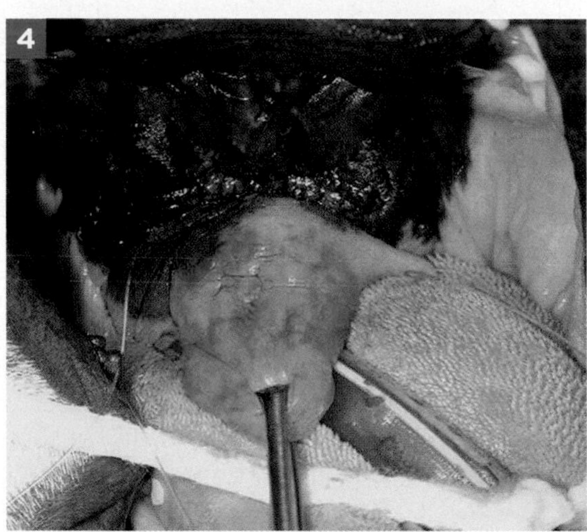

The forceps are grasping the tip of a greatly elongated soft palate of a 1-year-old English Bulldog with stertorous respirations.

5. To view the nasopharynx, pass the flexible endoscope caudally past the end of the soft palate, and flex the tip so that the light is directed down the nasopharynx. Optimal visualization of the nasopharynx is usually accomplished when the light is most apparent as it shines bright and central through the soft palate. In small dogs and cats, visualization of the nasopharynx can be improved if the base of the tongue, the endotracheal tube, and the scope are compressed ventrally to increase the dorsoventral dimension of the oropharynx, allowing the retroflexed scope tip to be directed into the nasopharynx. The image that is obtained through the retroflexed scope is inverted, with the dorsal surface of the soft palate seen at the top of the image, and the dorsal wall of the nasopharynx seen ventrally. In the dorsal roof of the nasopharynx is a mucous membrane covered bony ridge (vomer) that is continued forward (rostrally) as the membranous portion of the nasal septum on midline. Right and left orientations remain.

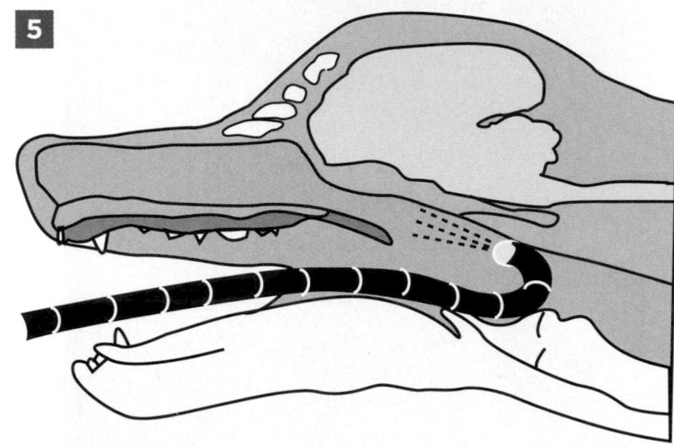

The tip of the endoscope is retroflexed so the light can be directed down the nasopharynx.

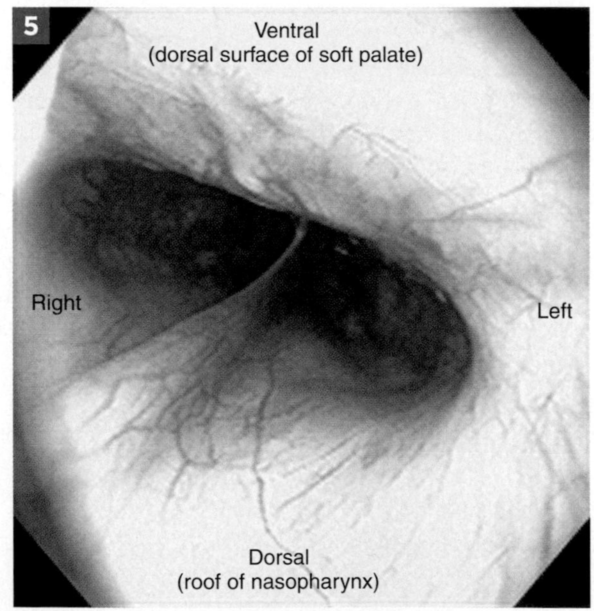

Retroflexed view down a normal nose through a flexed endoscope.

6. The nasopharynx should be examined for symmetry, discharge, and the presence of masses or foreign bodies. The caudal nasopharynx is a common location for foreign bodies, particularly grass and other plant material and food material that has been vomited by the patient. Nasopharyngeal polyps in cats and neoplastic masses in dogs and cats are often seen in this location. Nasal mites may be identified as small moving white dots as they crawl across the nasopharynx.

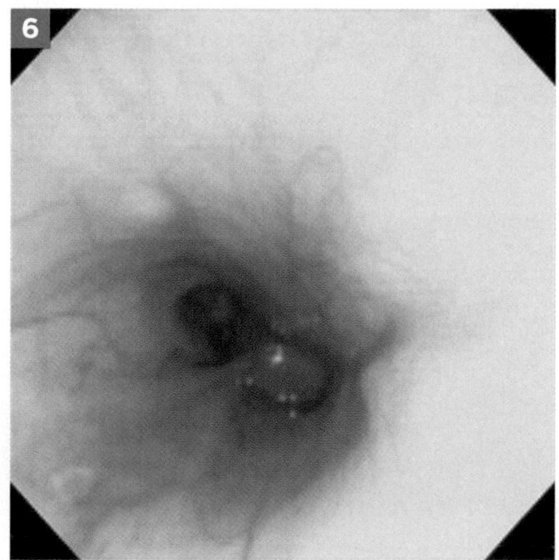

Retroflexed endoscopic view of the nasopharynx of a dog with an adenocarcinoma in the left nasal cavity.

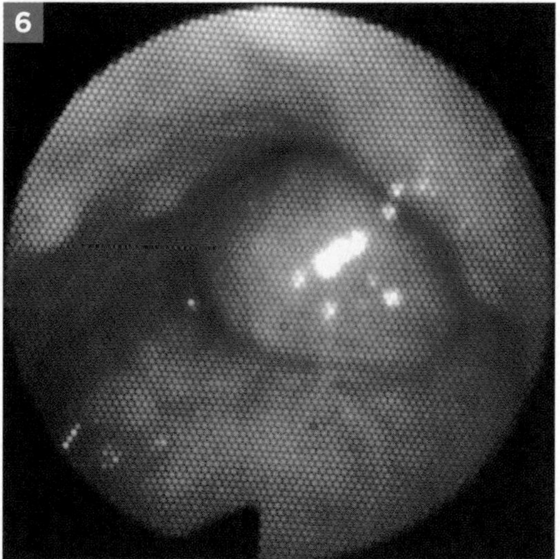

Retroflexed endoscopic view of a polyp in the caudal nasopharynx of a young cat with a long history of stertorous breathing.

7. Rarely nasopharyngeal stenosis is identified in cats. Affected cats have stertorous respiratory noise that may resolve when their mouth is held open, allowing them to mouth breathe. The retroflexed view of the nasopharynx, instead of revealing an ovoid orifice measuring approximately 5 mm wide by 6 mm tall, shows a pinhole-sized orifice in the center of a thin but tough web of tissue. Stertorous sounds during nasal breathing result from vibration of this web of tissue.

POTENTIAL COMPLICATIONS

1. Problems arising from general anesthesia
2. Animals with pharyngeal obstructive disease due to a mass or redundant soft tissues may develop total airway obstruction if sedated and left unattended before pharyngeal examination, or during anesthetic recovery if the pharyngeal obstruction was not resolved. A patent airway must be maintained and monitored from the time of induction until full recovery from anesthesia.

PROCEDURE 7-4

Laryngeal Examination

PURPOSE

To examine the larynx and assess its function in order to determine the cause of localizing clinical signs

INDICATIONS

1. Animals with inspiratory stridor (high-pitched noise and effort) suggesting laryngeal obstruction

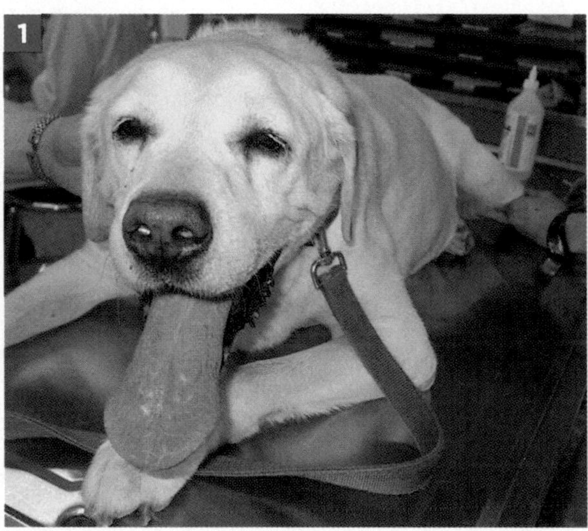

This 12-year-old Labrador Retriever with stridor and cyanotic mucous membranes was confirmed to have bilateral laryngeal paralysis using laryngoscopy.

2. Animals with unexplained aspiration pneumonia
3. Animals with chronic, unexplained cough, particularly on waking
4. Animals with loss of voice or a voice change

CONTRAINDICATIONS AND WARNINGS

1. Laryngeal examination requires a light plane of general anesthesia, so cannot be performed in animals that cannot be anesthetized.
2. Whenever possible, animals should have a complete neurologic examination before laryngoscopy. This should include assessment of their ability to swallow and thoracic radiographs or fluoroscopy to evaluate for megaesophagus. Corrective surgery for laryngeal paralysis has devastating consequences in animals with dysphagia or proximal esophageal dysfunction.
3. Personnel and equipment should be available to perform an emergency temporary tracheostomy if an endotracheal tube cannot be passed orally into the trachea past an obstructive laryngeal mass.
4. If anesthetic depth is excessive, laryngeal motion will be depressed or absent in a normal animal, potentially leading to a misdiagnosis of laryngeal paralysis.

EQUIPMENT

- Laryngoscope with light or flexible endoscope

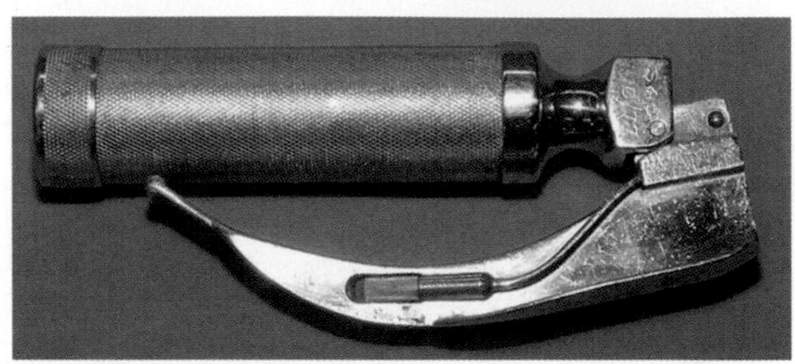

A laryngoscope is the only equipment required for laryngeal examination.

POSITIONING AND RESTRAINT

1. To evaluate laryngeal function, the patient needs to be in a light anesthetic plane, restrained in sternal recumbency while the mouth is held open and the tongue retracted.
2. The ideal drug or drug combination for evaluating laryngeal function provides relaxation of the jaw muscles while permitting normal arytenoid movement and range of motion.
   - A. Intravenous thiopental (10 to 20 mg/kg to effect) or propofol (6 mg/kg to effect) with no premedication may be the best anesthetic choice for evaluating laryngeal function in dogs.
   - B. Administration of acepromazine predication should be avoided if thiopental or propofol induction is planned because these drug combinations abolish laryngeal motion in some normal dogs.
   - C. Administration of doxapram (2 to 5 mg/kg IV) increases depth of respirations, making it easier to assess laryngeal function. Be aware that many dogs with laryngeal paralysis develop paradoxical movement (closing of the laryngeal opening during inspiration) following doxapram administration, making it critically important to correlate arytenoid movements with phase of respiration.

SPECIAL ANATOMY

1. The rima glottidis (laryngeal inlet) consists of the vocal folds and the corniculate processes of the arytenoid cartilages.

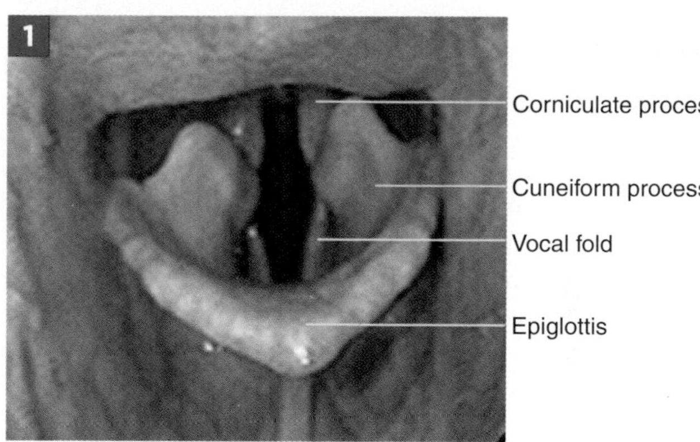

Labeled laryngeal anatomy.

2. During normal inspiration, the glottic opening is enlarged as abductor muscles (primarily the cricoarytenoideus dorsalis) contract and abduct the arytenoid cartilages. Motor and sensory innervation to the larynx is provided by branches of the vagus nerve (cranial nerve 10). Abductors of the larynx are innervated by the caudal laryngeal nerve—the terminal segment of the recurrent laryngeal nerve.
3. Relaxation normally results in passive adduction (coming together) of the cartilages, reducing the diameter of the rima glottidis but permitting adequate airflow for exhalation.
4. Active closing of the glottis by laryngeal adductors is controlled by the cranial laryngeal nerve, another branch of the vagus nerve.

TECHNIQUE: LARYNGEAL EXAMINATION

1. Following preoxygenation, the patient should be placed under a light plane of general anesthesia as described previously.
2. The mouth is held open and the tongue is gently pulled forward.

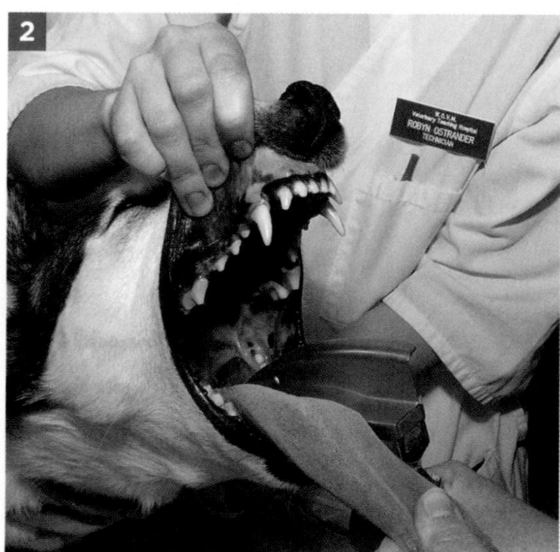

The mouth is held open and the tongue is gently pulled forward for laryngeal examination.

3. The caudal tongue just cranial to the epiglottis is depressed to provide a good view of the larynx. If necessary, the soft palate can be retracted dorsally with a cotton-tipped swab.
4. Observe the structure of the larynx and note any reddening, masses, or discharge. Masses of the larynx or diffuse thickening of laryngeal tissues should be biopsied.

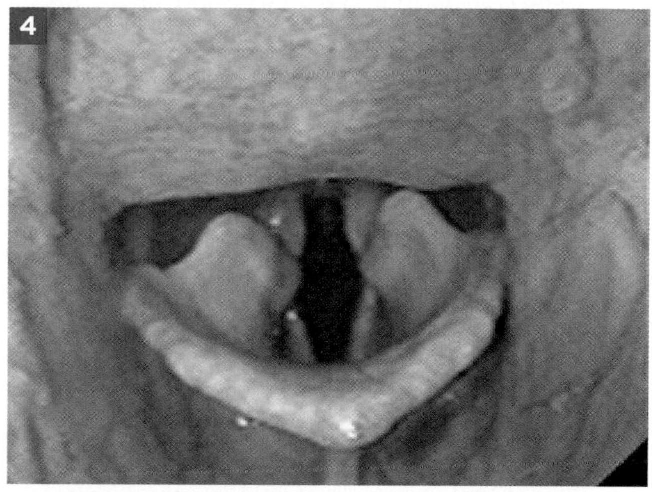

Normal canine larynx.

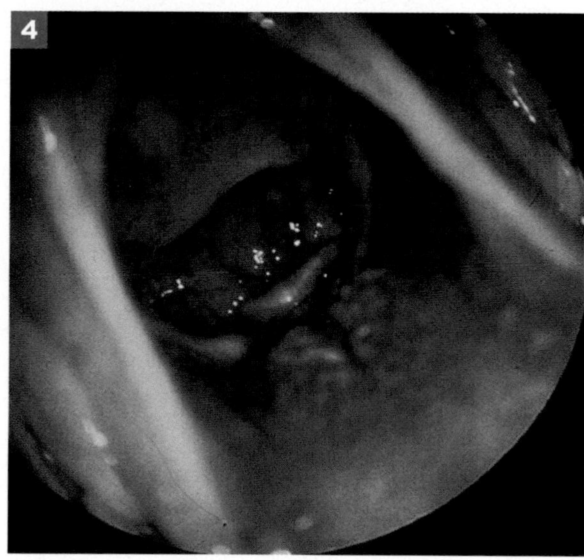

Obstructive mass of the larynx in a cat. Biopsy revealed lymphoma.

5. Observe the larynx during respiration.
   - A. Normally the arytenoids should abduct during inspiration, opening the laryngeal lumen. During exhalation they should return to a nearly midline position.
   - B. Laryngeal motion must be correlated with the phase of respiration. Observers should inform the examiner when the thorax is expanding (inhalation) because this should correspond with abduction of the laryngeal cartilages.

C. Fluttering of the vocal folds and arytenoid cartilages during breathing due to turbulent airflow must not be mistaken for purposeful abduction.
D. In some animals with laryngeal paralysis there is paradoxical movement, particularly after respiration is stimulated by doxapram administration. In animals with paradoxical movement the arytenoid cartilages are drawn inward by negative airway pressure during vigorous inhalation and subsequently forced apart by exhaled air. Thus there is movement of the arytenoid cartilages during respiration, but abduction occurs during exhalation not inhalation.
E. Whenever arytenoid movement is absent or questionable upon anesthetic induction, laryngeal function should be reassessed during anesthetic recovery, when the effects of the administered anesthetics have diminished.

POTENTIAL COMPLICATIONS

1. Problems arising from general anesthesia
2. If the airway is totally obstructed by a laryngeal mass, patients may require an emergency tracheostomy to establish an airway.
3. Patients with laryngeal paralysis, whether or not corrective arytenoid tie-back surgery is performed, are at some risk for aspiration during recovery from anesthesia. They should be propped upright and remain intubated until they are swallowing and objecting to the endotracheal tube.

PROCEDURE 7-5

Transtracheal Wash—Small and Large Dogs

PURPOSE

To collect a sample of secretions from the trachea and airways for cytologic and microbiologic analysis

INDICATIONS

1. Dogs with cough that is not the result of cardiac enlargement or cardiac failure
2. Dogs with disease localized to the airways or lungs

CONTRAINDICATIONS AND WARNINGS

1. Transtracheal wash is not necessary in dogs with cough caused by cardiac enlargement or cardiac failure (pulmonary edema)—the reason for cough in these dogs has already been determined.
2. Endotracheal wash is the preferred method for getting a sample in very small dogs that are stressed and dyspneic. These dogs may decompensate when struggling against the restraint required for transtracheal wash.
3. Cats do not tolerate the restraint required for transtracheal wash, so endotracheal wash is preferred.

POSITIONING AND RESTRAINT

1. The dog should be standing or sitting at the edge of a table or on the floor, with the nose raised and the feet restrained.

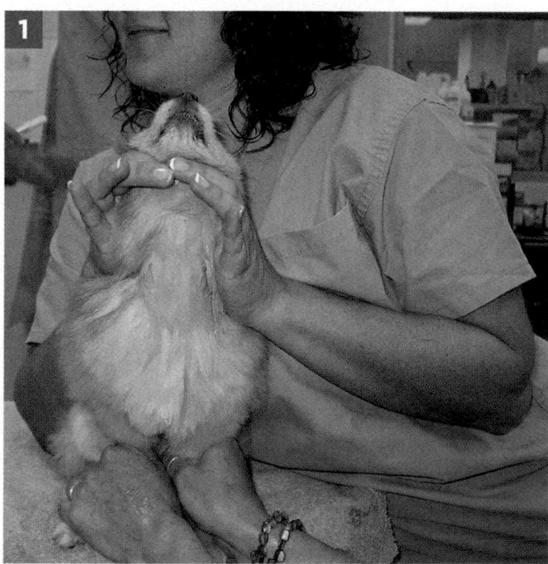

Restraint for transtracheal wash.

2. If necessary, the dog can be muzzled with a cage muzzle during the transtracheal wash to prevent injury to personnel while still allowing mouth breathing during the procedure.

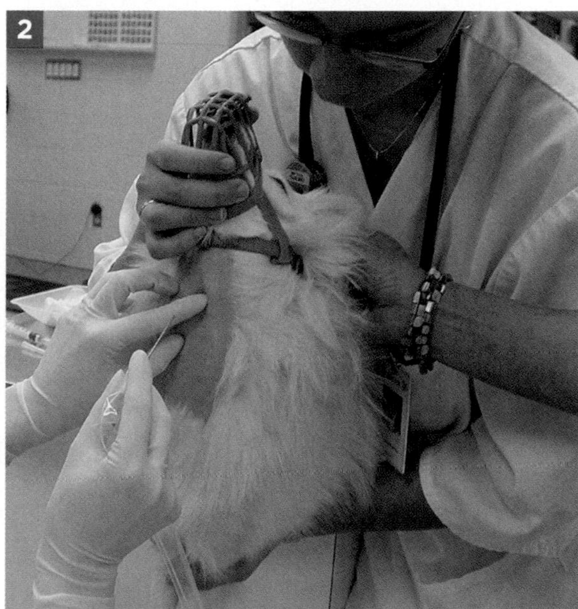

Cage muzzle during the transtracheal wash.

3. Chemical restraint or sedation is not recommended because it decreases the cough reflex and diminishes the quality of the sample obtained.
4. Lidocaine blocking solution (2% lidocaine mixed 9:1 with 8.4% sodium bicarbonate) can be used to block the skin at the site of needle entry. The addition of bicarbonate decreases the sting of injection and speeds the local analgesic effect of the lidocaine.

SPECIAL ANATOMY

1. In large and small dogs, access to the trachea for a transtracheal wash is best accomplished through the cricothyroid ligament. This is a tough membrane at the most cranial aspect of the trachea between the cricoid cartilage and the thyroid cartilage. The small, triangular cricothyroid membrane is entirely surrounded by cartilage, making it unlikely that significant laceration of tracheal tissues will occur, even if the dog struggles during the procedure. The cricoid cartilage completely encircles the lumen of the airway, so that even in dogs with soft tracheal cartilages due to the syndrome of tracheal collapse, the lumen of the trachea at the cricothyroid ligament remains cylindrical, facilitating catheter insertion at this site.

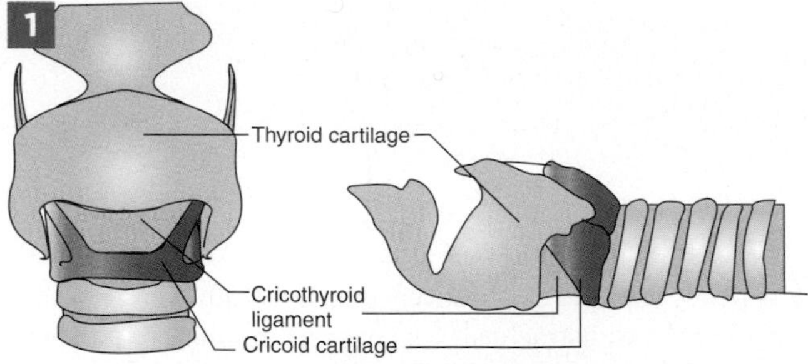

Anatomy of the cricothyroid ligament.

2. The cricothyroid ligament is palpated by restraining the dog with its nose pointing up toward the ceiling and palpating each individual tracheal ring on the anterior surface of the trachea, starting at the thoracic inlet and moving up toward the larynx. At the most cranial end of the trachea, a wide ring is palpated that protrudes more than the tracheal rings—this is the cricoid cartilage. The cricothyroid ligament is the small triangular membrane just rostral to (above) the cricoid cartilage, connecting this cartilage with the thyroid cartilage. In large dogs a triangular depression can actually be palpated just rostral to the cricoid cartilage, whereas in small dogs the only palpable landmark is the cricoid cartilage—the needle is inserted just barely above this larger ring.

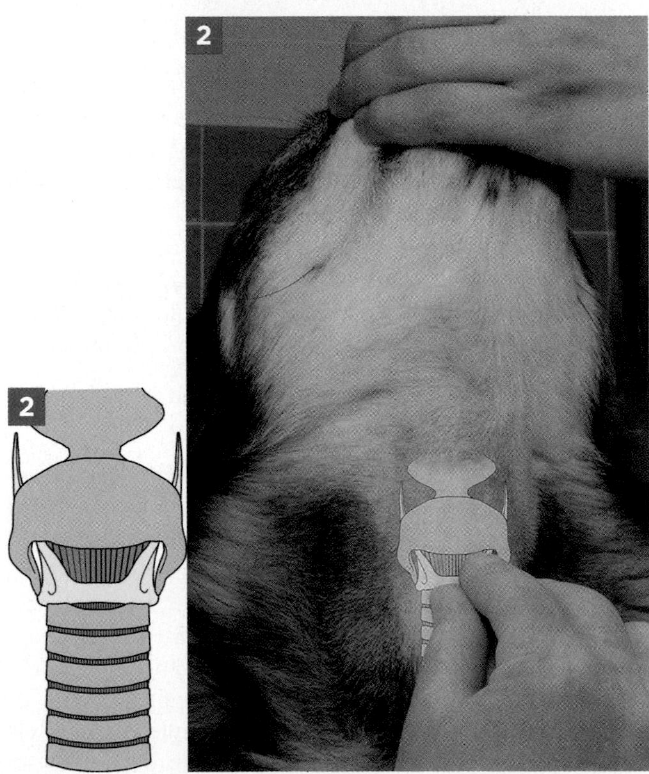

The cricoid cartilage is palpable as a wider ring above the smaller tracheal rings, and the cricothyroid ligament is the triangular depression immediately rostral to this cartilage.

3. The most diagnostic sample will be obtained if the catheter tip is located near the tracheal bifurcation (carina) over the base of the heart. Because of the length of the catheter required to reach this site, a slightly different technique is used to perform a transtracheal wash in a small dog when compared with a large dog.

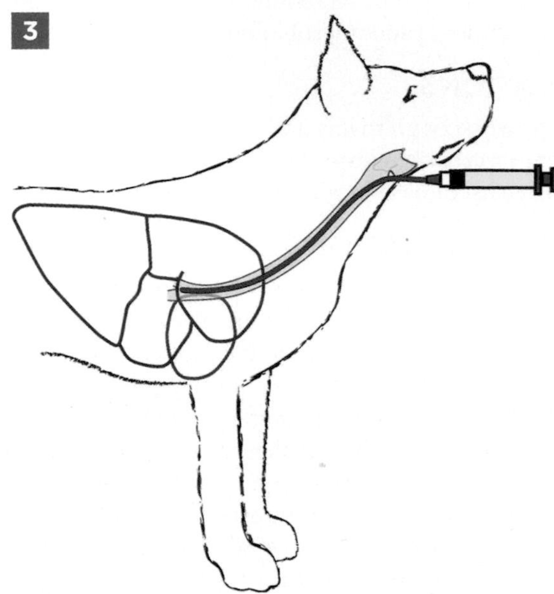

The most diagnostic sample can be obtained if the catheter tip is located near the tracheal bifurcation (carina) over the base of the heart.

POTENTIAL COMPLICATIONS

Rarely patients develop subcutaneous emphysema following a transtracheal wash. This is most likely to occur in a patient who repeatedly coughs after the procedure because air is forced from the trachea through the hole in the cricothyroid ligament and into the subcutaneous tissues. In most cases this can be prevented by applying a light wrap for an hour or two after the procedure.

SAMPLE HANDLING

The cells collected during a tracheal wash are fragile, so samples should be processed within 30 minutes of collection whenever possible. Direct smears of the fluid can be made, but most samples are poorly cellular and sediment or cytocentrifuge preparations are required for interpretation. Refrigeration may preserve cellular detail when cytologic analysis must be delayed. At least 0.5 mL of fluid should be submitted for bacterial culture. Fungal and *Mycoplasma* cultures also can be requested.

PROCEDURE 7-6

Small Dog Transtracheal Wash

EQUIPMENT REQUIRED

- Polyethylene 16- to 20-gauge through-the-needle catheter (Intra-Cath, sold for use as indwelling jugular vein catheter)
- Three 12-mL syringes with 6 mL saline in each
- 1 mL lidocaine blocking solution (2% lidocaine mixed 9:1 with 8.4% sodium bicarbonate), 3-mL syringe, 25-gauge needle
- Sterile gloves
- Bandage material

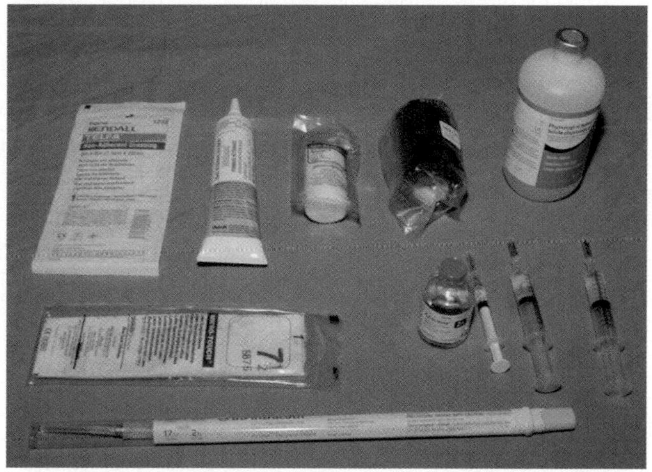

Equipment required for a small dog transtracheal wash.

TECHNIQUE: SMALL DOG TRANSTRACHEAL WASH

1. Restrain the dog on a table in a sternal position, with the nose pointing toward the ceiling. The front legs should be held down.
2. Identify the cricothyroid ligament by palpation.

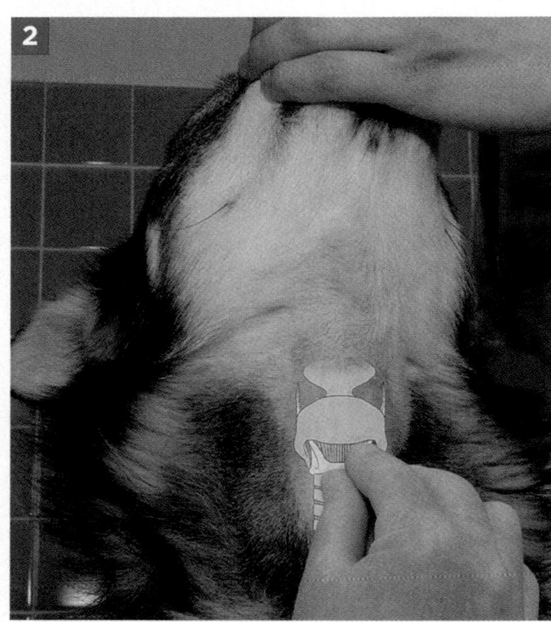

The cricothyroid ligament is identified by palpation.

3. Clip and prep the site over the cricothyroid ligament. Sterile gloves and aseptic technique are used for the procedure.
4. Block the site with 0.25 to 0.5 mL of lidocaine blocking solution; repeat final scrub.

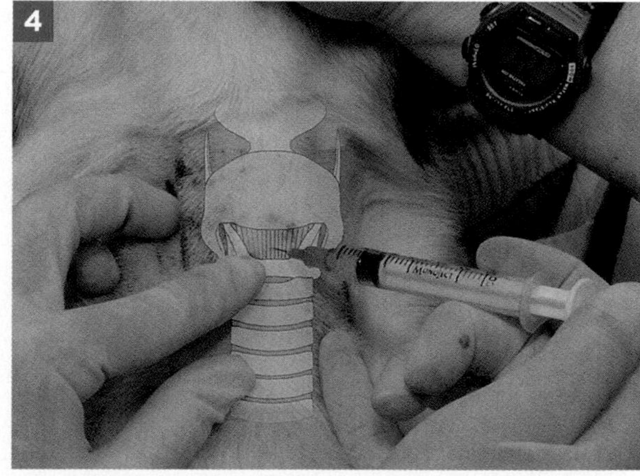

The skin over the cricothyroid ligament is blocked with lidocaine blocking solution.

PROCEDURE 7-6 Small Dog Transtracheal Wash—cont'd

5. Prepare the catheter for use. Separate the needle from the plastic hub and then reattach. Ensure that the catheter passes through the needle, then retract it into the needle. The catheter is now ready for use.

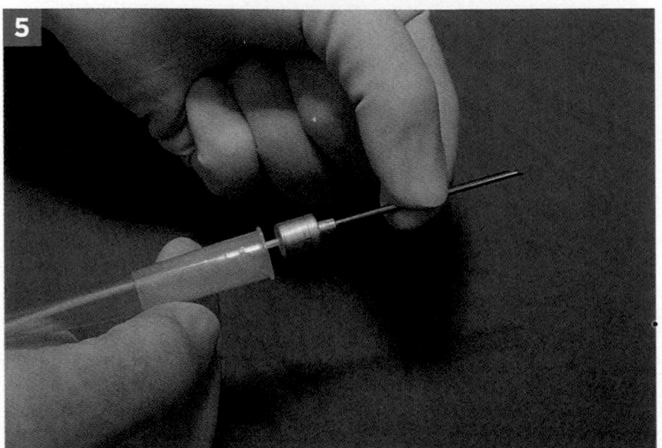

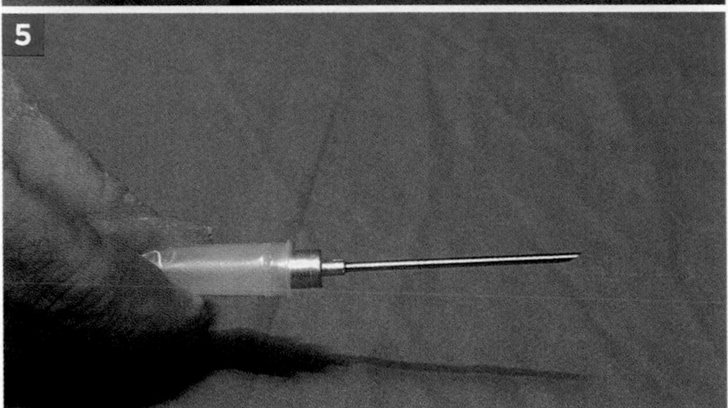

The needle is separated from the plastic hub and then reattached.

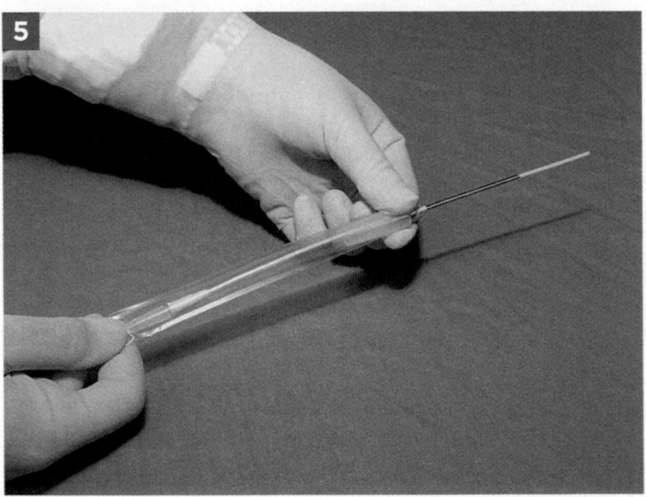

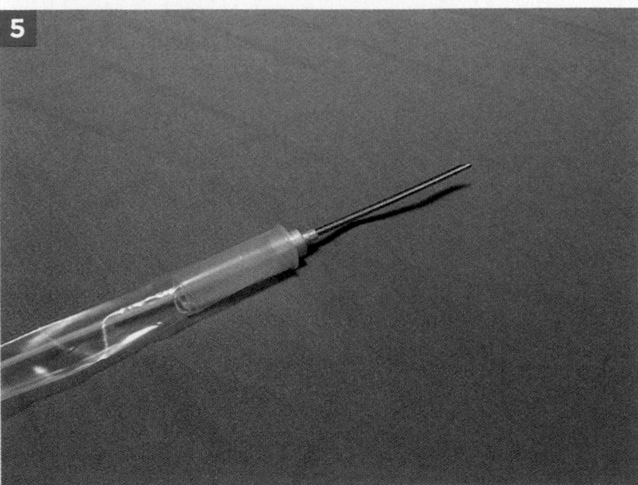

The catheter is passed through the needle and then retracted before use.

6. Stabilize the larynx and trachea by palpation to prevent side-to-side movement of these structures while attempting needle puncture.

7. Identify the cricoid cartilage, and place the tip of the needle (bevel down) at the level of the cricothyroid ligament (in the depression just above the cricoid cartilage) on the midline.

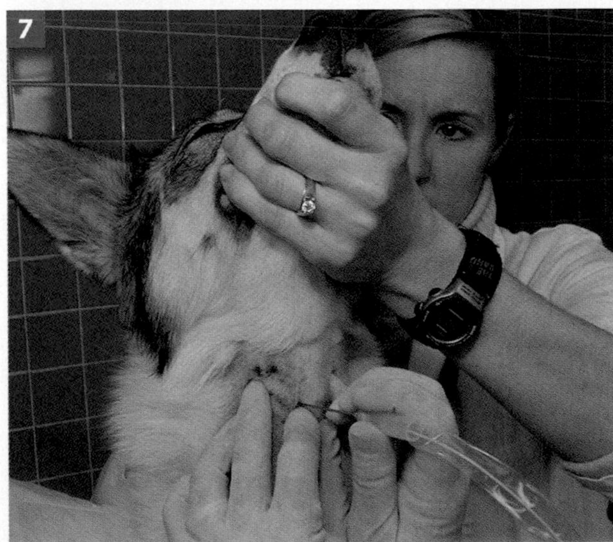

The needle is inserted bevel down through the cricothyroid ligament into the tracheal lumen.

8. Apply firm pressure inward and puncture the trachea, maintaining the needle perpendicular to the tracheal lumen. A "pop" may be felt as the needle enters the tracheal lumen.

9. Advance the needle a short distance into the trachea after the lumen is entered, until the needle tip is in approximately the center of the tracheal lumen.

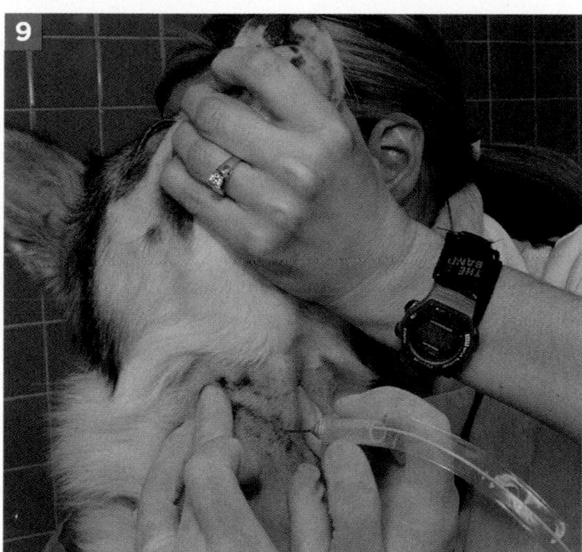
The needle is advanced a short distance, until the tip is in approximately the center of the tracheal lumen.

10. Tilt the needle approximately 45 degrees to direct the needle down the tracheal lumen and advance slightly.

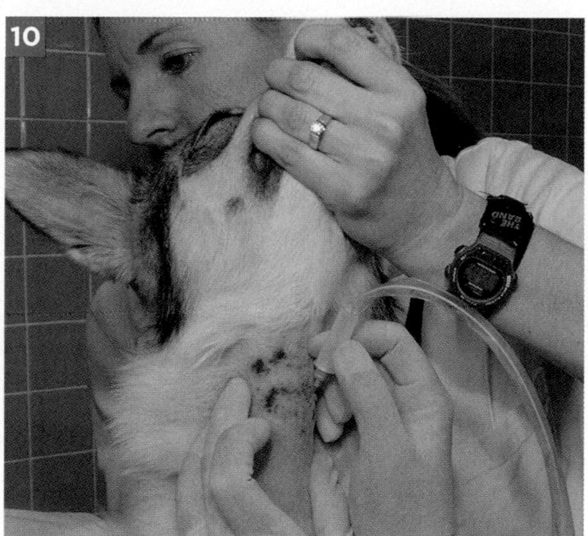
The needle is angled down the trachea approximately 45 degrees and advanced slightly.

11. Advance the catheter through the needle down the trachea to the level of the bifurcation. It is important that the tip of the catheter be at the bifurcation to collect the best sample. Note: The catheter should pass easily and the dog should cough. If the catheter does not pass easily, it is likely that the catheter is hitting the back or side wall of the trachea. Reassess the location of the needle tip and readjust so that the tip of the needle is in the center of the tracheal lumen. Most often the nose will need to be raised and the neck will need to be more fully extended to allow the needle and catheter to be directed more severely down the trachea.

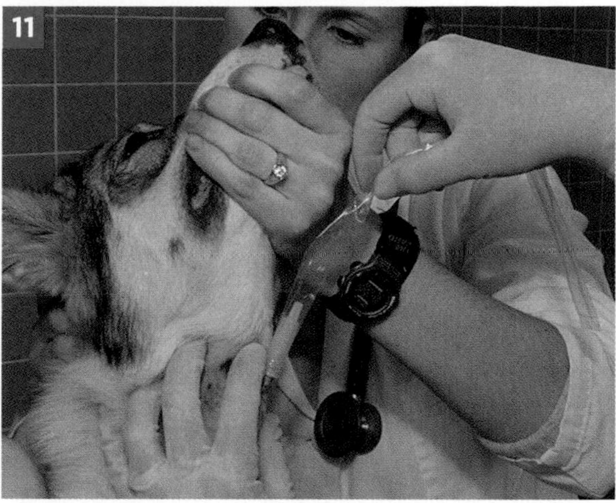
Advancing the catheter through the needle into the trachea.

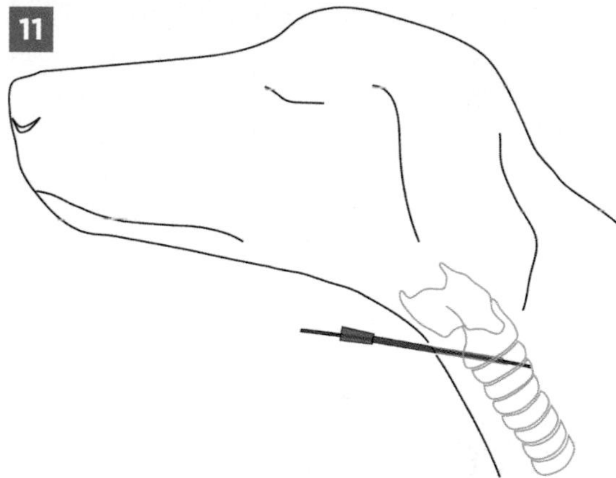
If the catheter does not advance easily, it is likely that it is hitting the back wall of the trachea.

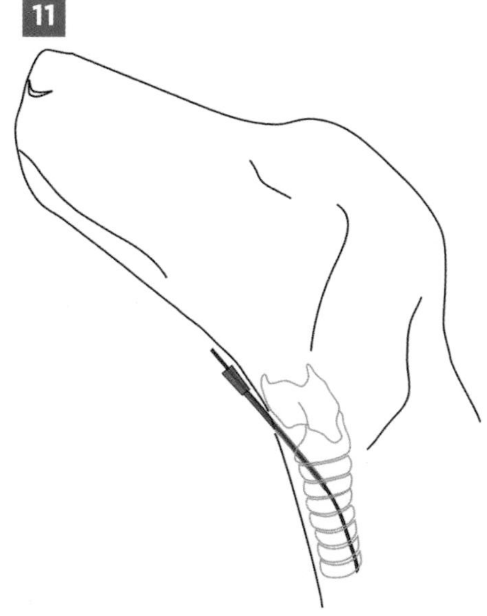
Raising the nose and angling the catheter down the trachea more severely allows the catheter to be passed.

PROCEDURE 7-6 Small Dog Transtracheal Wash—cont'd

12. Seat the catheter hub into the needle hub and remove the plastic sleeve.

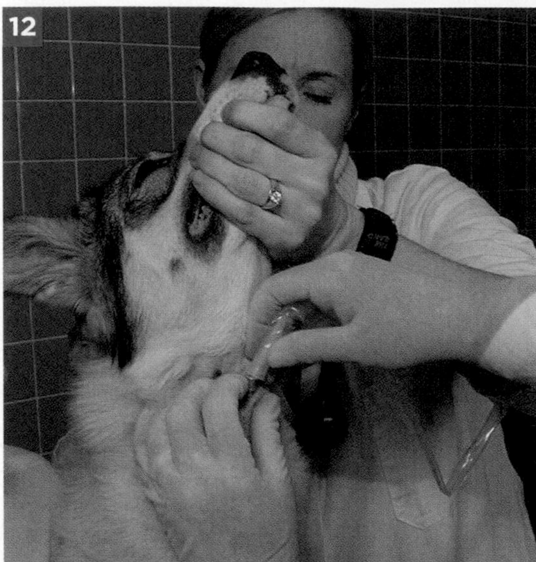

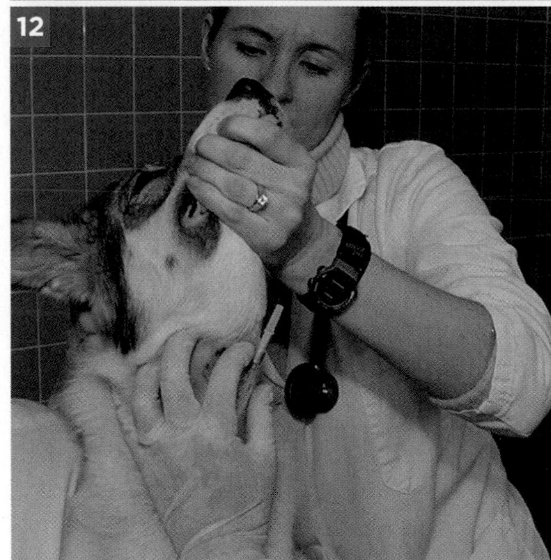

Seating the catheter hub into the needle hub and removing the plastic sleeve.

13. Once the catheter is passed to desired depth, back the catheter needle out of the trachea and skin, leaving the catheter in place.

14. Attach the needle guard to the catheter to prevent laceration of the catheter with the sharp tip of the needle. Be careful not to clamp the catheter in the needle guard.

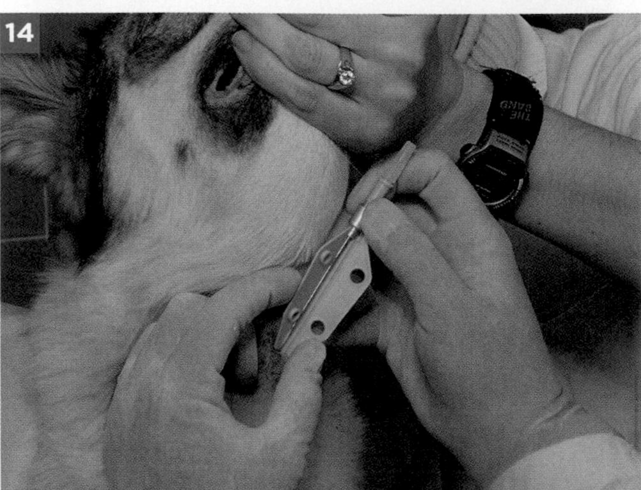

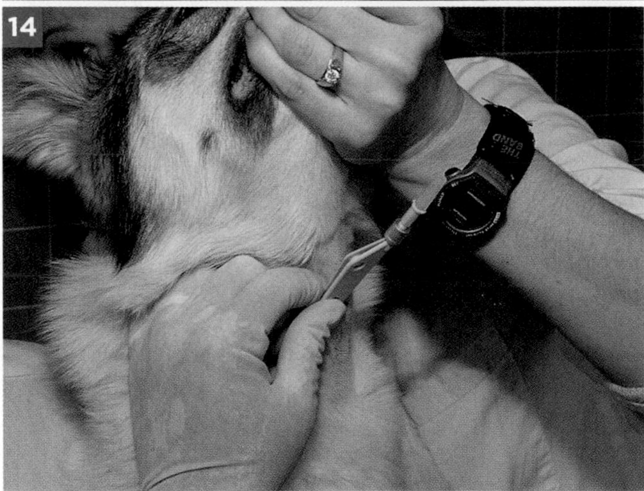

Attaching the needle guard to the catheter.

15. Remove the wire stylet from the catheter.

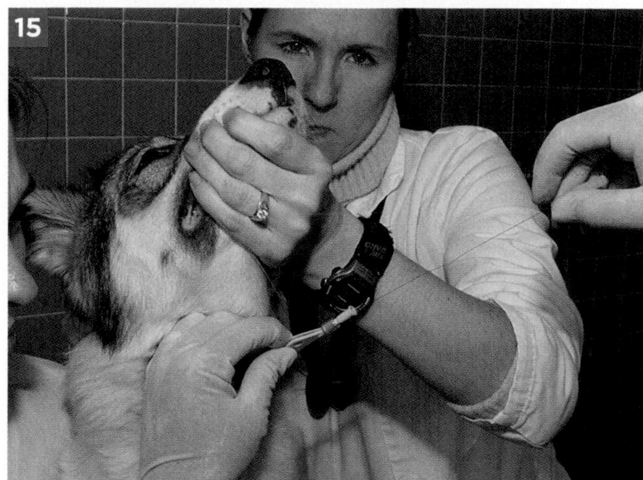

Removing the wire stylet from the catheter.

16. Attach a 12-mL syringe containing 6 mL of saline, inject 2 to 5 mL of the saline, then repeatedly aspirate to recover airway washings. Best recovery is during patient coughing. A total recovery of 1.5 to 3 mL of turbid fluid represents a good sample.

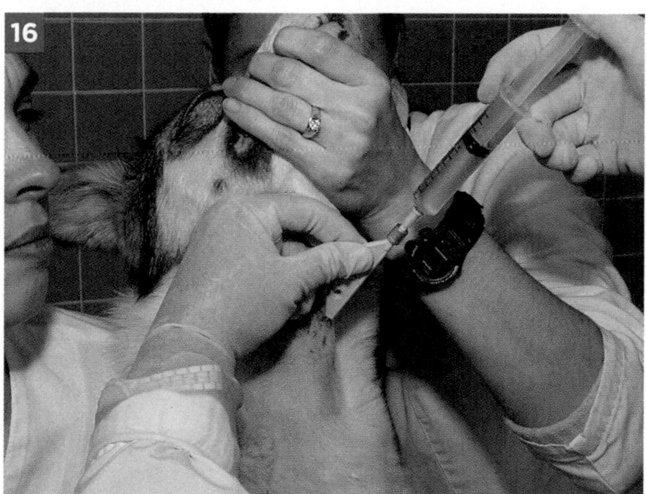

Saline is injected and repeatedly aspirated to obtain a sample.

17. If nothing is recovered, repeat the flush using a second 12-L syringe containing 6 mL of saline. Suction should be vigorously applied immediately after instilling the saline. If still nothing is recovered, have the patient lie down in sternal recumbency with the nose, head, and neck in a more neutral position and repeat the flush with a third syringe of saline.

18. Once a sample is recovered, withdraw the entire catheter. Submit samples for cytologic evaluation of a direct and concentrated sample as well as for culture.

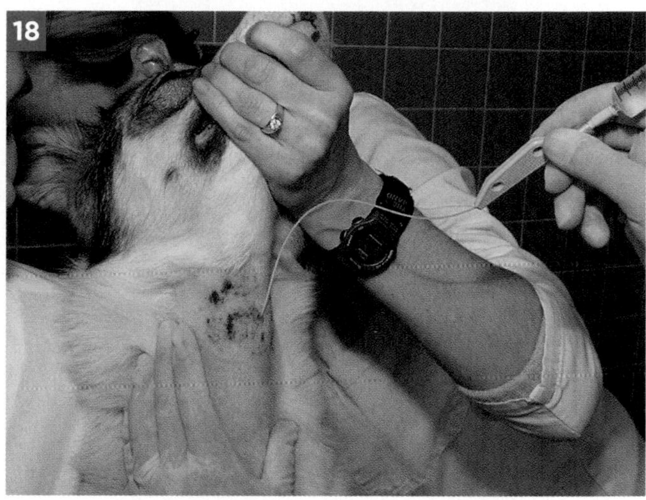

Once a sample is recovered, the entire catheter is withdrawn.

PROCEDURE 7-6 Small Dog Transtracheal Wash—cont'd

19. Place a light wrap around the neck to compress the tissues and minimize leakage of air from the trachea into the subcutaneous tissues if the dog coughs. Cover the skin entry wound with an occlusive ointment. Apply gauze sponges and then a light wrap, being careful to avoid restricting venous return or ventilatory efforts. Two fingers should fit easily beneath the wrap. The wrap can be removed after 1 to 2 hours.

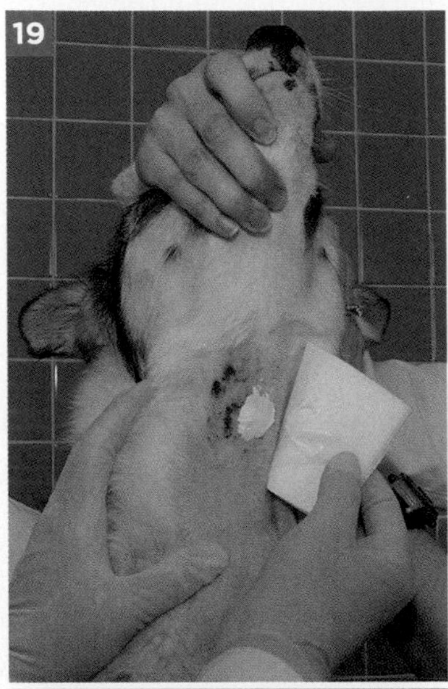

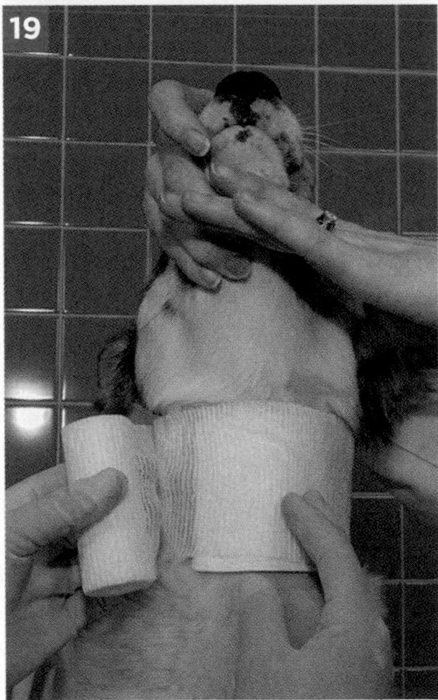

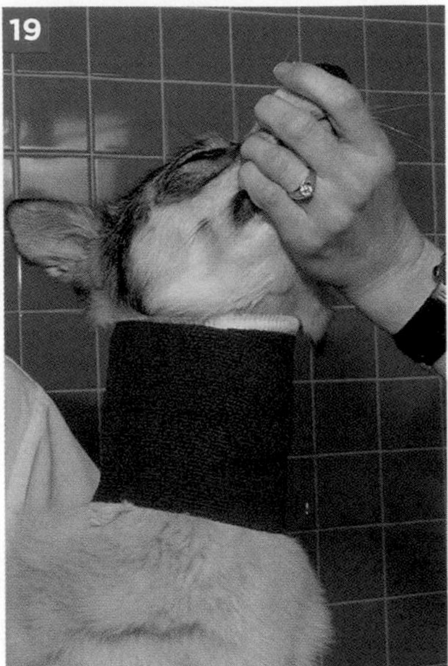

An occlusive ointment is placed over the needle entry site and a light bandage is applied.

20. Keep the patient quiet and monitor respirations for 1 to 2 hours following this procedure.

21. This technique is simple to perform, has a high diagnostic yield, and is minimally stressful for small dogs (Box 7-4, page 97).

BOX 7-4

Transtracheal Wash: Small Dog Technique Performed on an American Eskimo Dog

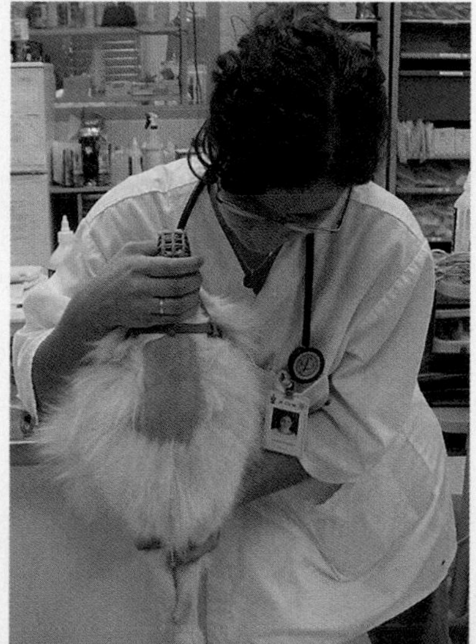

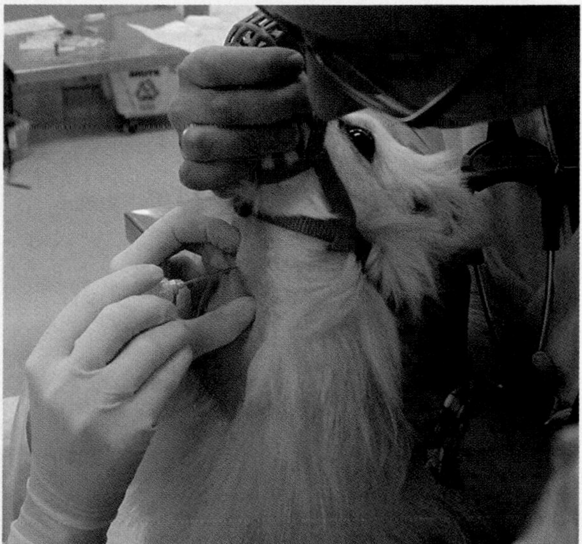

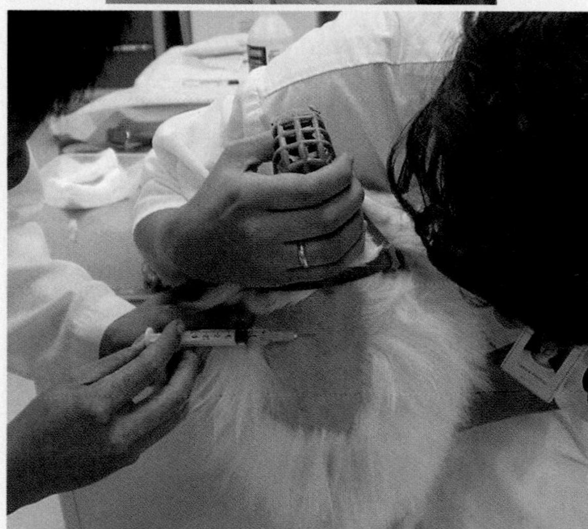

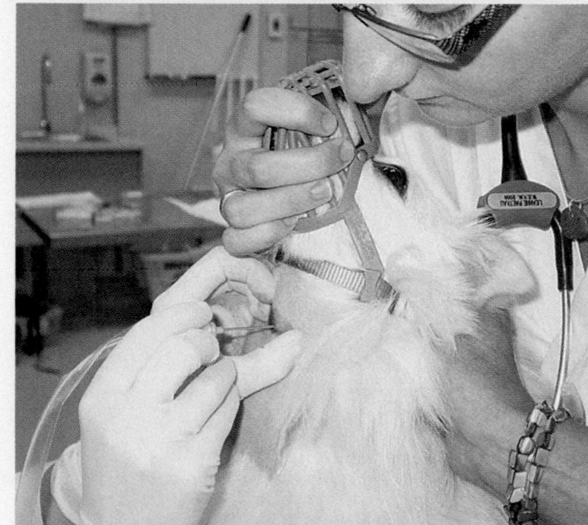

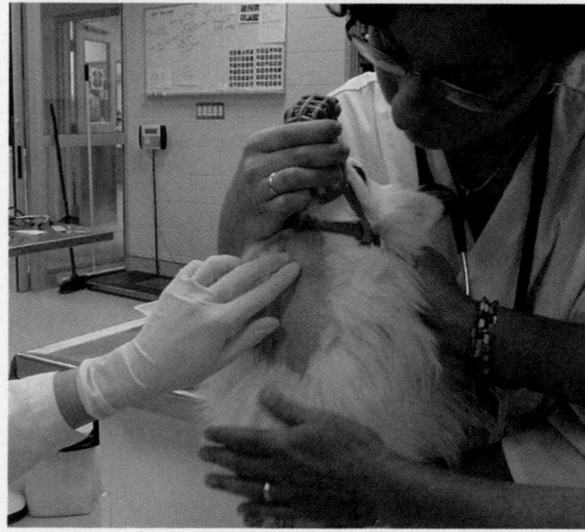

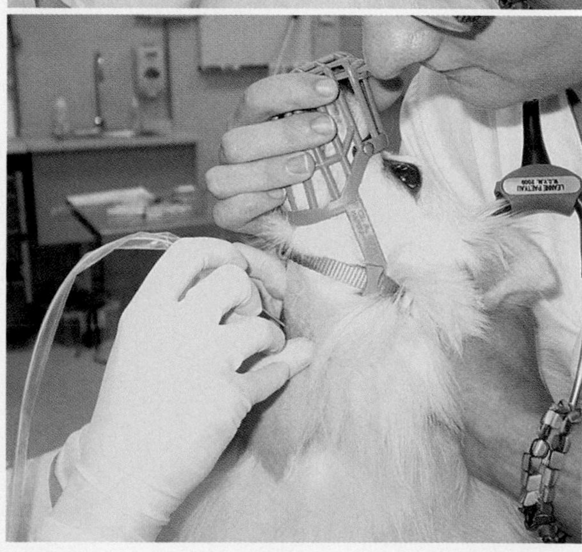

(Continued)

BOX 7-4

Transtracheal Wash: Small Dog Technique Performed on an American Eskimo Dog—cont'd

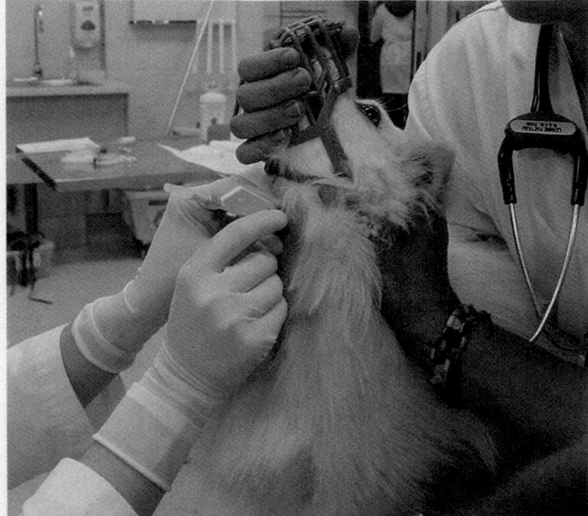

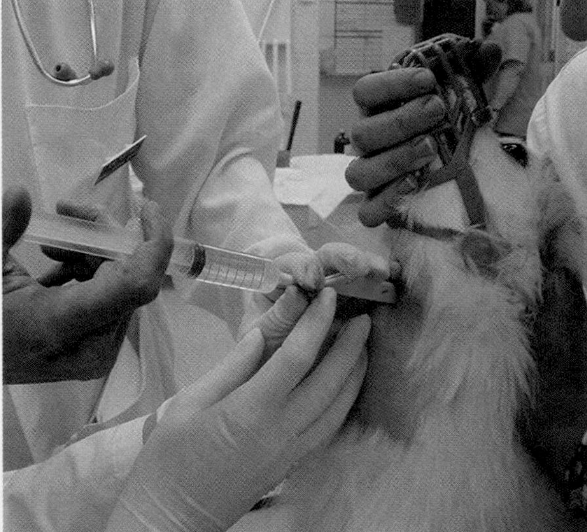

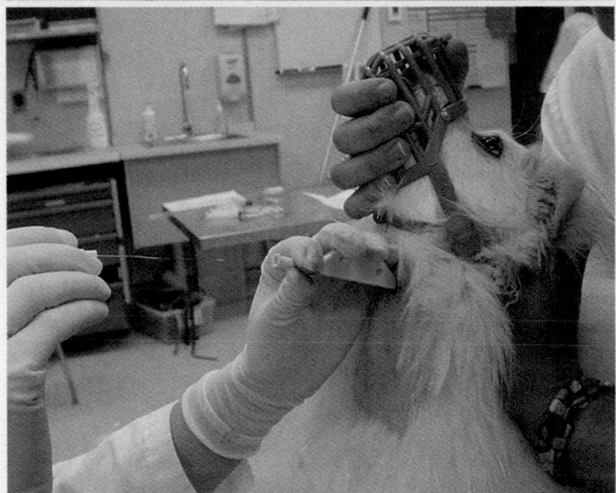

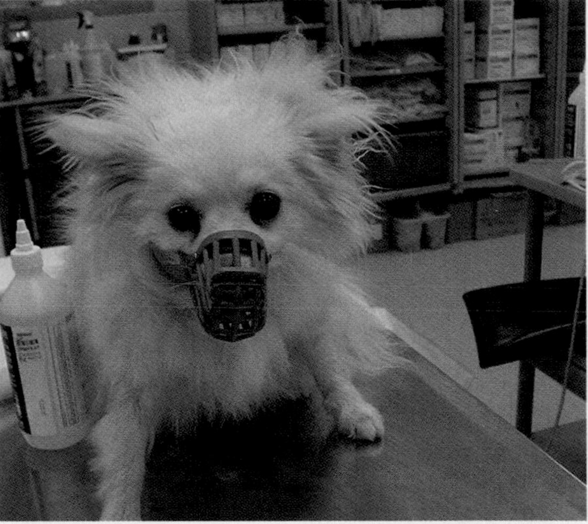

PROCEDURE 7-7

Large Dog Transtracheal Wash

EQUIPMENT

- 14-gauge Medi-Cut over the needle catheter. The Medi-Cut is an over-the-needle catheter, in which the needle acts as a large rigid stylet over which the catheter can be introduced into the tracheal lumen.
- 28-inch 3.5 or 5 French polypropylene catheter. Always check to ensure that the polypropylene catheter selected passes easily through the Medi-Cut catheter before starting the tracheal wash.
- Three or four 20-mL syringes with 10 mL saline in each
- 1 mL lidocaine blocking solution (2% lidocaine mixed 9:1 with 8.4% sodium bicarbonate), 3-mL syringe, 25-gauge needle
- Sterile gloves
- Bandage material

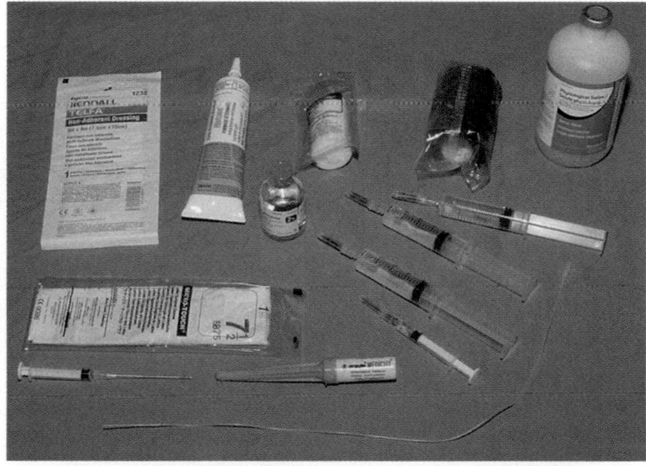

Equipment needed for a large dog transtracheal wash.

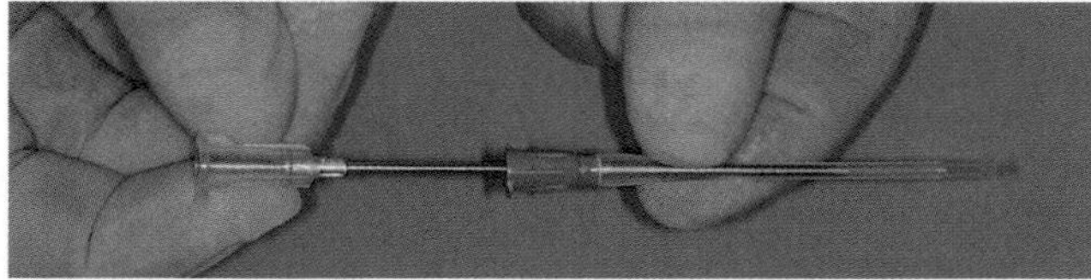

The Medi-Cut is an over-the-needle catheter, in which the needle acts as a large rigid stylet over which the catheter can be introduced into the tracheal lumen.

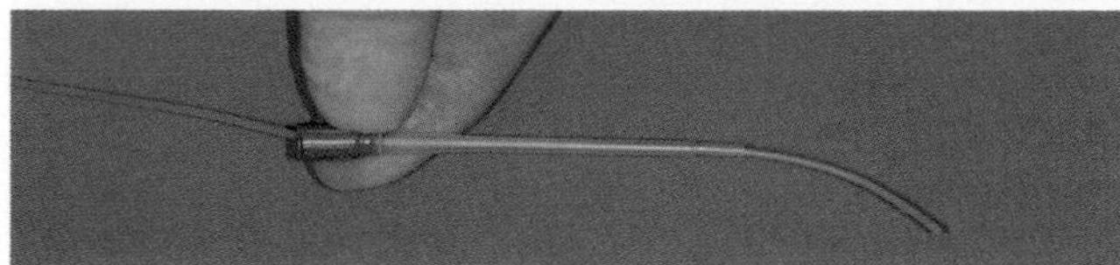

Always check to ensure that the polypropylene catheter selected passes easily through the Medi-Cut catheter before starting the tracheal wash.

TECHNIQUE: LARGE DOG TRANSTRACHEAL WASH

1. Restrain the dog on a table or on the floor in sternal position.
2. Extend the neck dorsally, pointing the nose toward the ceiling.
3. Have an assistant hold the front legs so that they cannot disrupt the procedure.
4. Identify the cricothyroid ligament by palpation.

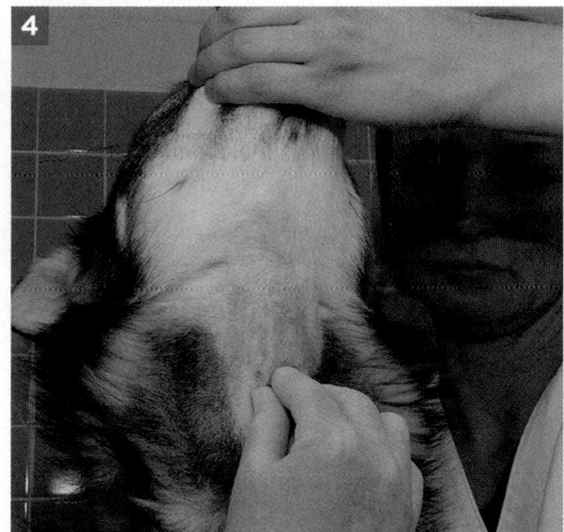

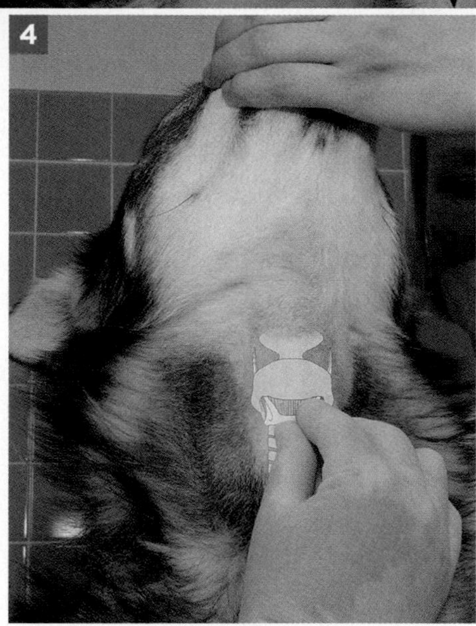

Identifying the cricothyroid ligament by palpation.

PROCEDURE 7-7 Large Dog Transtracheal Wash—cont'd

5. Clip and prep the site over the cricothyroid ligament. Sterile gloves and aseptic technique are used for the procedure.
6. Block the site with lidocaine blocking solution; repeat the final scrub.

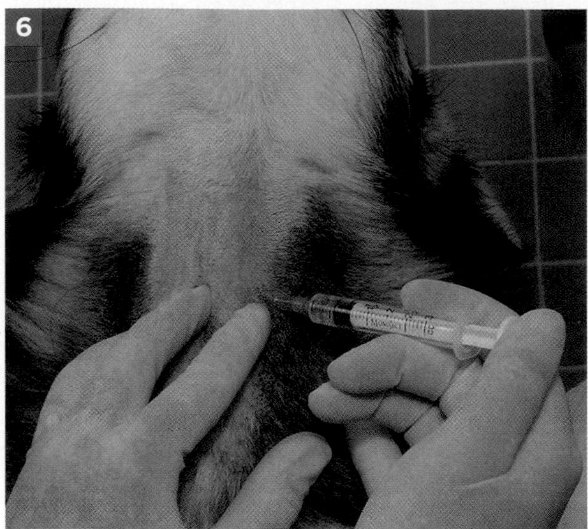

Blocking the region of the cricothyroid ligament with lidocaine blocking solution.

7. Prepare the catheters for use.
   A. Remove the Medi-Cut catheter from the needle, keeping both sterile.
   B. Make sure that the long polypropylene catheter passes easily though the short Medi-Cut catheter.
   C. Estimate how much of the long catheter will need to be advanced into the trachea in order to have the tip of the catheter sit at the tracheal bifurcation (over the heart base).
   D. Have an assistant hold on to the long catheter, keeping the tip sterile.
   E. Replace the needle inside the short catheter.
8. Stabilize the larynx and trachea by palpation to prevent side-to-side movement.
9. Maintaining the needle fully inside the short catheter, palpate the cricoid cartilage, and place the tip of the needle at the level of the cricothyroid ligament (just above the cricoid cartilage) on the midline.
10. Apply firm pressure inward and puncture the trachea, maintaining the needle perpendicular to the tracheal lumen. A "pop" may be felt as the needle enters the tracheal lumen.

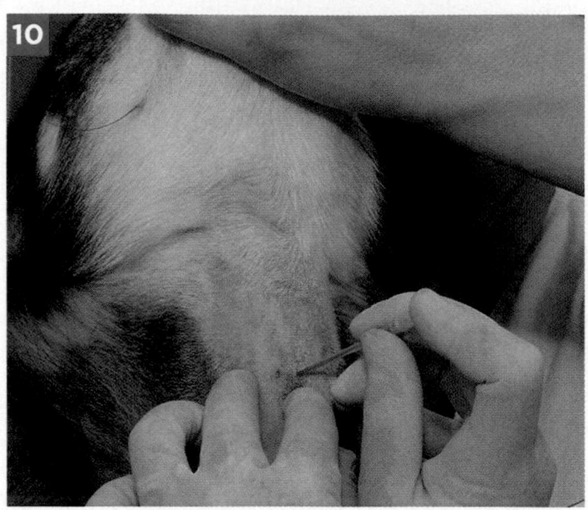

Advancing the needle into the trachea through the cricothyroid ligament.

11. Advance the needle a short distance into the trachea after the lumen is entered, until the needle tip is in approximately the center of the tracheal lumen.

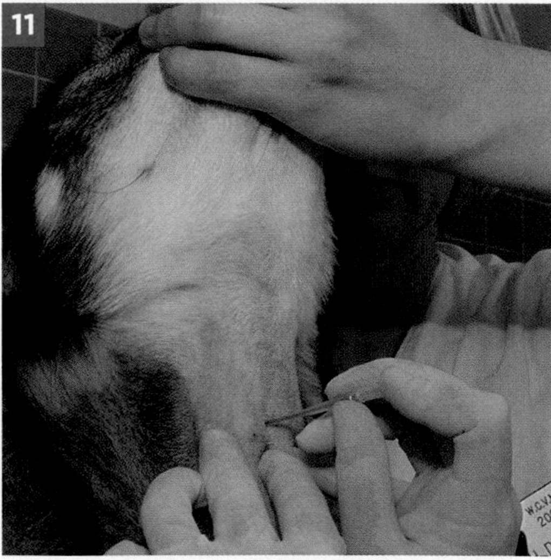

Advancing the needle until the needle tip is in approximately the center of the tracheal lumen.

12. Tilt the needle approximately 45 degrees to direct the needle down the tracheal lumen, and advance it slightly.

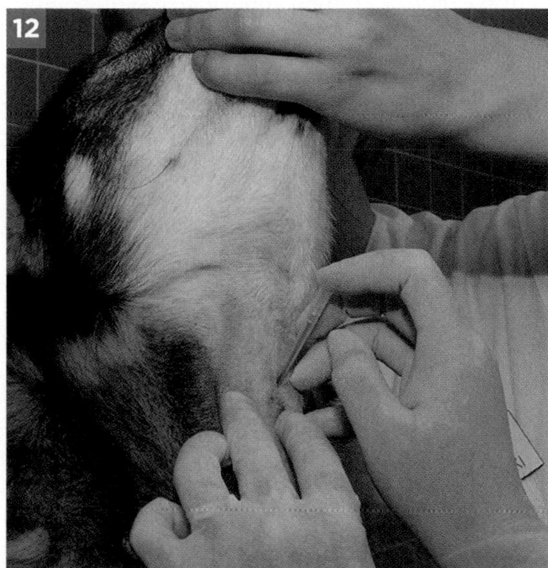

Tilting the needle approximately 45 degrees to direct the needle down the tracheal lumen while advancing it slightly.

13. Advance the short catheter over the needle as far down the trachea as it will advance, and then remove and discard the needle.

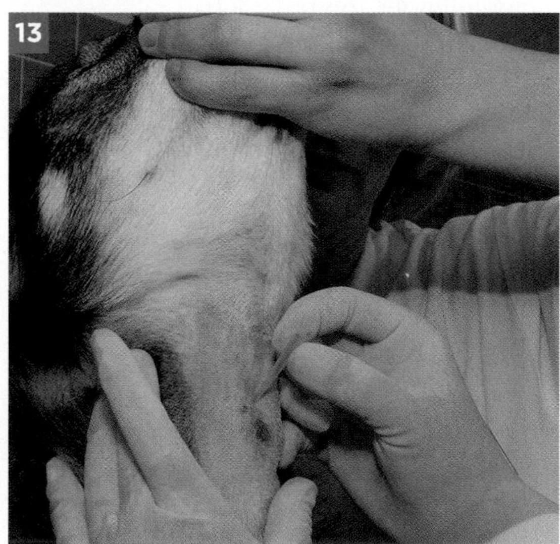

Advancing the catheter over the needle.

14. Grasp the long polypropylene catheter near its tip and pass the long catheter through the short one into the trachea. Continue advancing until the catheter tip is approximately at the level of the tracheal bifurcation (approximately the fourth intercostal space) to collect the best sample. The catheter should pass easily and the dog should cough. If the catheter does not pass easily, reassess the location of the tip of the short catheter—the patient position and angle of the short catheter may need to be modified to permit passage of the longer catheter without hitting the tracheal wall.

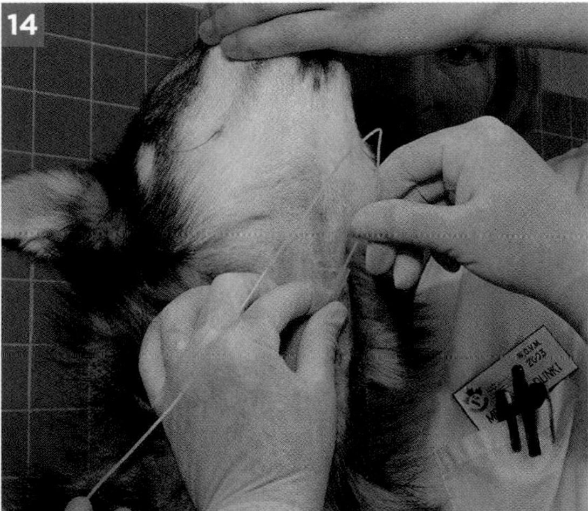

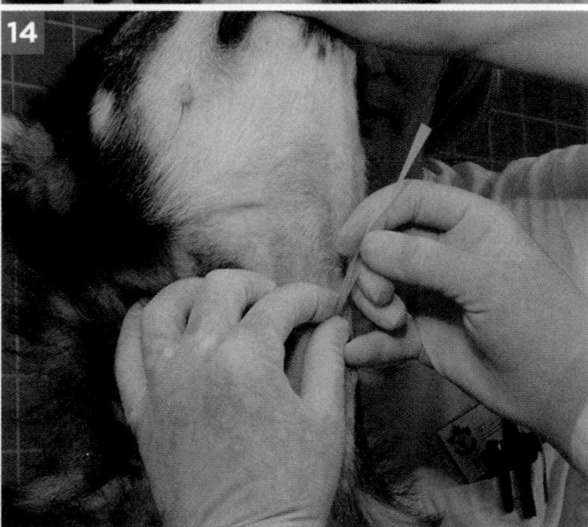

Advancing the long polypropylene catheter through the short catheter into the trachea until its tip is approximately at the level of the tracheal bifurcation.

PROCEDURE 7-7 Large Dog Transtracheal Wash—cont'd

15. Once the catheter is passed to the desired depth, attach a 20-mL syringe containing approximately 10 mL of saline, inject 7 to 8 mL of the saline, then repeatedly aspirate to recover airway washings. The best recovery is during patient coughing.

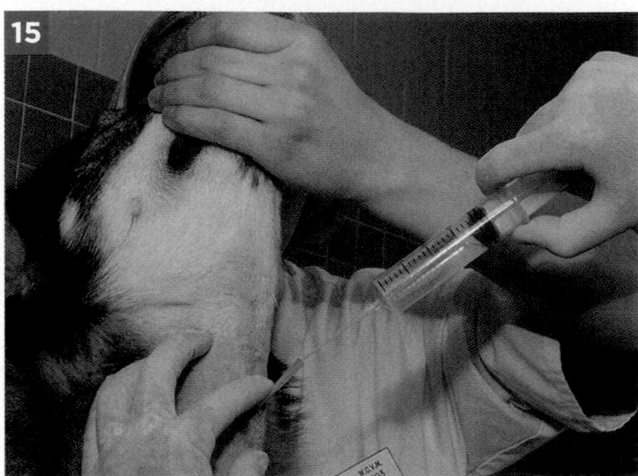

Flushing in and aspirating saline repeatedly until airway washings are recovered.

16. If nothing is recovered, repeat the washing using a second 20-mL syringe containing 10 mL of saline. Suction should be vigorously applied immediately after instilling the saline. If still nothing is recovered, restrain the dog in sternal recumbency with the nose and head in a more neutral position so that the instilled fluid pools at the carina rather than flowing into the caudal lung lobes, and repeat the wash with a third syringe of saline. Sometimes the catheter needs to be advanced or withdrawn slightly during suction to ensure that the catheter tip is at the tracheal bifurcation. The instilled fluid will be absorbed rapidly into the systemic circulation, so there is no concern that repeated washings will "drown" the patient.

17. Once a sample is recovered, withdraw the long catheter and then remove the short catheter.

18. Submit samples for cytologic evaluation of a direct and concentrated sample as well as for culture.

19. Place a light wrap around the neck to compress the tissues and minimize leakage of air from the trachea into the subcutaneous tissues. Cover the entry wound with an occlusive ointment, then apply gauze sponges and a light wrap, being careful to avoid restricting venous return or ventilatory efforts. Two fingers should fit easily beneath the wrap. The wrap can be removed after 1 to 2 hours.

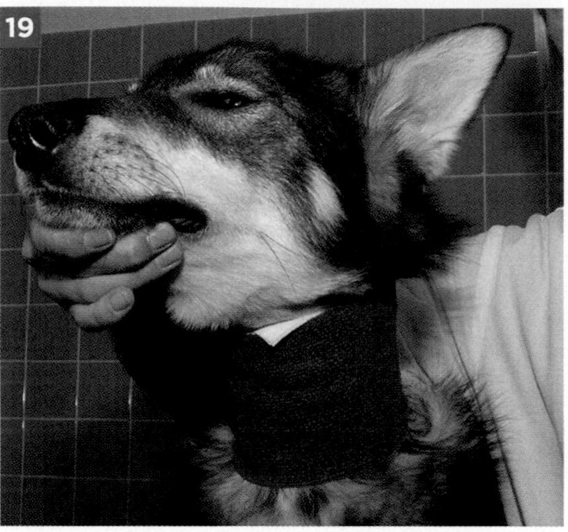

An occlusive ointment is placed over the needle entry site and a light bandage is applied.

20. Keep the patient quiet and monitor respirations for 1 to 2 hours following this procedure.

TRANSTRACHEAL WASH RESULTS

1. Eosinophilic inflammation in a transtracheal wash from a coughing dog reflects a hypersensitivity response most typical of allergic or parasitic disease.

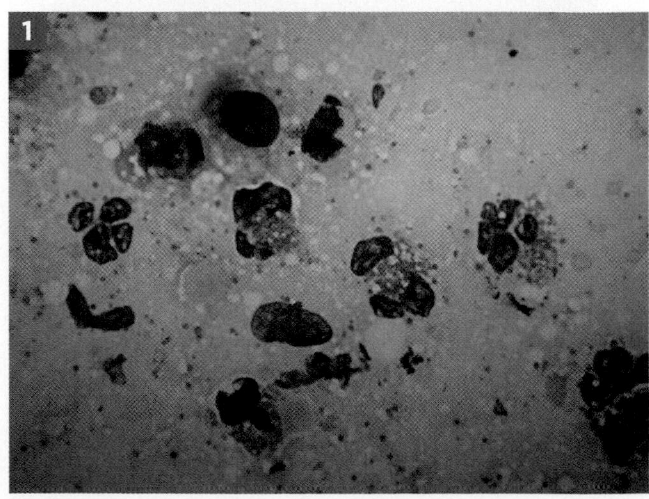

This dog had allergic tracheobronchitis.

2. A tracheal wash from a patient with metastatic neoplasia in the lungs may be normal or may reveal red blood cells, macrophages that have ingested red blood cells (erythrophagia), and hemosiderin-laden macrophages, indicating airway hemorrhage.

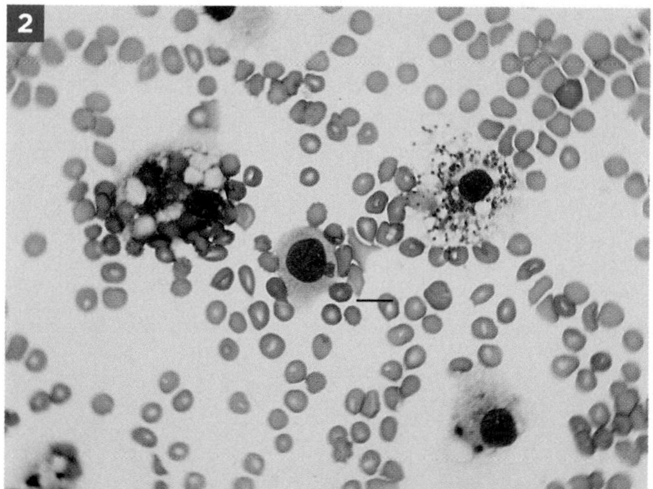

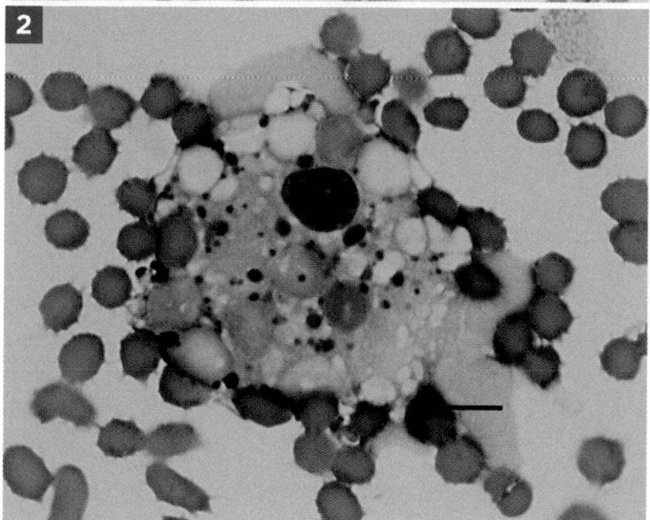

This transtracheal wash reveals red blood cells and highly vacuolated macrophages that have engulfed erythrocytes (erythrophagia) and hemosiderin pigment, indicating that airway hemorrhage is ongoing, not technique induced. This dog had pulmonary metastatic hemangiosarcoma. **(Courtesy Dr. Marion Jackson, University of Saskatchewan.)**

3. The presence of squamous epithelial cells and stacked *Simonsiella* bacteria in a tracheal wash indicate that oral contamination of the sample occurred. Either the needle was inadvertently inserted above the cricothyroid ligament, the dog coughed the catheter tip up into the pharynx during the procedure, or the dog aspirated saliva during the procedure.

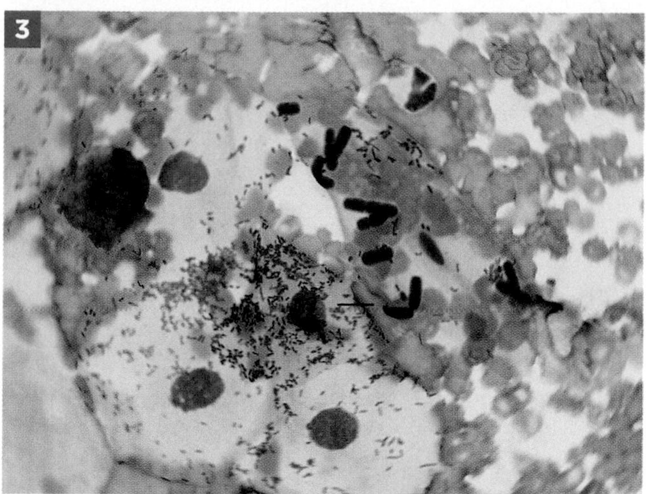

The presence of squamous epithelial cells and stacked Simonsiella bacteria in this tracheal wash indicates that oral contamination of the sample occurred. **(Courtesy Dr. Marion Jackson, University of Saskatchewan.)**

4. Transtracheal wash cytology can reveal a variety of infectious causes of cough.

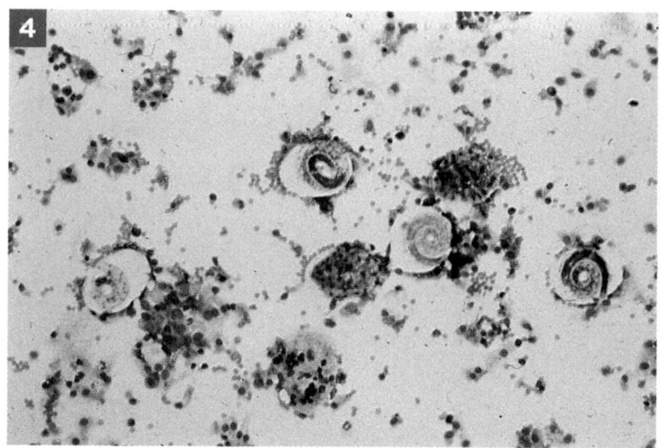

This transtracheal wash from a 19-month-old Jack Russell Terrier with a 3-month history of cough and normal thoracic radiographs reveals eosinophilic inflammation and numerous coiled larvae. This dog had Oslerus osleri tracheobronchitis.

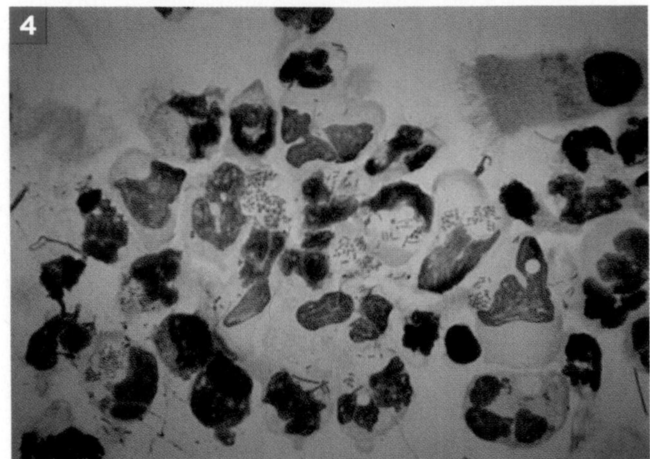

Transtracheal wash from a 3-year-old German Shorthaired Pointer with a 3-week history of cough and fever. Radiographs showed a focal region of consolidation within the right middle lung lobe. The tracheal wash is very cellular and reveals septic inflammation with degenerate neutrophils and pleomorphic bacteria. This dog had a bronchial foreign body (head of barley) removed endoscopically.

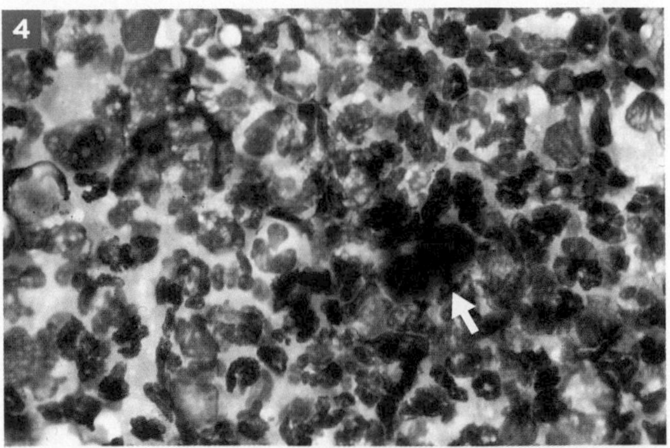

Transtracheal wash from a 4-year-old German Shepherd with a 2-week history of cough, lethargy, fever, and exercise intolerance. Auscultation revealed crackles over all lung fields, and radiographs revealed a diffuse mixed interstitial and alveolar infiltrate. Transtracheal wash revealed severe pyogranulomatous inflammation with occasional Blastomyces dermatitidis fungal organisms *(arrow)*.

PROCEDURE 7-8

Endotracheal Wash

PURPOSE

To collect a sample of secretions from the trachea and airways for cytologic and microbiologic analysis

INDICATIONS

1. Cats with cough. Most cats with cough have feline chronic bronchitis or asthma.
2. Cats with airway or lung parenchymal disease
3. Very small dogs with severe dyspnea or a nervous temperament, making restraint for awake transtracheal wash impossible or dangerous

CONTRAINDICATIONS AND WARNINGS

1. Endotracheal wash cannot be performed if an animal is not a candidate for general anesthesia.
2. Endotracheal wash should not be performed in severely dyspneic cats thought to have acute manifestations of feline asthma—these patients must be stabilized before anesthesia.

POSITIONING AND RESTRAINT

Animals are anesthetized and in sternal recumbency for this procedure.

SPECIAL ANATOMY

The best sample can be obtained if the catheter tip is at the tracheal bifurcation.

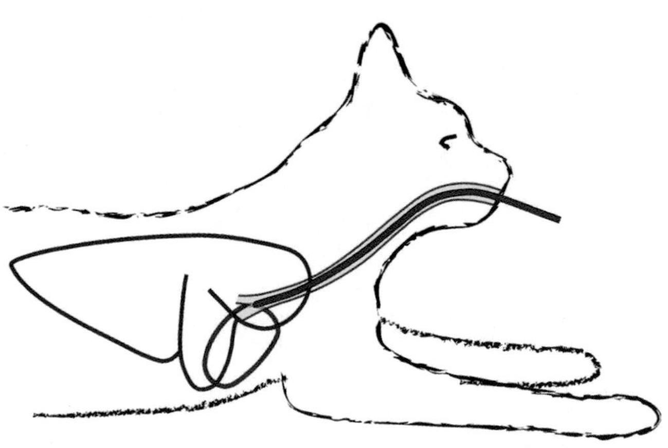

Catheter tip is at the tracheal bifurcation.

EQUIPMENT

- 28-inch 3.5 or 5 French sterile polypropylene catheter
- Sterile endotracheal tube or sheath from a spinal needle that passes through the glottal opening
- Three 12-mL syringes with 6 mL saline in each

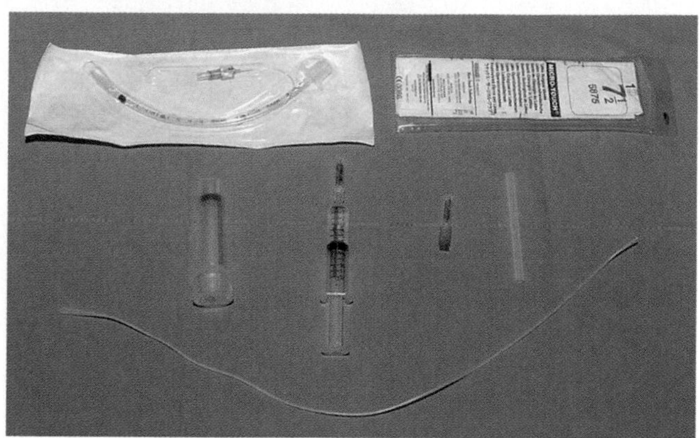

Equipment used for an endotracheal wash.

TECHNIQUE: ENDOTRACHEAL WASH

1. Preoxygenate by mask and then place the dog or cat under a light injectable plane of general anesthesia (propofol is often used).
2. Insert a sterile endotracheal tube or insert the sterile sheath from a spinal needle into the glottal opening to serve as a sheath for the long catheter.
3. Measure the length of the catheter needed to reach the tracheal bifurcation.

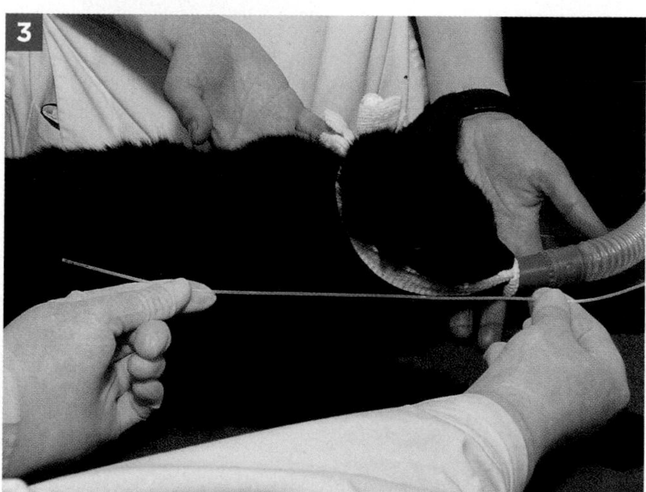

Determining the length of the catheter needed to reach the tracheal bifurcation.

4. Pass the polypropylene catheter down the trachea to the level of the tracheal bifurcation.

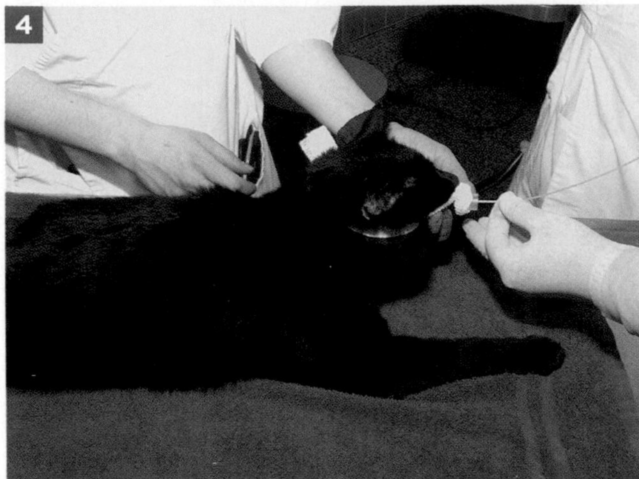

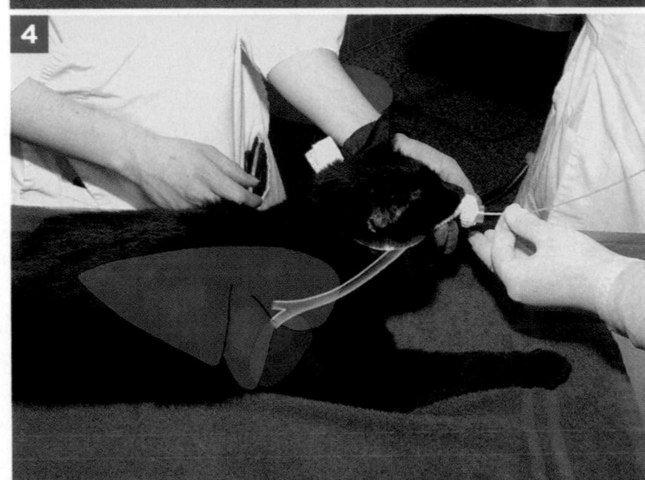

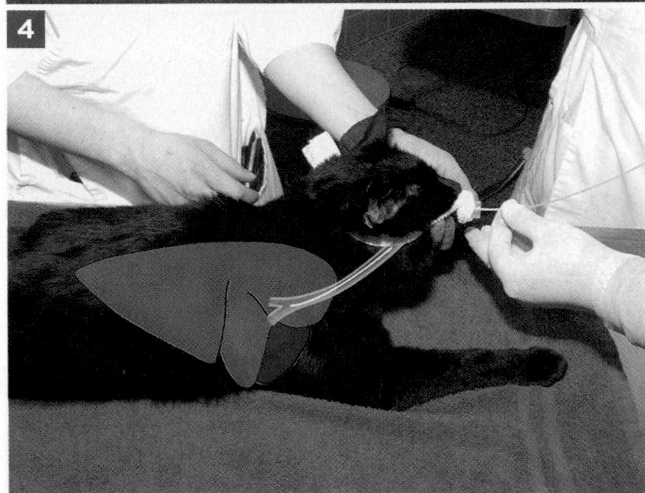

Passing the polypropylene catheter down the trachea to the level of the tracheal bifurcation.

5. Wait for the dog or cat to cough. The best samples are obtained when animals are coughing.

6. Attach a 12-mL syringe containing approximately 6 mL of saline. Inject 2 to 3 mL of saline, and then repeatedly aspirate to recover airway washings. If nothing is recovered, repeat until a sample is obtained.

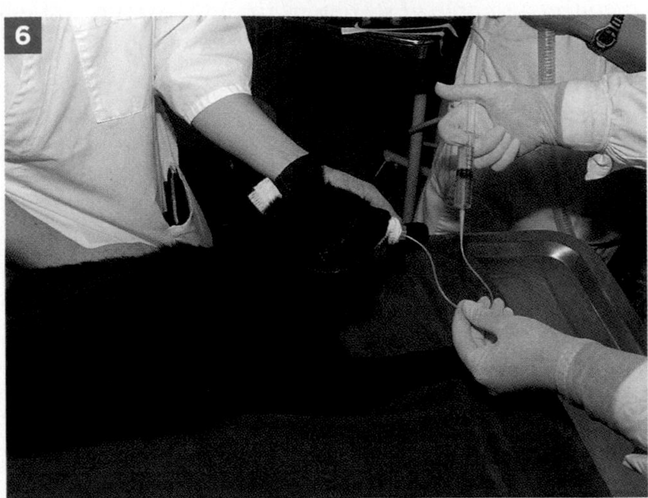

Saline is repeatedly injected and aspirated until a sample is recovered.

7. Once a sample is recovered, allow the patient to breathe oxygen until fully recovered.

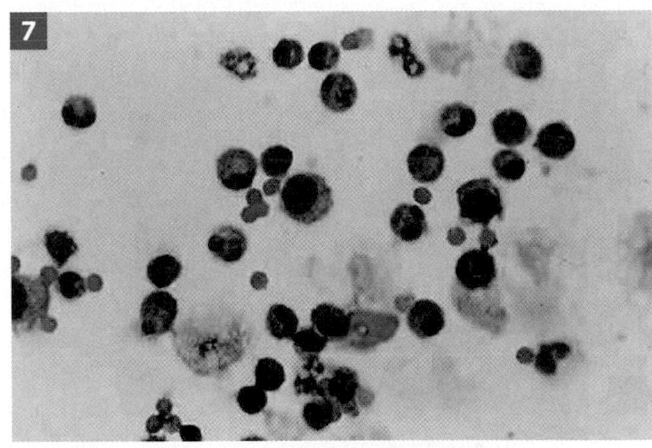

This endotracheal wash from a coughing cat with normal thoracic radiographs revealed abundant mucus and eosinophilic inflammation, consistent with a diagnosis of feline allergic tracheobronchitis (asthma).

PROCEDURE 7-9
Bronchoscopic Bronchoalveolar Lavage

PURPOSE

To collect a sample of secretions and cells from the small airways, alveoli and interstitium of the deep lung for cytologic and microbiologic analysis

INDICATIONS

1. Dogs and cats with disease involving the terminal airways, alveoli, or interstitium of the lung for which a diagnosis has not been achieved through awake procedures or diagnostic techniques.
2. Bronchoalveolar lavage (BAL) involves flooding of a defined region of the lung, then recovering the fluid that has filled the alveoli in that region. Results represent changes in the deep lung at the specific site that is flooded, so it is important that radiographs be used to select the lung lobe where BAL will be most likely to be diagnostic.

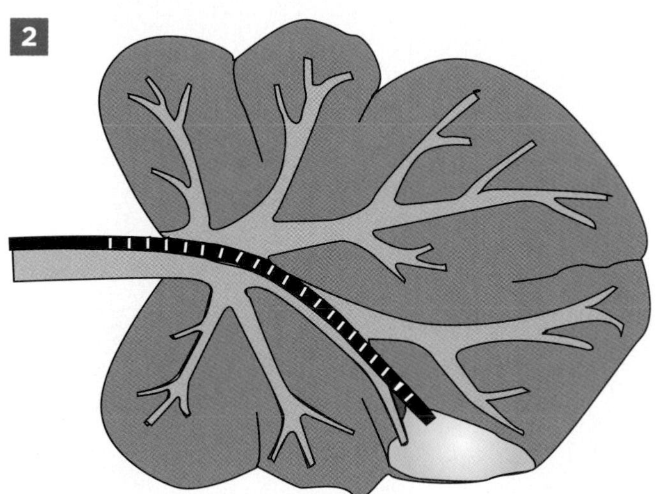

Diagram of bronchoscopic bronchoalveolar lavage showing the region of lung flooded during this procedure.

CONTRAINDICATIONS AND WARNINGS

1. BAL cannot be performed if an animal is not a candidate for general anesthesia.
2. Although nonendoscopic BAL techniques have been reported, bronchoscopic BAL is necessary when it is important to select the lobe of the lung to be sampled. A bronchoscope is required for this technique.
3. The primary complication of BAL is significant hypoxemia during the procedure. This usually resolves quickly, but animals that are significantly hypoxemic at rest in room air are probably not good candidates for BAL. Monitoring of patient oxygenation and ability to supplement with oxygen during and following BAL are prerequisites for performing the procedure.
4. Some animals, especially cats, have reactive airways and may develop bronchospasm as a complication of BAL. Pretreatment with bronchodilators is recommended in these patients.
5. BAL is not the most appropriate technique for animals with disease that primarily involves the airways—transtracheal or endotracheal wash are better techniques to recover samples from the trachea and airways. BAL is used to sample the interstitium and alveoli of the lung.

POSITIONING AND RESTRAINT

Animals are anesthetized and in sternal recumbency for this procedure.

EQUIPMENT

- A small-diameter flexible endoscope. A pediatric bronchoscope (4.8 mm outer diameter, 2-mm biopsy channel) can be passed in most dogs and cats.
- Aliquots of sterile 0.9% sodium chloride (saline) solution that has been warmed to body temperature
- Syringes for aspirating BAL fluid

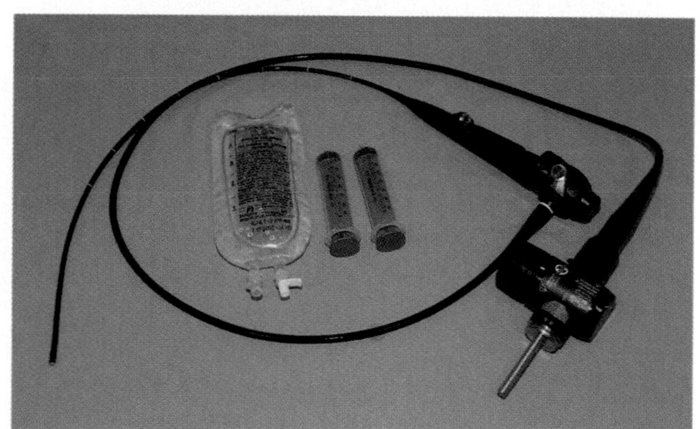

Equipment required for endoscopic bronchoalveolar lavage.

TECHNIQUE: BRONCHOSCOPIC BRONCHOALVEOLAR LAVAGE

1. Preoxygenate by mask for several minutes, then place the dog or cat under a light injectable plane of general anesthesia (propofol is often used).
2. Insert a sterile endotracheal tube and administer inhalant anesthesia. In cats and in very small dogs, extubation is required during bronchoscopy and bronchoscopic

BAL. In larger dogs the scope can be passed through an adapter on the endotracheal tube, allowing ventilation during the procedure.

3. Perform routine diagnostic bronchoscopy, evaluating the trachea and the length of the major bronchi entering each lung lobe that can be accessed with the scope.
4. Pass the bronchoscope into the lobe to be lavaged until the tip is lodged snugly into an airway. If a snug fit is not achieved, sampling will come from the airways rather than the deep lung, and fluid recovery will be poor.
5. Ensure that the suction line of the bronchoscope is clamped off.
6. In medium and large dogs, 25 mL of sterile 0.9% saline solution that has been warmed to body temperature is instilled by syringe into the lung through the biopsy channel of the scope. In very small dogs and cats 10 mL per aliquot may be used.
7. Immediately after the saline is instilled, gentle suction is applied to the syringe and the fluid is recovered. When air fills the syringe it is eliminated and additional suction attempts are made until no more fluid can be obtained.
8. A second 25 mL (or 10 mL) aliquot of saline is instilled into the lung and retrieved in the same manner, with the scope in the same position. If desired a third aliquot also can be instilled.
9. If desired, the scope is repositioned and BAL is performed in another lobe in the same manner.

SPECIMEN HANDLING

1. BAL fluid should be grossly foamy—a result of the surfactant from the alveoli.
2. BAL fluid should be placed on ice immediately after collection and processed quickly.
3. The fluid obtained should be analyzed cytologically and microbiologically.

PROCEDURE 7-10
Transthoracic Lung Aspiration

PURPOSE

To collect a sample of cells or fluid from the lung parenchyma for cytologic and microbiologic analysis

INDICATIONS

1. Animals with solitary lung parenchymal lesions located adjacent to the body wall
2. Animals with diffuse, multifocal, or focal disease of the lung parenchyma in which a transtracheal or endotracheal wash was inconclusive or yielded a negative result
3. In animals with multifocal or diffuse disease, aspirate the region of lung that appears most severely affected radiographically, or if disease is truly diffuse, aspirate the superficial parenchyma of a caudal lung lobe.

CONTRAINDICATIONS

1. Masses deep within the lung parenchyma adjacent to the heart or major blood vessels and masses separated from the body wall by a large volume of aerated lung present a high risk for complications from this procedure. Noninvasive alternative techniques such as transtracheal wash should always be performed first in these patients to attempt to reach a diagnosis.
2. Lung aspiration should not be performed in animals with a coagulopathy, known pulmonary hypertension, or a suspected lung abscess.
3. Severely dyspneic patients with diffuse lung disease are at increased risk for developing pneumothorax following lung aspiration, and this complication can be fatal.

EQUIPMENT

- 22-gauge spinal needles, 1½ or 2½ inches
- 6-mL syringes
- Glass microscope slides on a tray
- Sterile gloves
- Lidocaine blocking solution (2% lidocaine mixed 9:1 with 8.4% sodium bicarbonate)

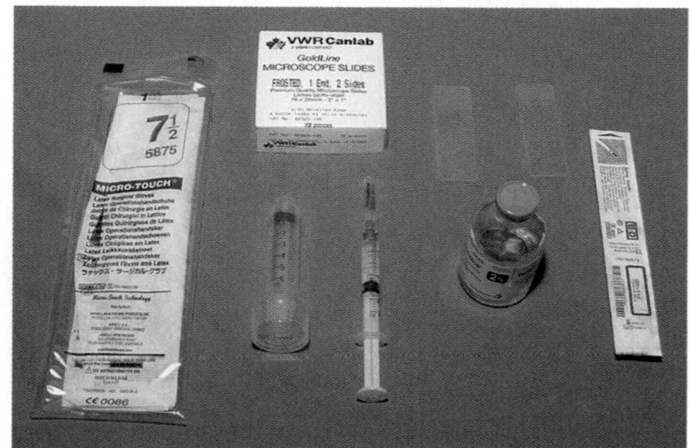

Equipment required for transthoracic lung aspiration.

POSITIONING AND RESTRAINT

1. Have the patient standing or lying in sternal recumbency, with restraint to prevent movement. An assistant needs to occlude the nares while the needle is within the thorax.
2. No sedation is administered so that changes in the animal's respiratory pattern after the procedure can be monitored.

PROCEDURE 7-10 Transthoracic Lung Aspiration—cont'd

SPECIAL ANATOMY

1. Radiographs are used to locate the precise region within the lung that will be aspirated. Determine the correct intercostal space, the distance above the costochondral junction, and the depth (length of needle insertion) required.

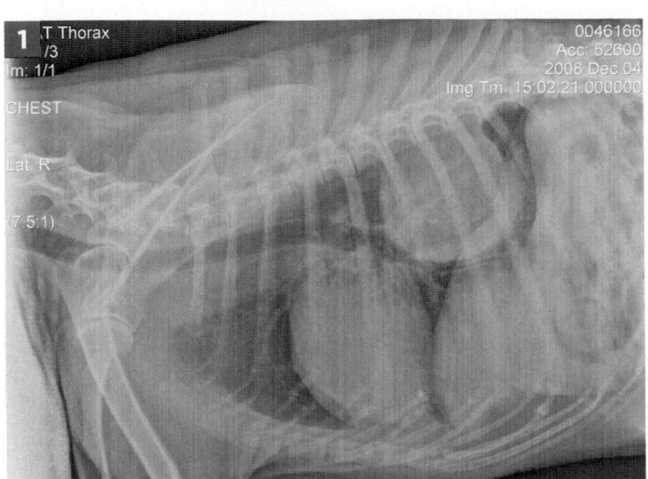

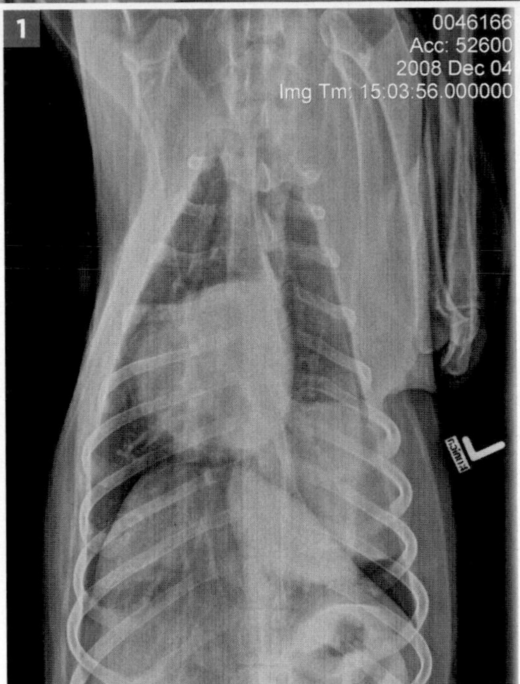

Lateral *(top)* and ventrodorsal *(bottom)* radiographs from a dog with a large solitary mass within the left caudal lung lobe. Evaluation of these radiographs suggests that aspiration should take place from the left side in the sixth or seventh intercostal space, in the dorsal 25% of the chest cavity. The appropriate depth of needle insertion can be determined from the ventrodorsal radiograph. **(Courtesy Dr. Elisabeth Snead, University of Saskatchewan.)**

2. When a focal mass is in contact with the body wall, ultrasound can be used to guide the needle placement.

TECHNIQUE

1. Identify the area to be aspirated based on radiographs.
2. Have the patient standing or restrained in sternal recumbency. Clip and prep the skin over the region. Sterile gloves and aseptic technique are used for the procedure.

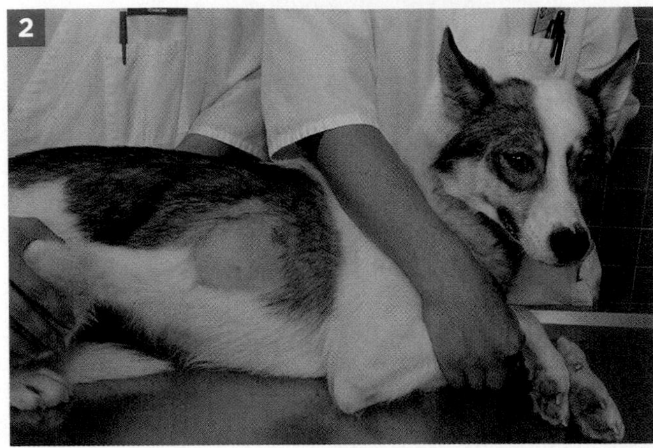

Restraint of a dog for lung aspiration.

3. Instill lidocaine blocking solution to block the skin and underlying tissues to the pleura at the site of entry.

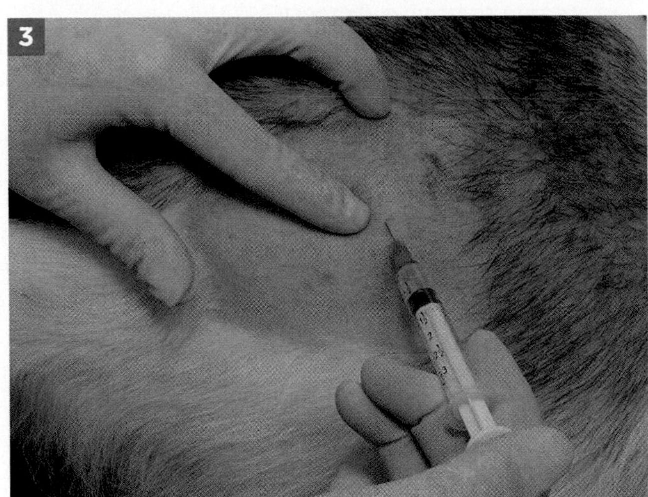

Injecting lidocaine blocking solution.

4. Insert a needle with a stylet through skin, subcutaneous tissues, and approximately to the pleura. Avoid puncture of the intercostal vessels, which are located at the caudal margin of each rib.

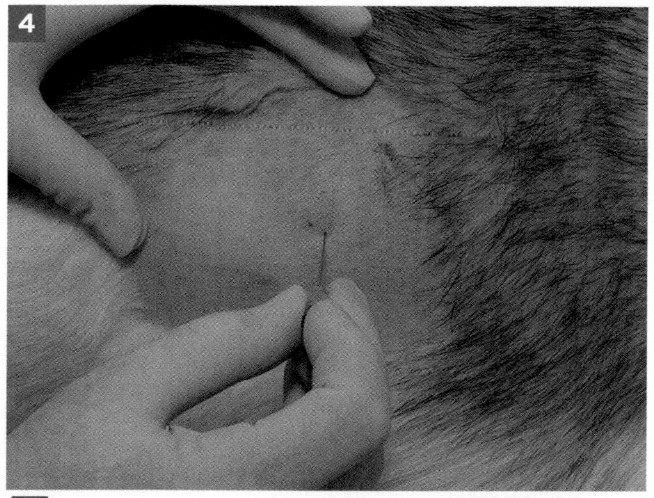

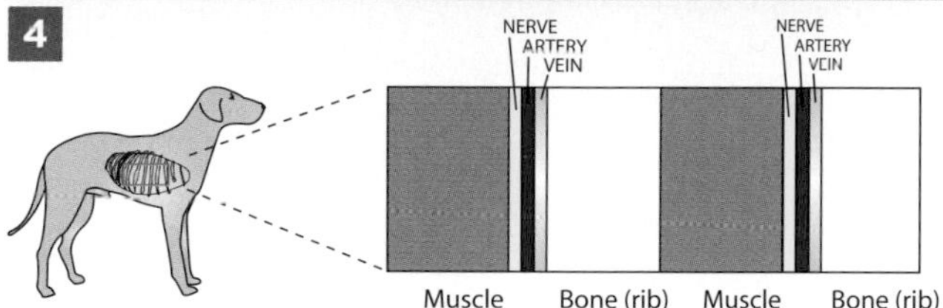

Inserting a needle with a stylet to approximately the pleura, avoiding puncture of the intercostal vessels that are located at the caudal margin of each rib.

5. Have an assistant hold off the patient's mouth and nose to prevent respiratory chest excursions.

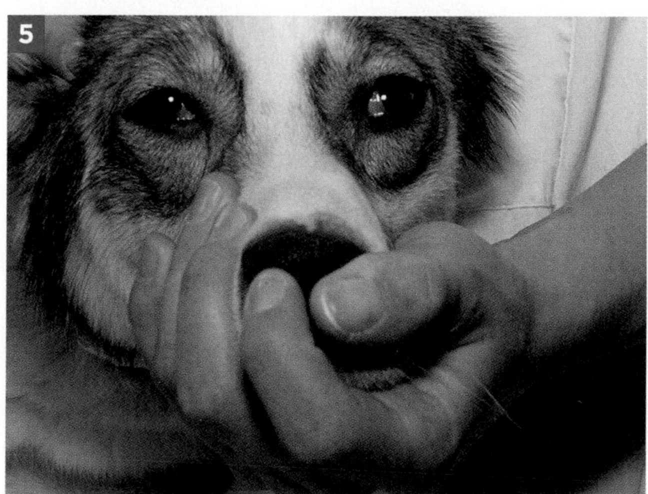

An assistant holds off the patient's mouth and nose to prevent respiratory chest excursions.

6. Remove the stylet and attach the syringe.
7. Apply suction and plunge the needle to the desired depth. Release suction and then reapply 5 to 8 mL of suction two or three times, moving quickly so that the needle is only within the lung parenchyma for a total of 1 to 2 seconds.

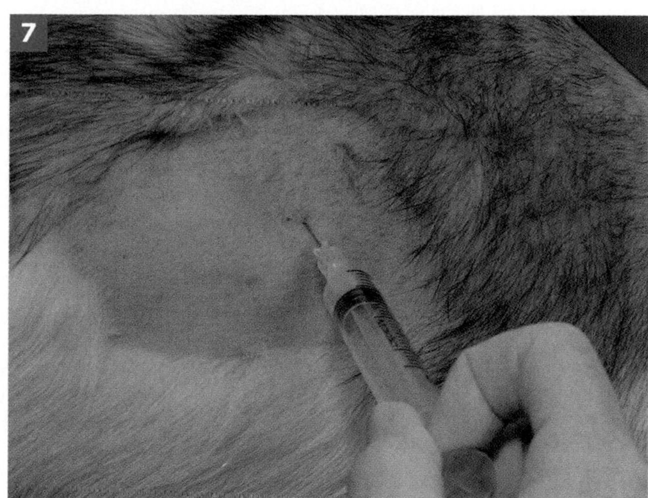

Inserting the needle into the lung to be sampled.

8. Release suction and withdraw the needle from the chest; make slides immediately.
9. Monitor respirations and color for 30 to 60 minutes following the procedure.

POTENTIAL COMPLICATIONS

1. Pneumothorax may occur, especially if there is aerated lung between the mass being aspirated and the body wall. In most cases this is mild and does not require treatment, but occasionally it can be severe. Animals that are repeatedly coughing and animals that are severely dyspneic before the procedure are at highest risk for this complication.
2. Hemothorax or pulmonary hemorrhage can occur when there is hemorrhage from the aspirated site. This is usually mild.
3. Occasionally animals die acutely following transthoracic lung aspiration. Most often these are very dyspneic dogs or cats with diffuse severe pulmonary disease, and they are unable to tolerate the added stress of a pneumothorax or hemothorax.

SAMPLE HANDLING

1. Typically the recovery of cells is not very large using transthoracic lung aspiration. Often all the aspirated material is within the needle and not visible in the needle hub. Slides must be made promptly or the sample will clot and be unavailable. Once the needle has been withdrawn from the chest, the needle should be removed from the syringe and the syringe reattached with 4 mL of air inside so that the needle contents can be expelled onto a slide, and smeared immediately. Slides are routinely stained and examined cytologically.

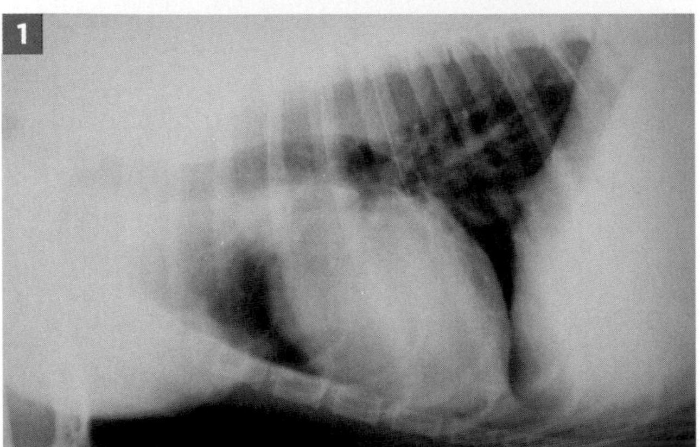

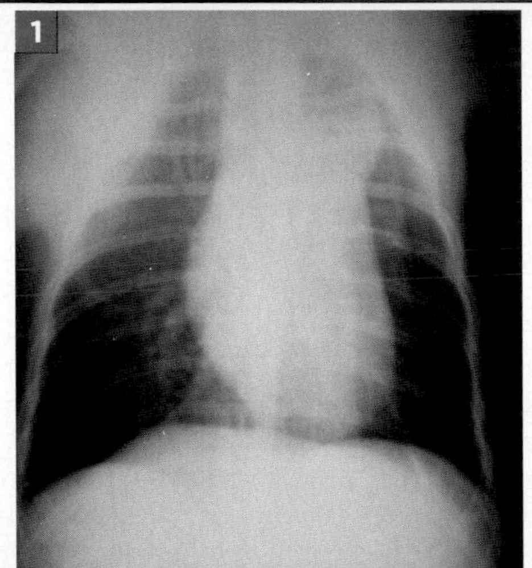

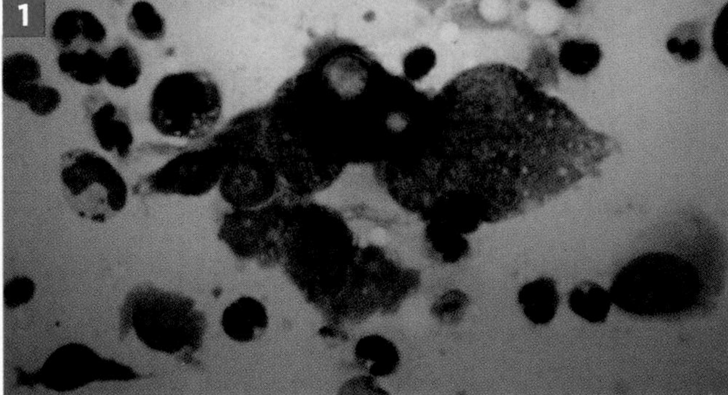

Thoracic radiographs from a 3-year-old Labrador Retriever with fever, anorexia, and anterior uveitis showed a solitary mass within the lung parenchyma. Transtracheal wash cytology yielded evidence of inflammation but no organisms. Fine-needle aspiration revealed blastomycosis.

2. Rarely a lung aspirate yields 0.5 to 1 mL of a bloody fluid. If this occurs, place the fluid immediately into an ethylenediaminetetraacetic acid (EDTA) tube to prevent clotting, then make direct smears and concentrated preparations for examination.

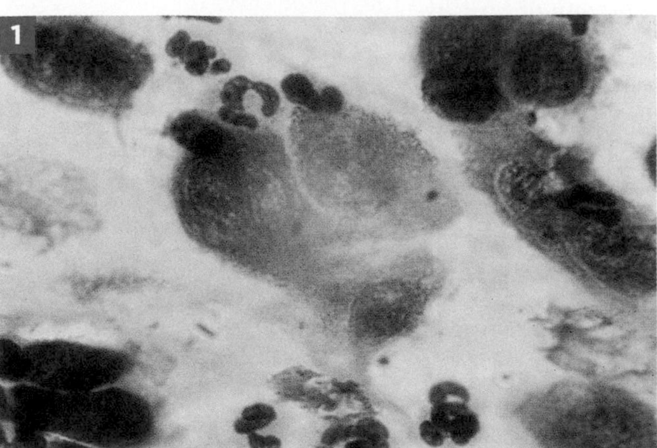

Cytology obtained from a fine-needle aspirate of a solitary left caudal lung lobe mass identified in a coughing 8-year-old German Shepherd. There is a population of large cells with many criteria of malignancy. The diagnosis is carcinoma.

PROCEDURE 7-11
Thoracentesis

PURPOSES

1. To collect fluid that has accumulated in the pleural space for cytologic and microbiologic analysis
2. To relieve clinical signs of dyspnea caused by the accumulation of fluid or air in the pleural space

INDICATIONS

1. Dogs or cats with pleural effusion
2. Dogs or cats with dyspnea due to significant air accumulation within the pleural space (pneumothorax)

CONTRAINDICATIONS AND WARNINGS

1. Pleural effusion should be suspected on physical examination in a dog or cat with rapid shallow respirations and muffled heart and lung sounds ventrally. When dyspnea is severe, it is advised to perform therapeutic thoracentesis before restraining the animal for diagnostic radiography.
2. Cats with chronic thoracic effusions commonly develop fibrinous pleuritis that prevents their lung from expanding normally and prevents normal elastic recoil of the lung. Inadvertent needle puncture of the lung in these animals may result in a severe, nonresolving pneumothorax.
3. When a hemothorax is present, only use thoracentesis to remove sufficient blood to relieve dyspnea and restore the animal's ability to ventilate effectively. Blood that is left behind will be reabsorbed.

POSITIONING AND RESTRAINT

Minimal restraint is required in most cases. Thoracentesis can be performed with the animal standing or in sternal or lateral recumbency. If the animal is dyspneic, administration of supplemental oxygen during the procedure is advised to decrease the animal's anxiety. Sedation is rarely required or advised.

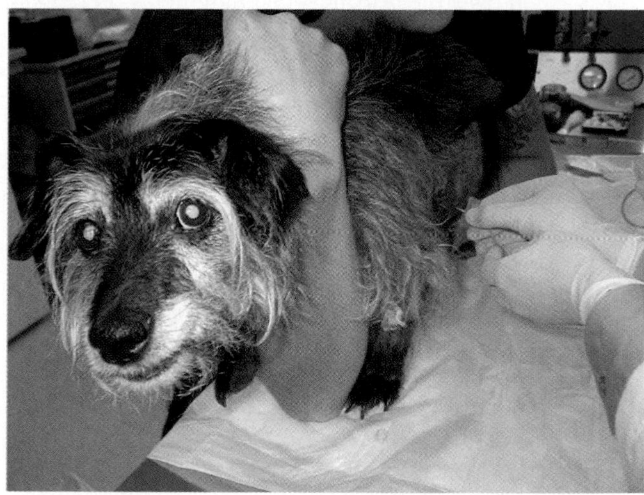

Restraint for thoracentesis.

SPECIAL ANATOMY

1. The pleural space in the normal animal is only a potential space as the visceral and parietal pleura are in contact. A number of disorders can lead to fluid accumulation within this space (pleural effusion).
2. Most cats and dogs with a pleural effusion develop fluid in both sides of the chest. The best site to perform thoracentesis depends on the amount and location of pleural fluid identified on physical examination or with radiographs. Needle insertion between the sixth and ninth intercostal spaces just above the costochondral junction is usually successful. Fluid has a tendency to accumulate ventrally when the animal is standing or in sternal recumbency. Therapeutic thoracentesis is usually performed bilaterally.

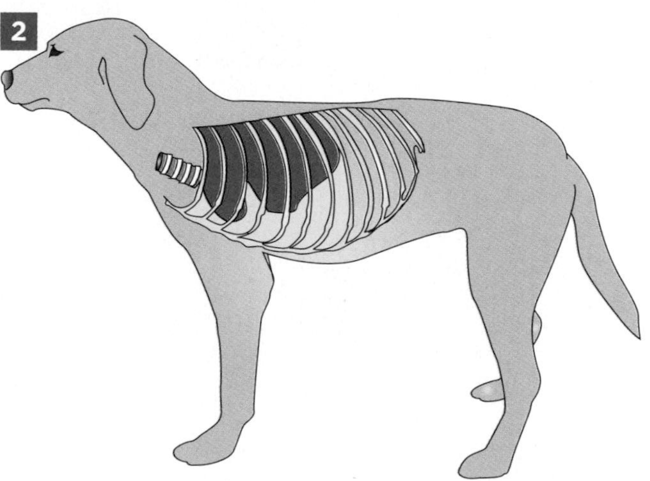

Pleural fluid accumulates ventrally in the standing or sternal patient.

PROCEDURE 7-11 Thoracentesis—cont'd

3. Animals with pneumothorax have air that accumulates dorsally when the patient is standing or in sternal recumbency. Thoracentesis in these animals should be performed over the dorsal caudal lung fields. Percussion can be used to identify the most resonant site for thoracentesis to relieve a pneumothorax.

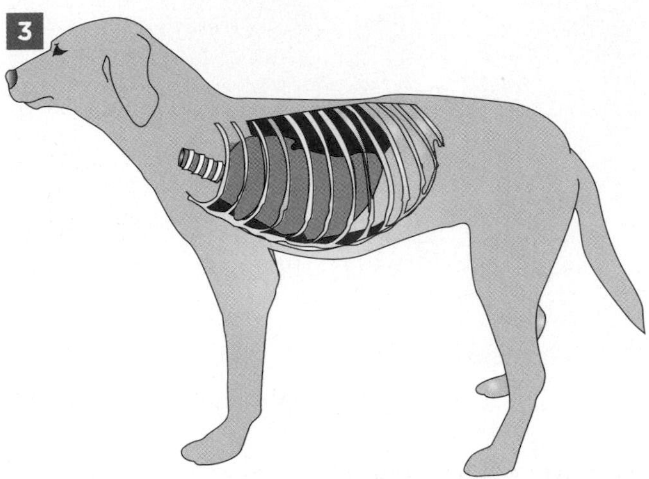

Pleural air accumulates primarily in the dorsal and caudal thorax in the standing or sternal patient.

4. The blood supply to the thoracic wall is provided by the intercostal arteries that lie just caudal to each rib in conjunction with a vein and a nerve. Whenever thoracentesis is performed, the needle should be inserted at the cranial edge of a rib to avoid puncture of an intercostal vessel.

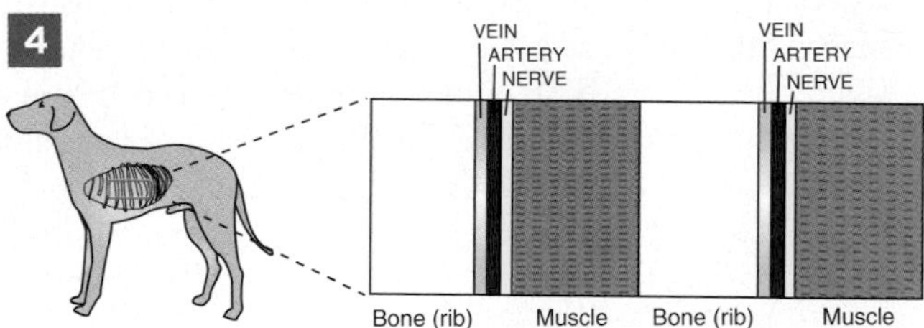

The intercostal vessels are located immediately caudal to each rib.

EQUIPMENT

- 19-gauge or 21-gauge butterfly catheter
- Three-way stopcock
- Syringe
- In large dogs or in animals with thick effusions, a larger-gauge needle or catheter (14- to 18-gauge) can be used instead of the butterfly catheter, but the needle should be connected to the syringe and stopcock using extension tubing to minimize movement of the needle or catheter during movement of the collecting syringe.
- Lidocaine blocking solution (2% lidocaine mixed 9:1 with 8.4% sodium bicarbonate), 3-mL syringe, 25-gauge needle
- Sterile gloves

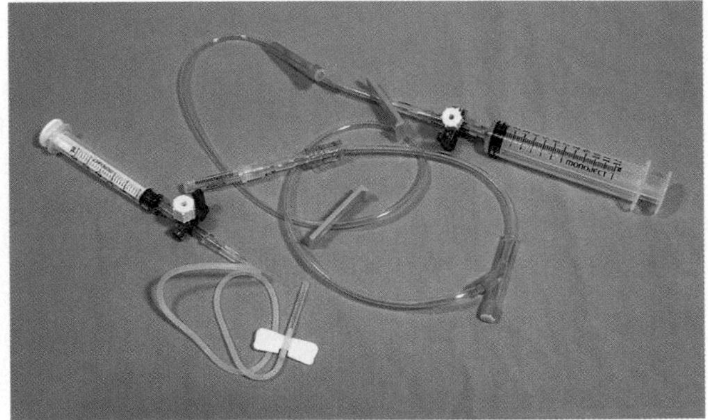

Equipment used for thoracentesis.

TECHNIQUE

1. Gently restrain the animal standing or in sternal or lateral recumbency. Administer supplemental oxygen if the animal is dyspneic.

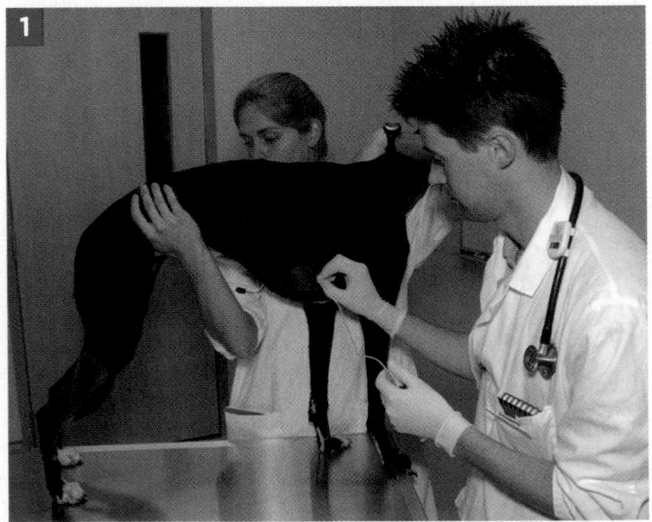

Dog restrained while standing for thoracentesis.

2. Determine the site where thoracentesis should be attempted. When a pleural effusion is present, this is usually between the sixth and eighth intercostal spaces near the costochondral junction.
3. Clip and prep the site. Sterile gloves and aseptic technique should be used for thoracentesis.
4. Block the site with lidocaine blocking solution if the needle is to remain inserted for several minutes for therapeutic thoracentesis. Diagnostic thoracentesis (removal of 1 to 6 mL of fluid), rarely requires local anesthetic.
5. With the syringe attached, the bevel directed cranially, and the stopcock open between the needle or catheter and the syringe, the needle is advanced through the skin and the intercostal muscles just cranial to a rib. The needle is held with a hand resting against the chest wall so that it will not move relative to the respirations or movement of the animal.

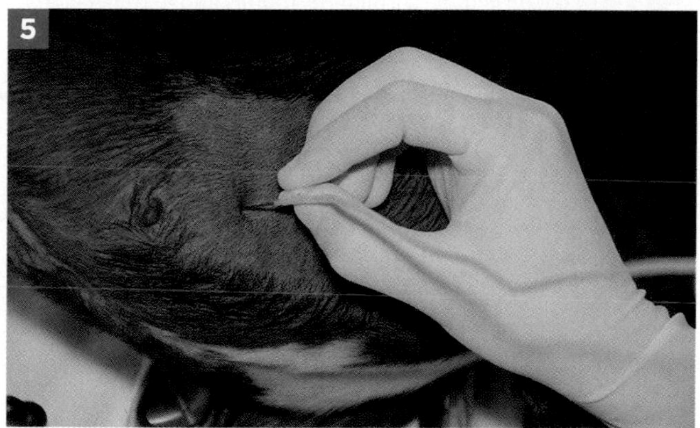

The needle is advanced through the skin and the intercostal muscles just cranial to a rib, with the hand holding the needle resting against the chest wall for stability.

6. Apply gentle suction to the syringe so that entry into the pleural space is immediately identified by the recovery of fluid or air.
7. As the pleural space is entered, continue to advance the needle while directing the tip slightly caudally so that the needle rests against the parietal pleura with the bevel toward the inside of the chest. This will allow aspiration of fluid or air from the chest without lacerating the lung.

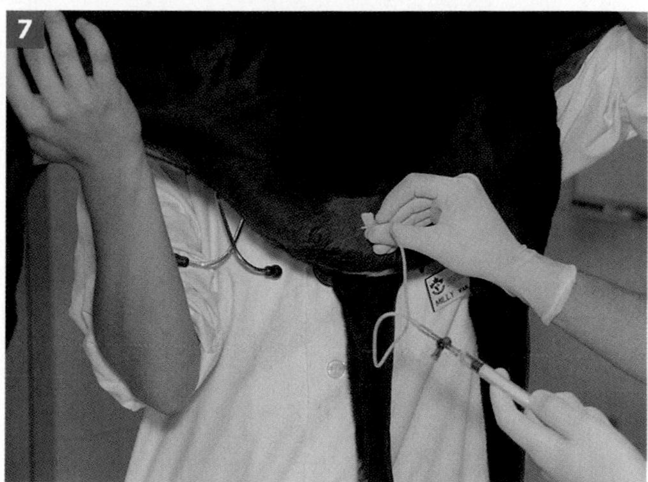

Advancing the needle while directing the tip slightly caudally as the pleural space is entered.

8. If no fluid or air is obtained, or if the flow stops, try an alternate site.

POTENTIAL COMPLICATIONS

Iatrogenic pneumothorax may occur due to needle puncture of the lung. This is usually mild and rarely requires specific treatment, except in animals with fibrosing pleuritis or pulmonary neoplasia preventing normal elastic recoil of the lung.

SAMPLE HANDLING

Fluid collected should be submitted for cytologic and microbiologic analysis.

RESULTS

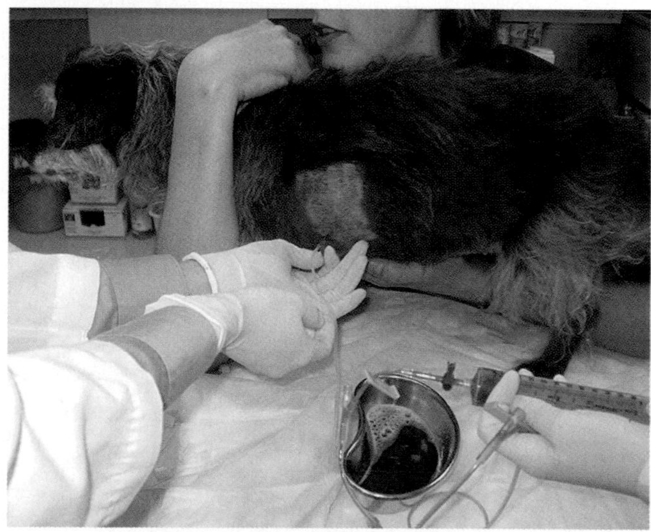

Collection of a modified transudate from the pleural space of a dog with right heart failure.

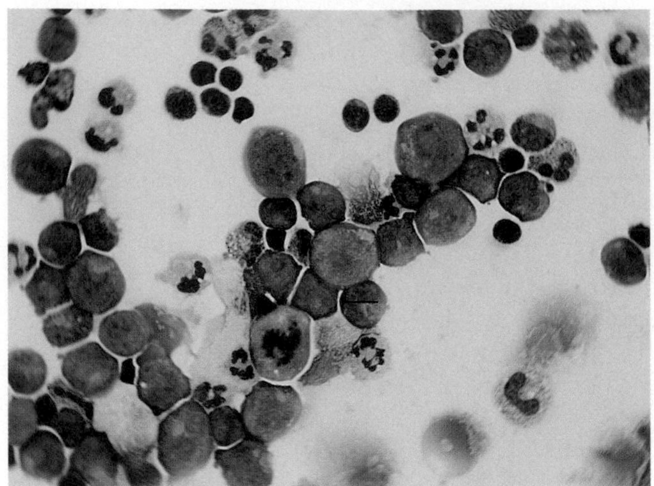

Pleural fluid collected from a 6-year-old spayed female Golden Retriever with a short history of dyspnea and lethargy. The fluid is dominated by a population of large round atypical lymphocytes. This dog has thymic lymphoma. **(Courtesy Dr. Marion Jackson, University of Saskatchewan.)**

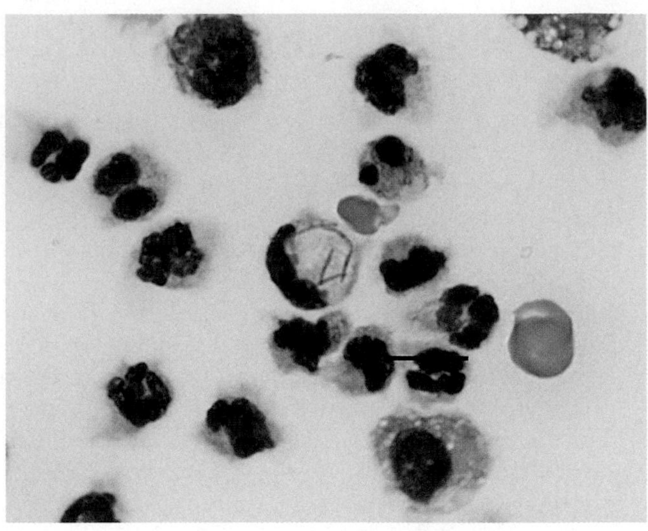

Pleural fluid collected from a 5-year-old male German Pinscher with a 4-week history of lethargy and weight loss, and a 2-day history of dyspnea. The fluid is highly cellular and contains primarily neutrophils, many of which are degenerate. There was a pleomorphic population of bacteria both within neutrophils and extracellularly, including thin filamentous forms (shown), cocci, and rods. This is a pyothorax. **(Courtesy Dr. Marion Jackson, University of Saskatchewan.)**

8 Pericardiocentesis

PROCEDURE 8-1 Pericardiocentesis

PURPOSE

To remove fluid that has accumulated within the pericardial sac surrounding the heart

INDICATIONS

Dogs or cats with significant accumulation of pericardial effusion causing decreased cardiac output (cardiac tamponade).

CLINICAL CONSIDERATIONS

1. Pericardial fluid accumulation compresses the heart, limiting cardiac filling and decreasing cardiac output. Low cardiac output, arterial hypotension and poor perfusion of the heart and other organs can lead to cardiogenic shock, cardiac dysrhythmias, and death. Pericardiocentesis is often performed as an emergency procedure. Removal of even small amounts of pericardial fluid can relieve cardiac tamponade and improve cardiovascular function.
2. Acute cardiac tamponade should be suspected in animals with exercise intolerance, tachycardia, weak femoral arterial pulses (especially during inspiration), and muffled heart sounds. Jugular venous distention may also be evident. In animals with chronic cardiac tamponade, pleural and peritoneal effusion may also occur. Radiographs typically reveal a globoid-shaped enlarged heart, whereas an electrocardiogram (ECG) reveals small-voltage QRS complexes and electrical alternans (the height of the QRS complex varies with every other beat). Fluid accumulation between the pericardium and the heart can best be documented by echocardiography. Tamponade is confirmed by finding compression or collapse of the right atrium and sometimes the right ventricle during diastole.

CONTRAINDICATIONS AND CONCERNS

1. Pericardiocentesis is usually performed from the right side in the cardiac notch to minimize the risk of trauma to the lungs and the major coronary vessels. There is still some risk of lung laceration, leading to pneumothorax, or myocardial puncture, leading to hemorrhage or dysrhythmias.
2. Whenever possible, an ECG should be monitored during pericardiocentesis. Needle or catheter contact with the heart can induce ventricular dysrhythmias, signaling that the needle has been inserted too deeply.

POSITIONING AND RESTRAINT

Minimal restraint is required in most cases. Pericardiocentesis is usually performed with the animal in sternal or in left lateral recumbency, and the tap is performed on the right side.

SPECIAL ANATOMY

Pericardiocentesis should be performed from the right side. The lungs on the right side have a more prominent cardiac notch, so inserting the needle on the right decreases the chance of lung puncture or laceration. The major coronary vessels are located mostly on the left side, so tap on the right also minimizes the risk of lacerating these vessels. The puncture site is located by palpating where the cardiac impulse is strongest. Generally, pericardiocentesis is performed between the fourth and sixth ribs just below the costochondral junction on the right side.

PROCEDURE 8-1 Pericardiocentesis—cont'd

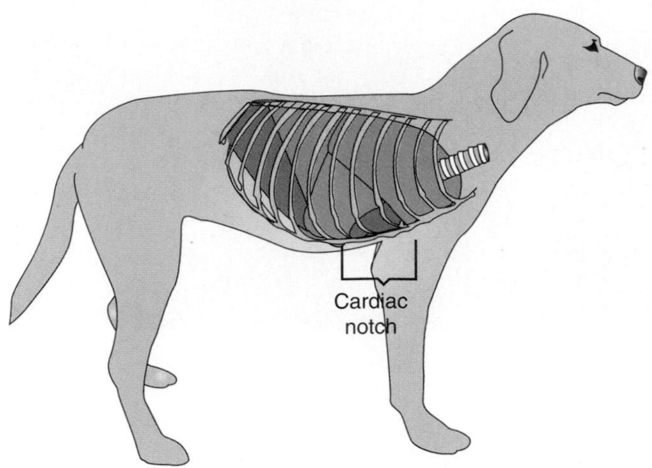

During pericardiocentesis the needle is inserted on the right side in the cardiac notch to decrease the risk of lung puncture or laceration.

EQUIPMENT

- For small dogs or cats, a 19- or 21-gauge butterfly catheter
- For larger dogs, a large (14- to 16-gauge) over-the-needle catheter (Medi-Cut catheter) and extension tubing
- Three-way stopcock
- Collection syringe (12- to 35-mL) and extension tubing
- Lidocaine blocking solution (2% lidocaine mixed 9:1 with 8.4% sodium bicarbonate), 1 mL in 3-mL syringe, 25-gauge needle
- Bowl for collecting the fluid

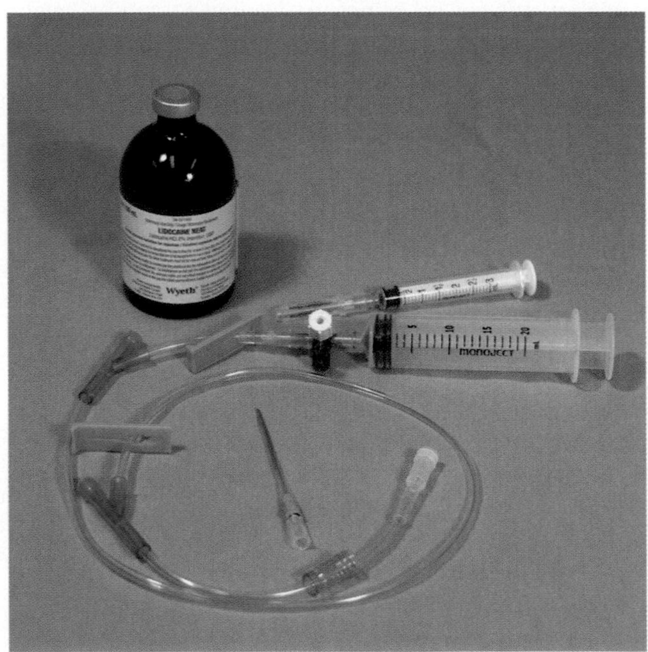

Equipment required for pericardiocentesis.

TECHNIQUE

1. Gently restrain the animal in sternal or lateral recumbency. Administer supplemental oxygen if the animal is dyspneic. Intravenous access is desirable, and fluid administration may improve cardiac filling.
2. Determine the site where pericardiocentesis should be attempted by palpating where the cardiac impulse is strongest. If the heart cannot be palpated, pericardiocentesis should be performed between the fourth and sixth ribs just below the costochondral junction on the right side.
3. Clip and prep over the ventral third of the right hemithorax from the third to the seventh intercostal space. Sterile gloves and aseptic technique are used for the procedure.
4. Block the site with lidocaine blocking solution from the skin to the pleura.
5. Advance the catheter through the skin and the intercostal muscles just cranial to the rib to avoid injury to the intercostal vessels. Angle the catheter and needle slightly dorsally while holding the needle with a hand resting against the chest wall for added stability.

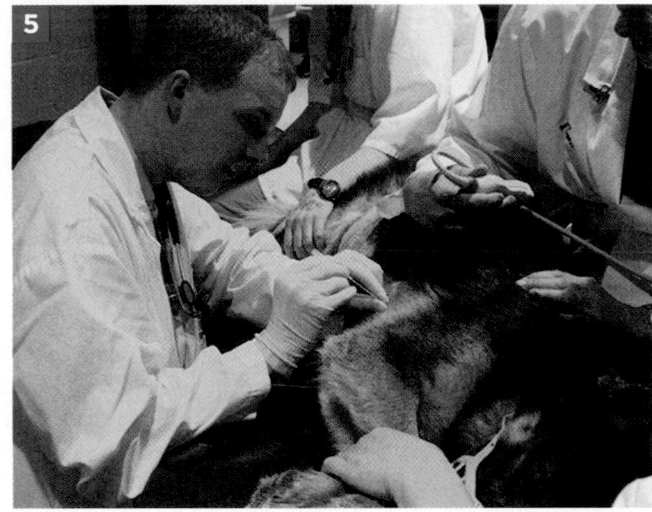

Advancing the catheter through the skin, intercostal muscles, and chest cavity to the pericardial sac.

6. With long-standing effusions there is often increased resistance and a scratching sensation when the pericardial sac is first encountered. This is followed by a distinct "pop" when the fibrous pericardial sac is penetrated and pericardial fluid under pressure begins to flow from the catheter.
7. Where pericardial fluid and a large volume of pleural effusion coexist, pleural fluid may appear in the hub of the needle immediately on entering the pleural space. When this is the case, advance the catheter and needle until the beating of the heart is palpable against the needle, and then advance into the pericardial space.

8. When the pericardial sac is entered, advance the catheter over the needle, remove the needle, and connect an IV extension set that is already connected to a stopcock and syringe to the catheter.
9. ECG monitoring is recommended to detect needle contact with the myocardium. Ventricular premature complexes (VPCs) usually suggest that the needle or catheter is touching the heart.
10. Fluid is drained slowly until the heart can be palpated against the needle. During fluid removal, the ECG complexes should increase in amplitude, the femoral pulses should get stronger, and the animal's tachycardia should diminish.

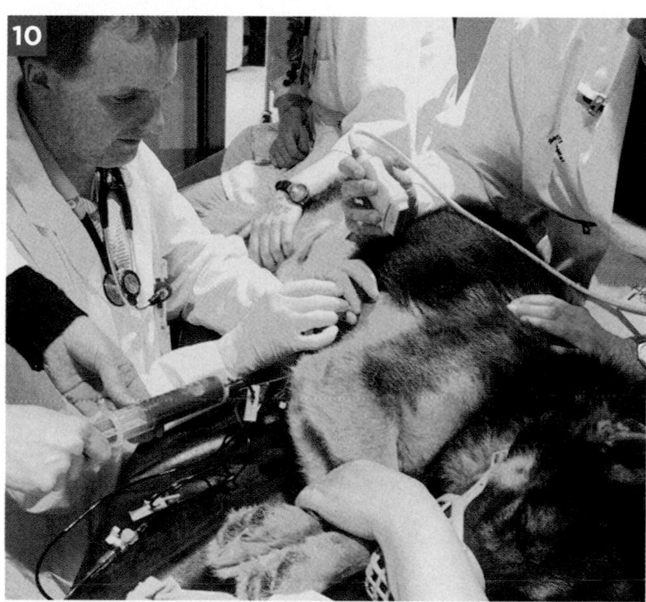

Fluid is drained slowly from the pericardial sac until the heart can be palpated against the catheter.

11. Pericardial fluid is typically quite hemorrhagic in dogs, and dark, bloody fluid is often aspirated into the tubing. This fluid should not clot when it is placed in a bowl. If it does, there should be some concern that there may be acute hemorrhage from rupture of a cardiac chamber, vessel, or neoplasm or that the tip of the catheter is within a chamber of the heart.

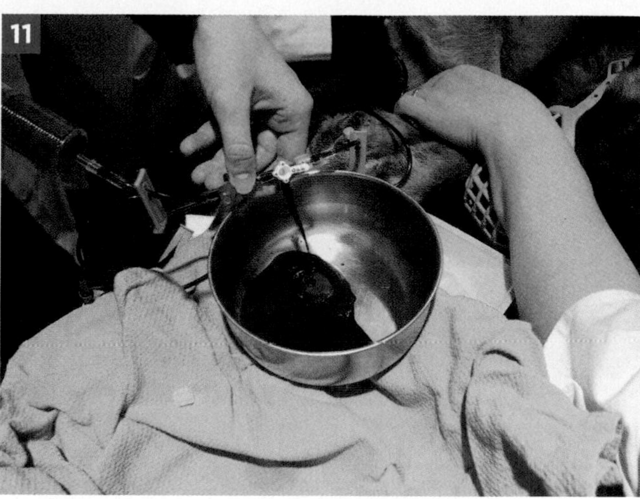

Draining hemorrhagic pericardial fluid causing cardiac tamponade from a dog with a right atrial hemangiosarcoma.

POTENTIAL COMPLICATIONS

1. If the needle contacts the heart, a marked scratching or tapping sensation is felt, and the needle will move with each heartbeat. Ventricular premature complexes often are apparent on the ECG. The needle should be retracted slightly if cardiac contact occurs.
2. If a sustained ventricular dysrhythmia develops and persists after the catheter is retracted slightly, administer lidocaine intravenously (without epinephrine) 2 mg/kg.
3. Rarely, a pneumothorax occurs due to lung puncture during pericardiocentesis.

SAMPLE HANDLING AND ANALYSIS

1. Fluid collected should be submitted for cytologic and microbiologic analysis.
2. Cytologic differentiation of neoplastic pericardial effusion from benign hemorrhagic pericarditis in dogs may be difficult or impossible because of the failure of tumor cells to exfoliate into the pericardial fluid and the common presence of very reactive mesothelial cells exhibiting many criteria of malignancy.
3. Neoplastic lymphoid cells may occasionally be identified in dogs and cats with lymphoma.

9 Gastrointestinal System Techniques

PROCEDURE 9-1
Oral Examination

PURPOSE

To examine and evaluate the oral cavity

INDICATIONS

An oral examination should be performed as part of every physical examination.

EQUIPMENT

- Penlight

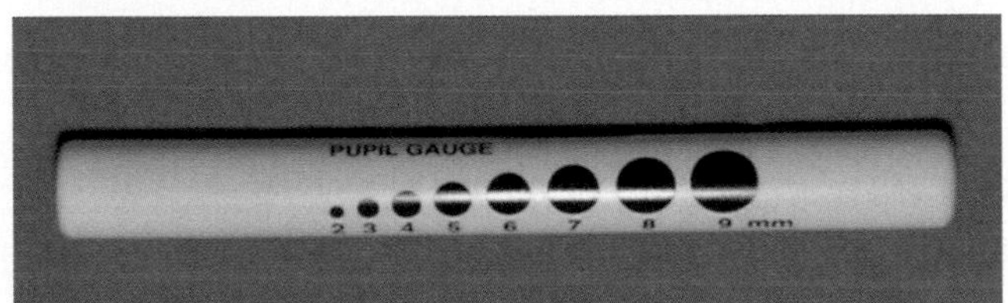

A light source is required for oral examination.

TECHNIQUE

1. Restrain the patient on a table in standing or sitting position.

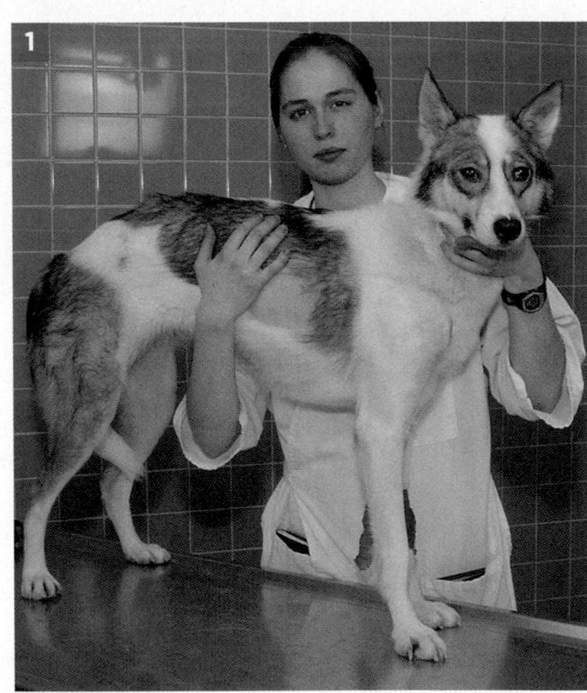

Restraining the patient on a table in a standing or sitting position.

2. Retract the lips to visualize the teeth and gingiva. Look for loose teeth, excessive tartar and tooth fractures, as well as for oral masses. In puppies and kittens, assess occlusion and look for retained deciduous teeth or cleft palate.

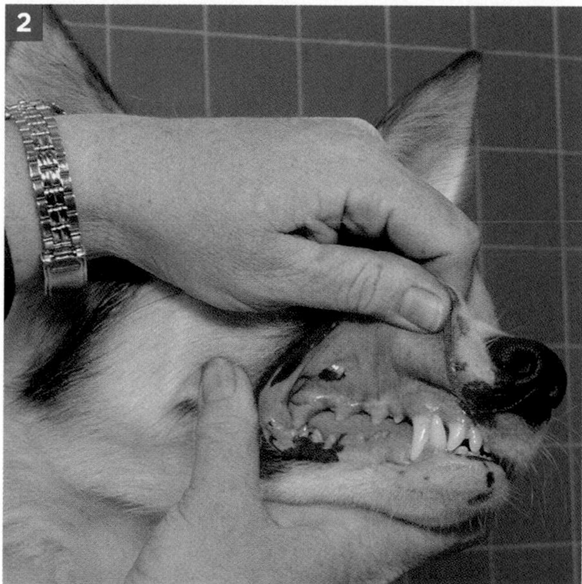

The lips are retracted to visualize the teeth and gingiva, revealing mild dental calculus in this 3-year-old Husky.

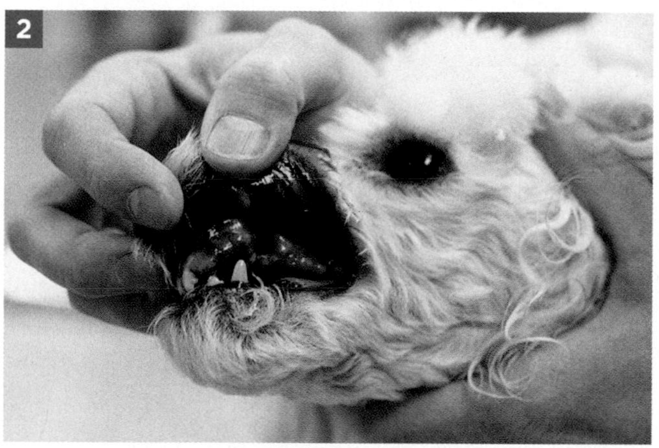

Oronasal fistula in an 11-year-old Poodle.

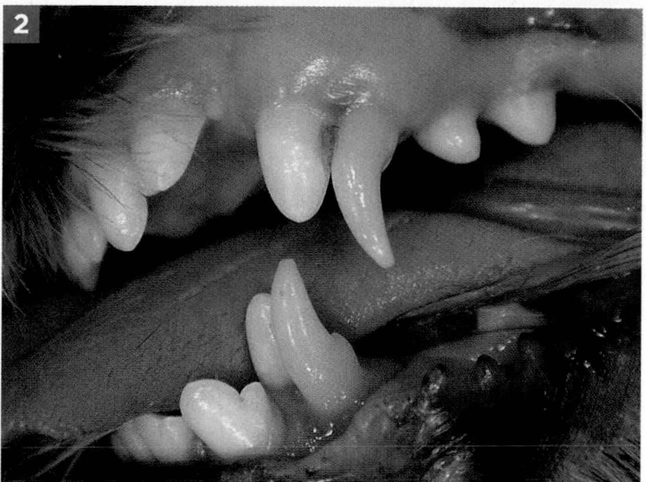

Retained deciduous canine teeth in a terrier.

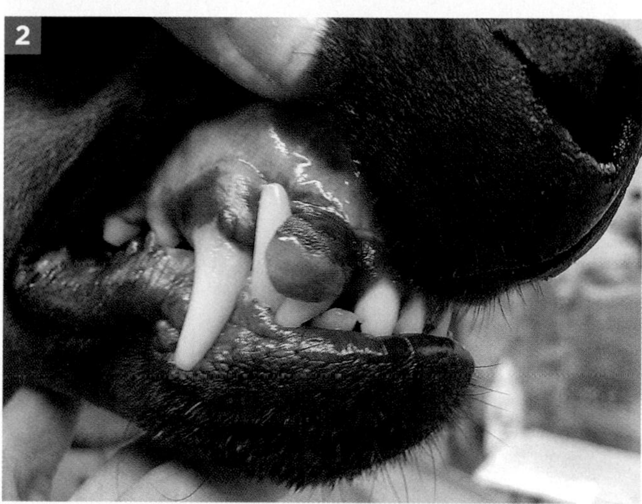

Gingival mass (epulis) in a Doberman Pinscher.

PROCEDURE 9-1 Oral Examination—cont'd

3. Examine the gums and the buccal mucosa (inside of lips) for evidence of anemia, icterus, or petechiation.

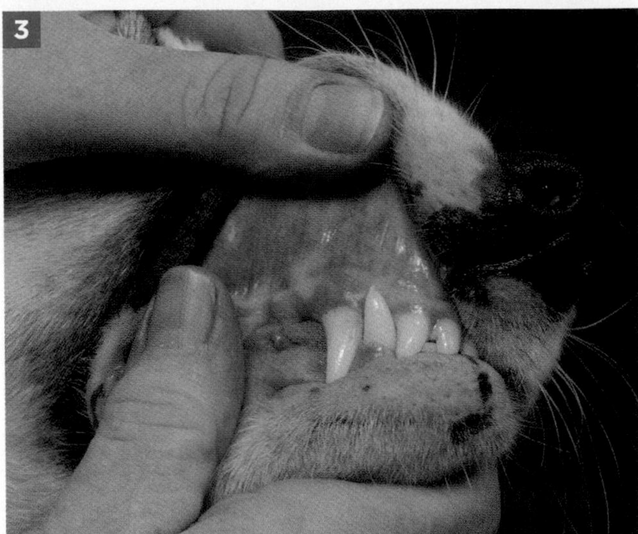

Pink mucous membranes in a normal dog.

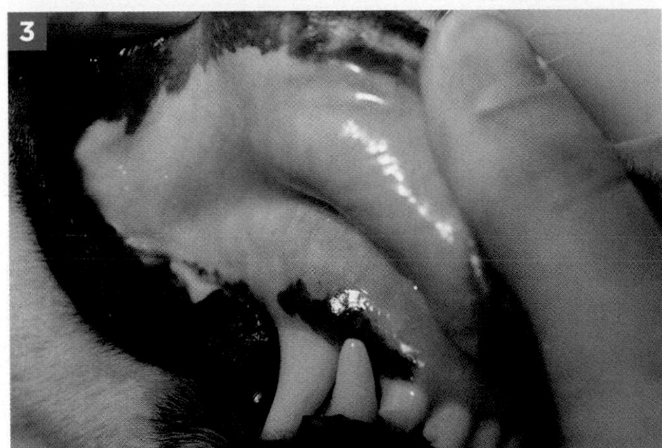

Pale yellow mucous membranes in a dog with hemolytic anemia.

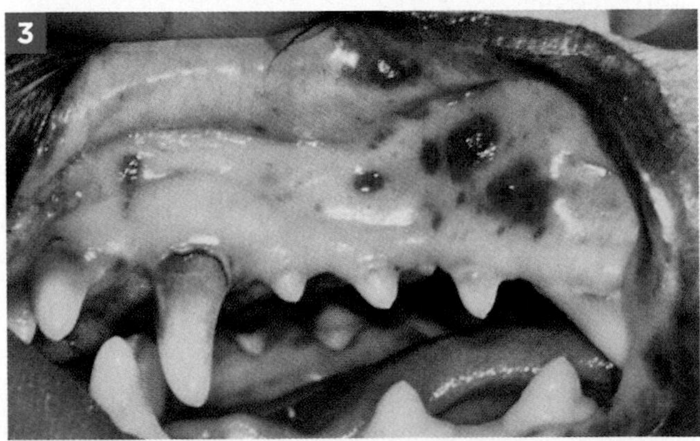

Oral petechiae and pallor in a dog with immune-mediated thrombocytopenia.

4. Examine the tonsils for color, size, or discharge and check for foreign bodies or masses. If the dog is sedated you can probe the tonsillar crypt, palpate the hard palate, and examine the sublingual salivary glands.

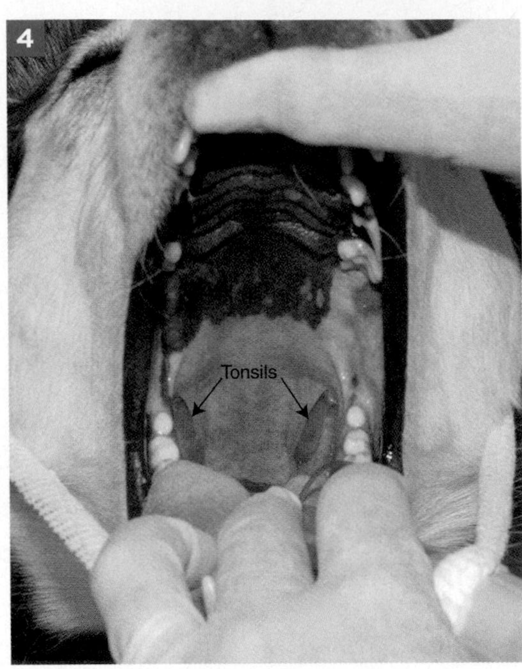

Examining the tonsils and the pharynx.

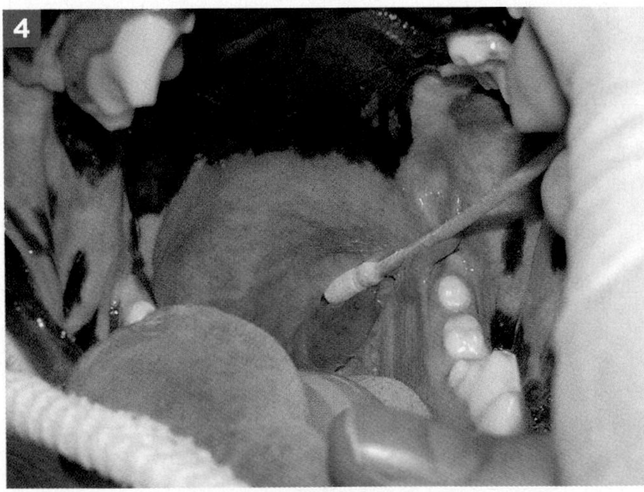

Probing the tonsillar crypt.

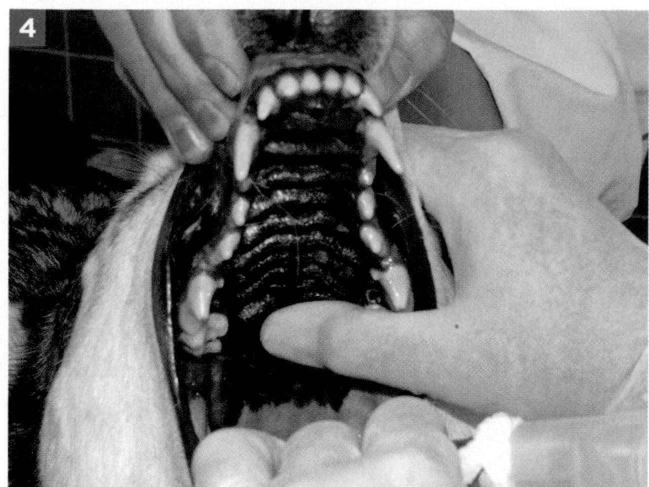

Palpating the hard palate.

5. Examine the tongue for ulcers, burns, or tumors. Lift the tongue to see the frenulum and to exclude a mass or a string foreign body wrapped around the base of the tongue.

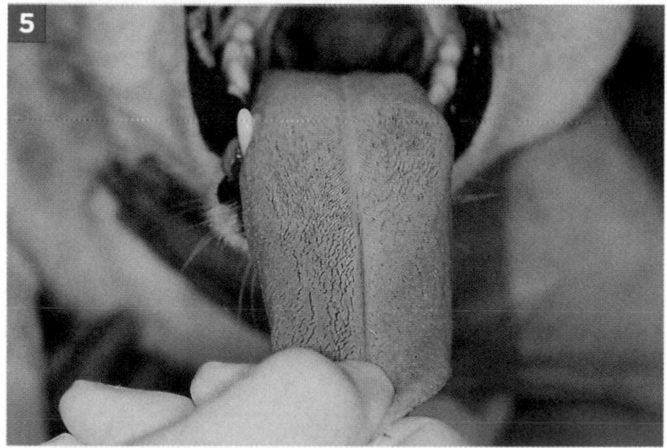

Examining a normal dog tongue for ulcers, burns, or tumors.

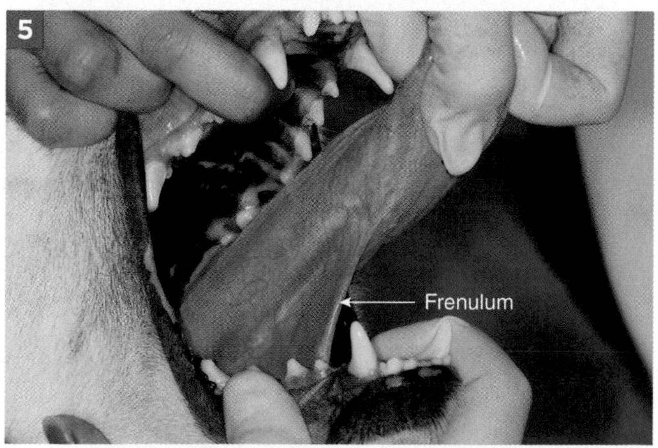

Lifting a dog's tongue to see the frenulum.

6. The normal cat tongue, used for grooming, is covered with firm spines (papillae).

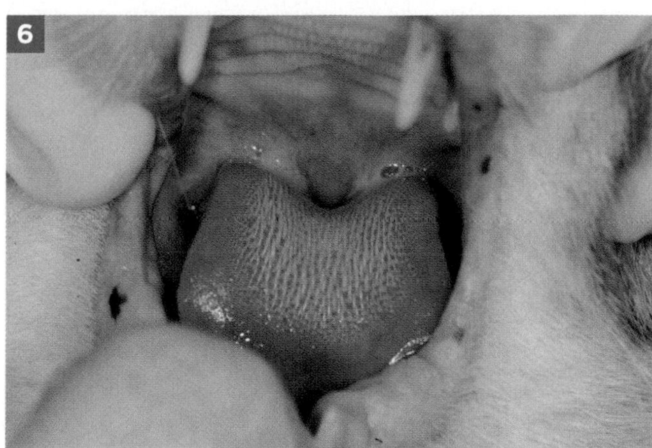

The normal cat tongue.

7. The figure shows a 7-year-old German Shepherd that developed tongue ulcers due to vasculitis. This dog had systemic lupus erythematosus (SLE).

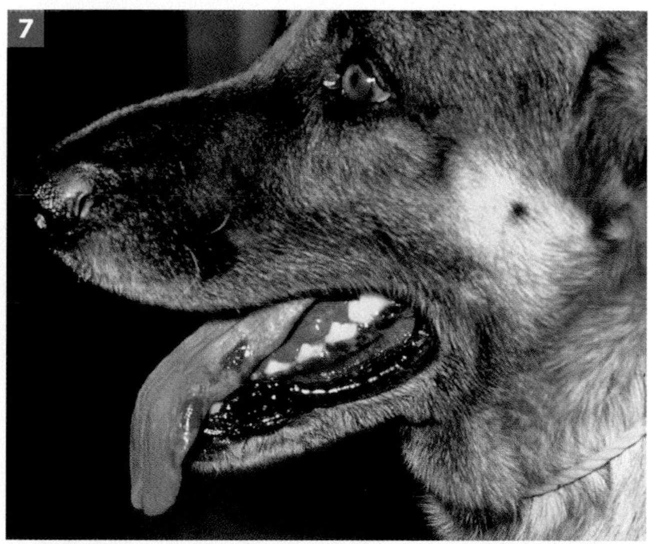

A 7-year-old German Shepherd developed tongue ulcers due to vasculitis. This dog had systemic lupus erythematosus (SLE).

PROCEDURE 9-1 Oral Examination—cont'd

8. This figure shows tongue ulcers caused by calici virus infection in a cat.

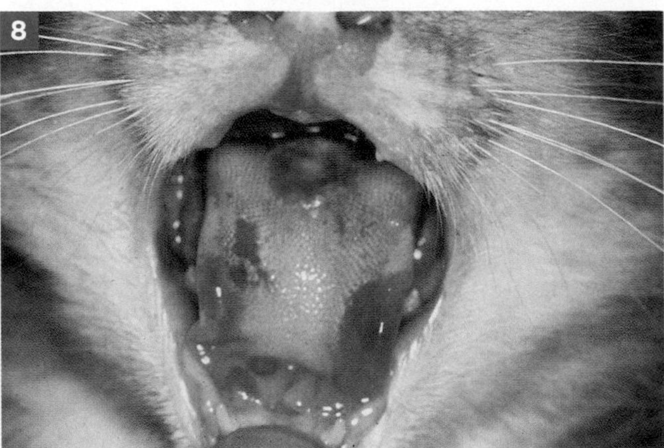

Tongue ulcers caused by calicivirus infection.

9. Cats very commonly get string foreign bodies. To look under the tongue of a cat:
   A. Restrain the head and use a thumb to push up in the intermandibular space.

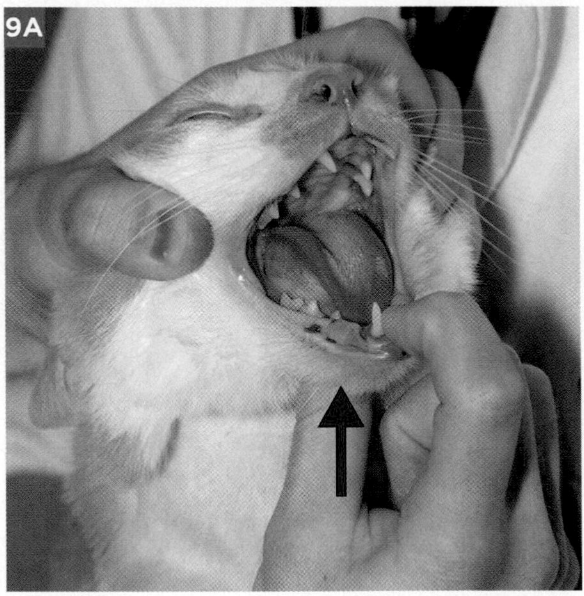

Restraining the head and using a thumb to push up in the intermandibular space.

   B. Open the cat's mouth and flip the tongue up with a finger, exposing the frenulum.

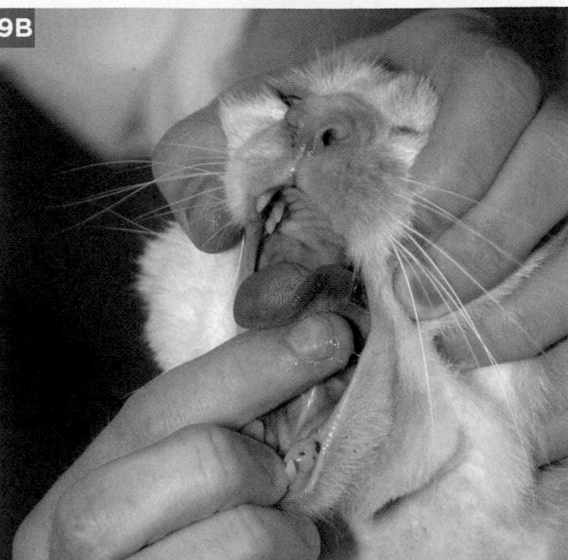

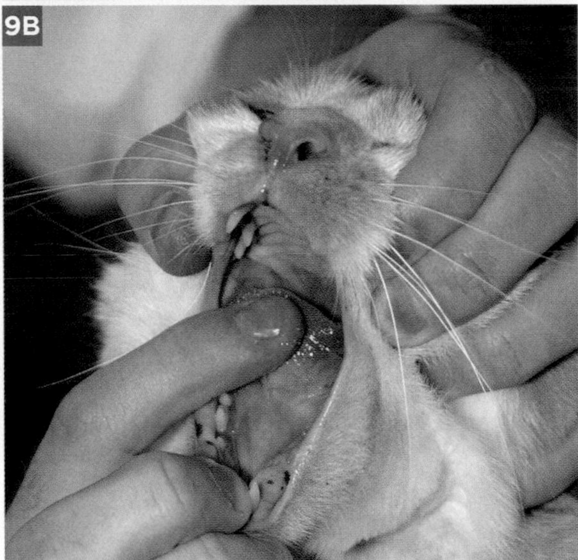

The cat's mouth is opened and the tongue is flipped up with a finger.

   C. The frenulum must be visualized as a straight, uninterrupted membrane in order to rule out a string foreign body.

D. In some cats, lifting the tongue is better accomplished using a cotton-tipped swab.

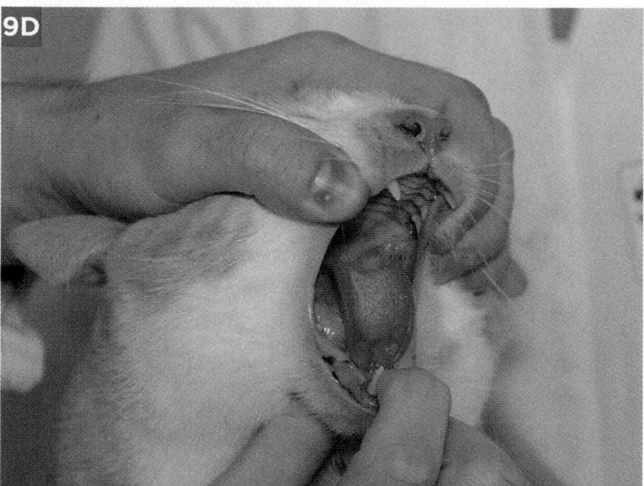

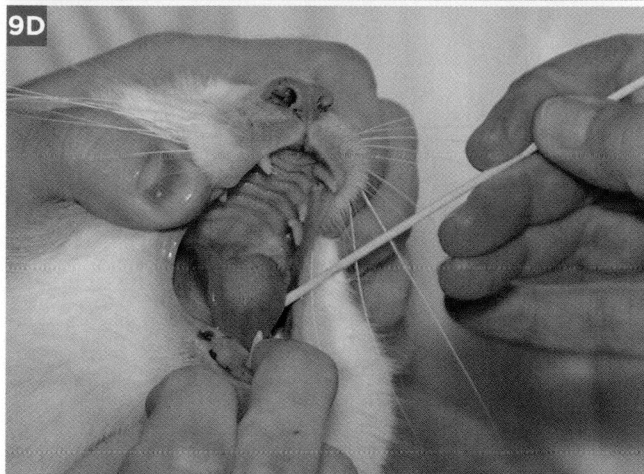

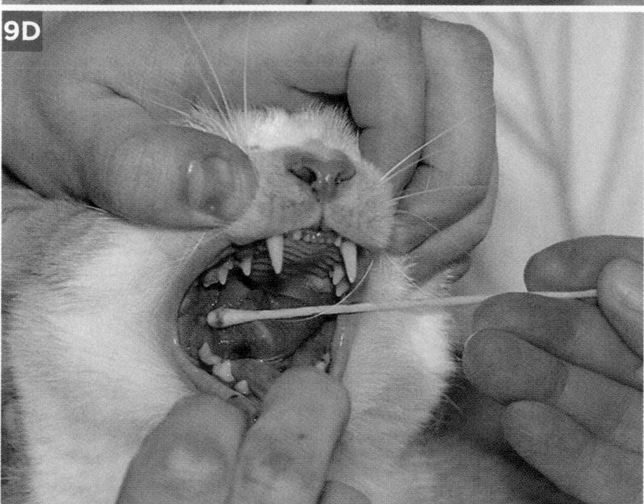

Lifting the tongue using a cotton-tipped swab.

10. This figure shows a string foreign body under the tongue of a 1-year-old cat presented for a 3-day history of vomiting.

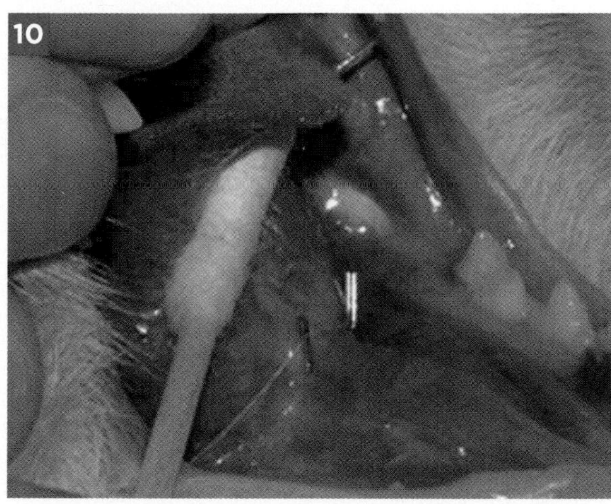

String foreign body under the tongue of a 1-year-old cat presented for a 3-day history of vomiting. **(Courtesy Dr. Anthony Carr.)**

PROCEDURE 9-2

Orogastric Intubation (Passing a Stomach Tube)

PURPOSE

To establish temporary direct access to the stomach of an animal

INDICATIONS

1. To administer medication, radiographic contrast material, or nutrition directly into the stomach as a bolus
2. To remove or sample stomach contents after a suspected poisoning and to perform gastric lavage
3. To attempt decompression of a gas-dilated stomach

CONTRAINDICATIONS AND WARNINGS

1. Adequate restraint is essential.
2. Careful attention must be made to ensure that a tube is correctly placed before anything is administered through the tube. Administration of most substances into the trachea can be fatal.

EQUIPMENT

- Stomach tube:

10-12 French rubber or polypropylene infant feeding tube for puppies and kittens
18 French rubber or polypropylene tube for adult cats and dogs up to 18 kg
Foal stomach tube (9.5-mm outside diameter) for dogs more than 18 kg

- Speculum: commercial canine mouth speculum
- Roll of 2-inch-wide adhesive tape
- Speculum: use a commercial canine mouth speculum, a roll of 2-inch wide adhesive tape, a syringe case, or a dowel with center holes and holes for canine teeth
- Adhesive tape or marking pen for marking stomach tube
- Lubricating jelly
- Syringe containing 5 mL of sterile saline
- Syringe or funnel for material to be administered

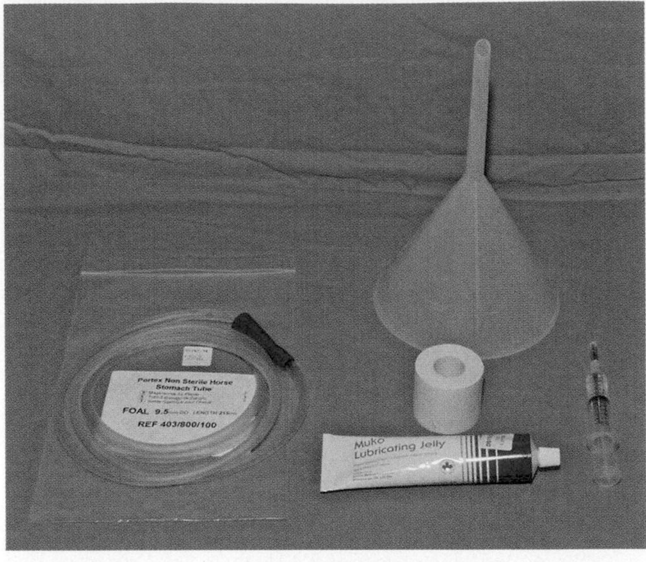

Equipment required to pass a stomach tube.

POSITIONING AND RESTRAINT

Restrain the animal sitting or in sternal recumbency (cats and small dogs) on a table. For large dogs, allow them to sit on the floor against a corner wall straddled by an assistant.

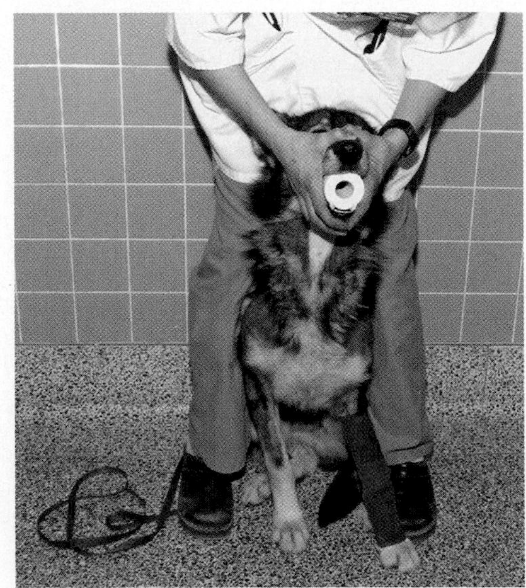

Restraining a large dog by allowing it to sit on the floor against a corner wall straddled by an assistant.

SPECIAL ANATOMY

The length of a tube required to reach the stomach can be measured from approximately the canine tooth to the last rib.

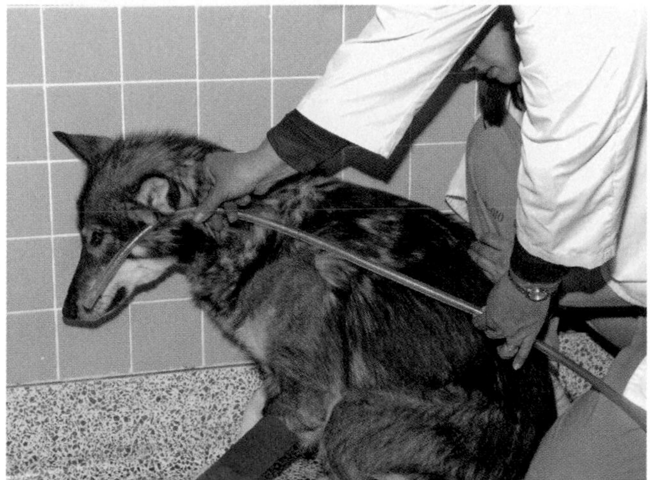

Measuring the length of a tube required to reach the stomach from approximately the canine tooth to the last rib.

TECHNIQUE

1. Premeasure the stomach tube by holding it next to the animal. When the tip is at the level of the last rib, mark the point on the tube at oral opening with a piece of tape or a marker.

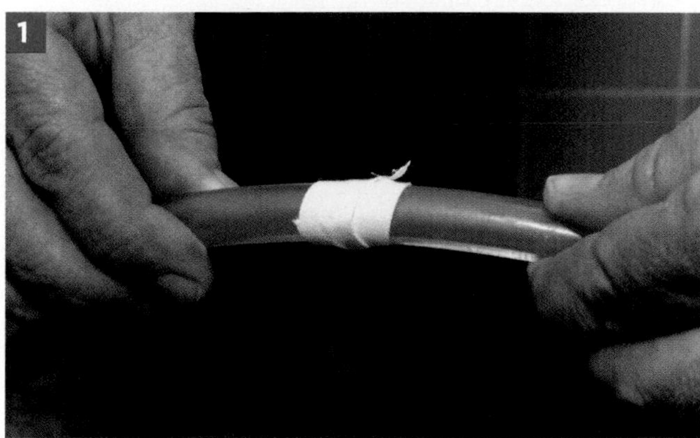

Marking the location on the tube indicating that the tube should have reached the stomach.

2. Moisten the tip of the tube with lubricating jelly.

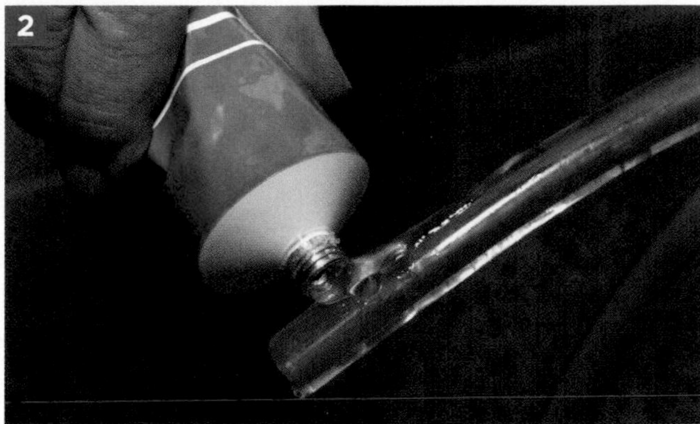

Lubricating the tip of the tube.

3. Insert the speculum into the animal's mouth and hold the jaws closed on the speculum.

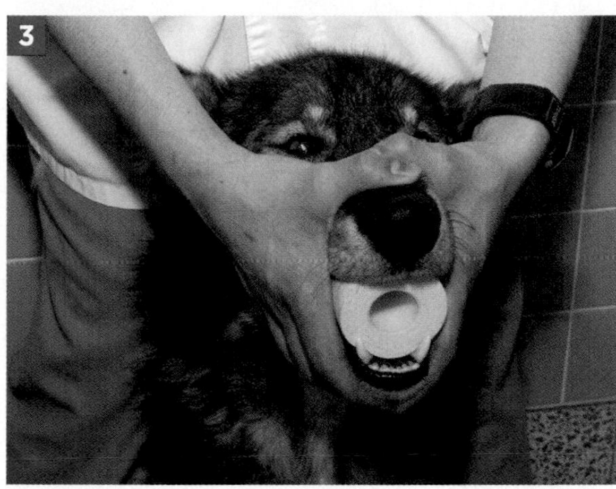

A speculum is placed in the animal's mouth and the jaws held closed around the speculum.

PROCEDURE 9-2 Orogastric Intubation (Passing a Stomach Tube)—cont'd

4. Pass the lubricated tube through the speculum and advance to the premarked point.

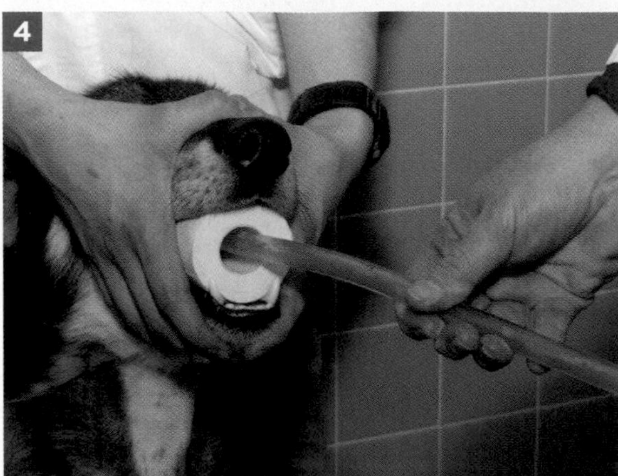

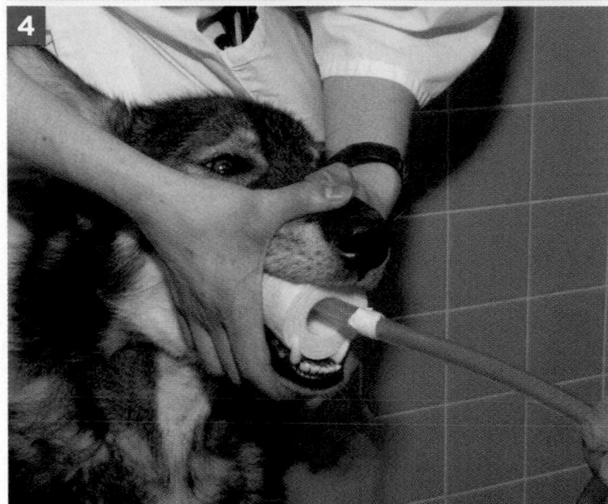

The lubricated tube is passed through the speculum to the premarked point.

5. Check proper placement of the stomach tube. This is a critical step because administration of material into the lungs instead of into the stomach is often fatal. To check tube placement:
   A. Palpate the tube in the cervical region. In medium-sized and large dogs, the tube will be palpable adjacent to the tubular trachea, so two tubular structures will be palpable in the neck. In smaller animals this is not reliable because the tube that has been passed is often not palpable.
   B. Administer 5 mL of sterile saline through the stomach tube and observe for coughing. This is the most reliable method to determine if the tube is properly placed, and the only method that is effective in small dogs and cats.

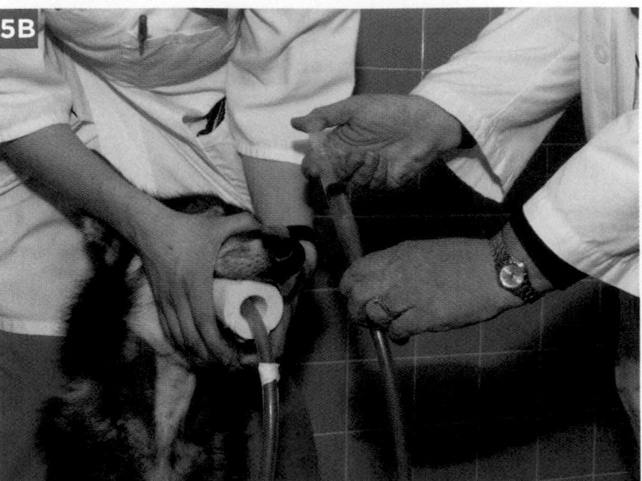

Administering 5 mL of saline through the tube to check for proper placement.

6. Administer materials prescribed or remove gastric contents through the tube. Before removing the tube, flush it with 3 to 8 mL of water, seal the end of the tube with the thumb to prevent leaking of tube contents back into the esophagus, and withdraw it in one motion.

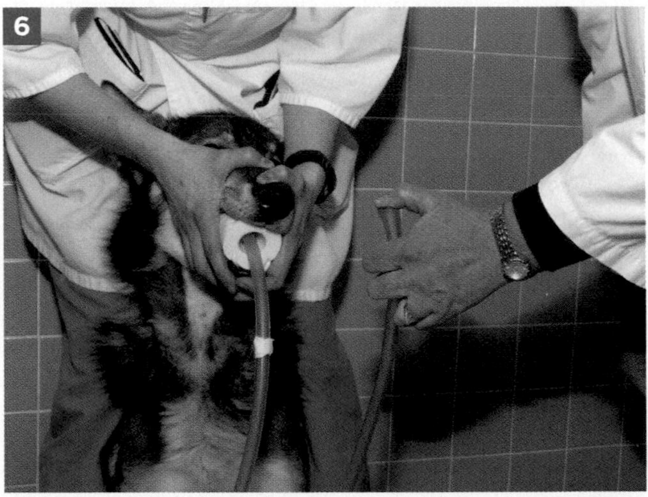

The end of the tube is sealed with the thumb before the tube is withdrawn.

POTENTIAL COMPLICATIONS

Inadvertent administration of material into lungs
Esophageal trauma
Gastric irritation
Gastric perforation

PROCEDURE 9-3

Nasogastric Intubation

PURPOSE

To establish direct access to the stomach or esophagus

INDICATIONS

1. To administer medications, radiographic contrast material, or nutrition and water as a bolus
2. To administer medications or nutrition and water as a continuous infusion, bypassing the requirement for the patient to swallow or eat voluntarily
3. To perform gastric decompression in patients with gastric atony

CONTRAINDICATIONS AND WARNINGS

1. Careful attention must be made to ensure that a tube is correctly placed before anything is administered through the tube. Administration of most substances into the trachea can be fatal.
2. Bolus administration of medications or other liquids can be made directly into the stomach, but maintaining the end of the tube in the stomach promotes gastroesophageal reflux and esophagitis. For long-term use, the tube should only be passed into the caudal esophagus.

EQUIPMENT

- Infant feeding tube of appropriate size
  - o In cats, use a 3.5 to 5 French tube
  - o In dogs less than 15 kg, use a 5 French tube
  - o In dogs greater than 15 kg, use an 8 French tube
- Topical ophthalmic anesthetic
- Lubricating jelly
- Syringe with 1 to 2 mL of sterile saline
- Bandaging material if the tube is to remain in place

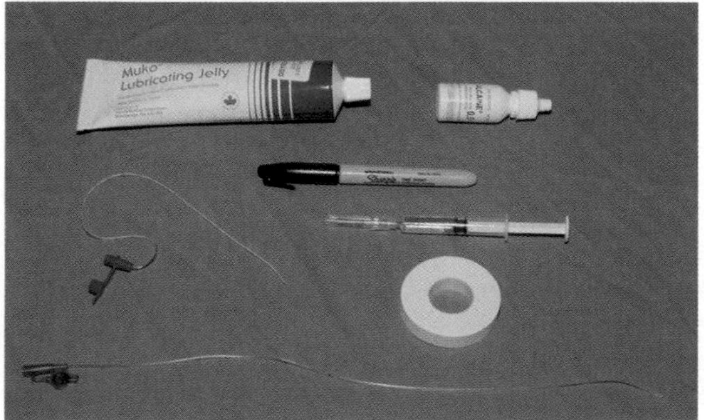

Equipment required to pass a nasogastric tube in a cat.

POSITIONING AND RESTRAINT

Hold the animal in a sternal or sitting position on a table. Fractious cats are best restrained in a cat bag for this procedure.

SPECIAL ANATOMY

1. The length of a tube required to reach the stomach for bolus administration of medications or feeding can be measured from approximately the canine tooth to the last rib.

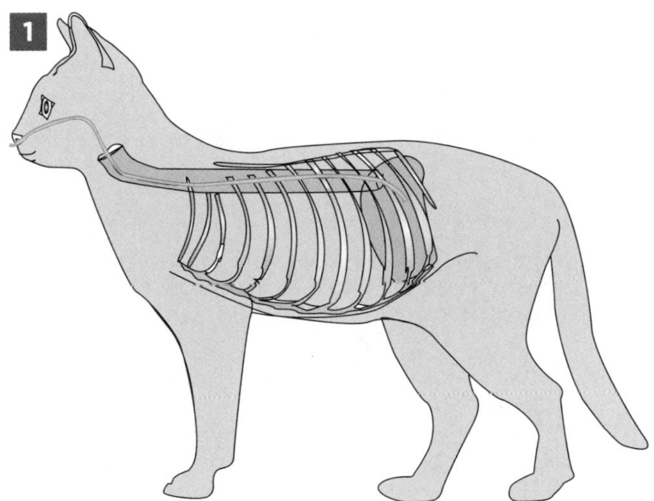

The length of a tube required to reach the stomach is measured from approximately the canine tooth to the last rib.

PROCEDURE 9-3 Nasogastric Intubation—cont'd

2. The length of the tube to be inserted for administration of a continuous infusion can be measured from the canine tooth to the seventh or eighth intercostal space.

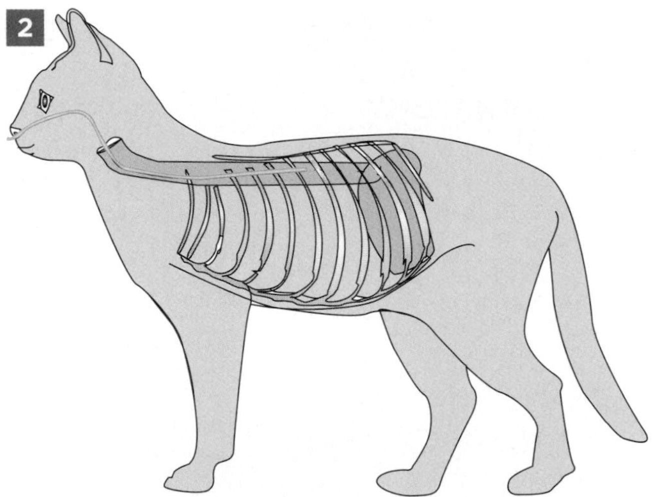

The length of the tube to be inserted for administration of a continuous infusion is measured from the canine tooth to the seventh or eighth intercostal space.

PROCEDURE

1. Premeasure the tube from the nostril to the level of the last rib (for bolus use) or to intercostal space 7 or 8 (for continuous use), and mark with adhesive tape or marker.

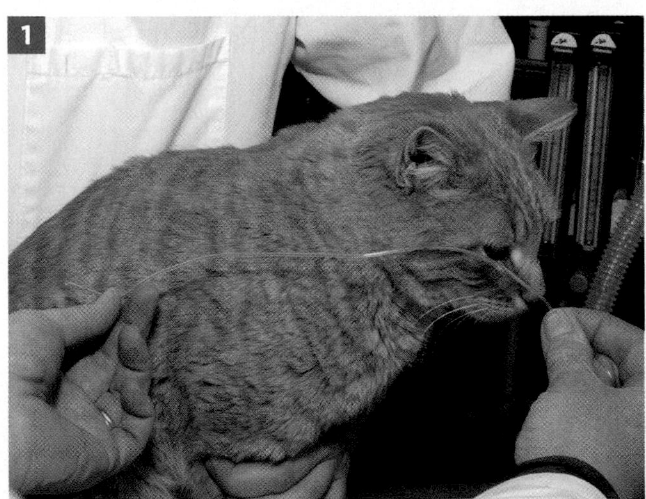

Measuring the length of the tube to be inserted.

2. Instill 4 or 5 drops of topical anesthetic into one nostril, tilting the head to allow the nasal mucosa to be coated and anesthetized. Wait 2 to 3 minutes, then instill 2 more drops.

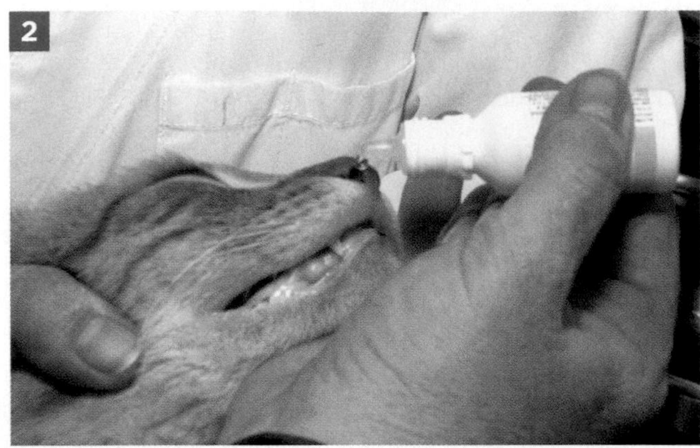

Topical anesthetic is instilled into one nostril, tilting the head to allow the nasal mucosa to be coated and anesthetized.

3. Apply a small amount of lubricating jelly to the tip of the nasogastric tube.

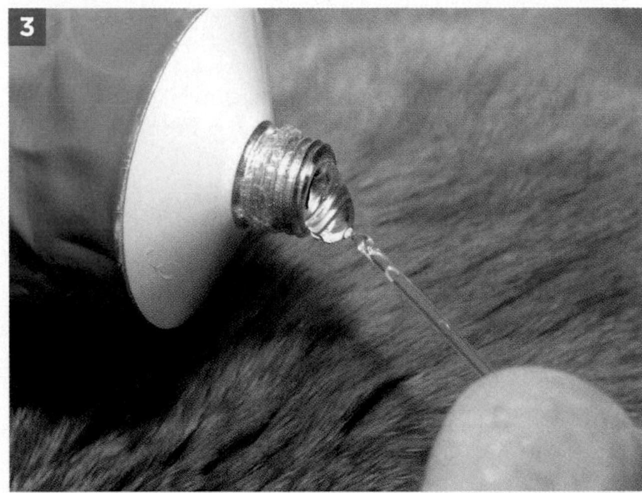

Applying a small amount of lubricating jelly to the tip of the nasogastric tube.

4. Holding the animal's head with one hand, use the other hand to insert the tube into the ventromedial aspect of the anesthetized nostril. Hold the tube close to the nose to prevent the patient from sneezing the tube out during insertion. Advance the tube to the premeasured mark.

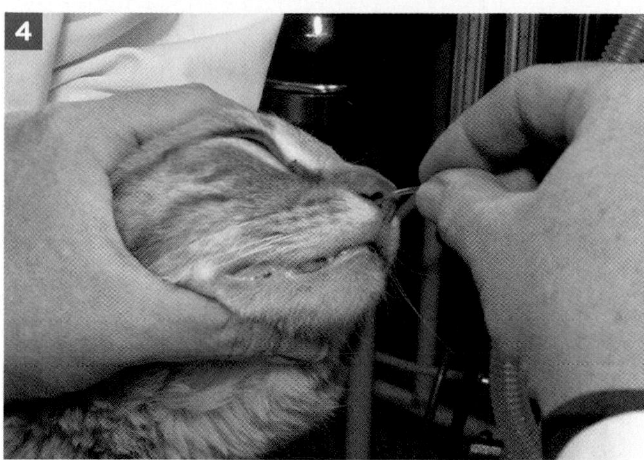
Inserting the tube into the ventromedial aspect of the anesthetized nostril and advancing it to the premeasured mark.

5. Check proper placement of the tube by instilling 1 to 2 mL of sterile saline into the tube. If the tube was inadvertently placed in the trachea, this will cause the animal to cough. Alternatively, a lateral thoracic radiograph can be performed to check tube placement.

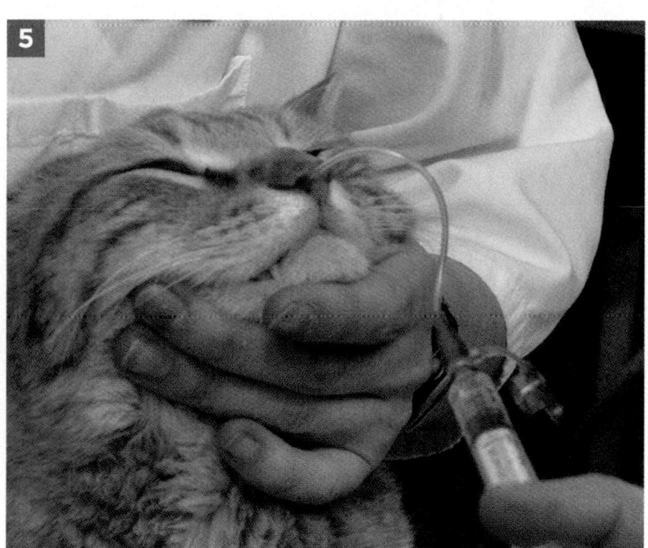
Assessing tube placement by instilling 1 to 2 mL of sterile saline into the tube and observing for cough.

6. For bolus administration into the stomach, administer prescribed materials, flush the tube with 1 to 2 mL of water, then before removing the tube, seal the end with your thumb or finger.

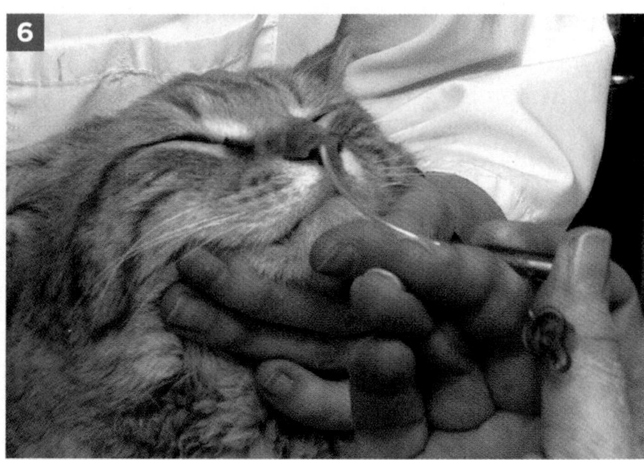
Before removing the tube, seal the end with a finger.

7. If the tube is to be maintained in place, it should be passed into the esophagus only to the level of approximately the seventh or eighth intercostal space. It should then be attached (suture, staple, glue) to the animal's nose and forehead. Avoid contact with whiskers because this will annoy the patient. An Elizabethan collar is useful to prevent the patient from dislodging the tube by pawing or facial rubbing.

POTENTIAL COMPLICATIONS

Inadvertent administration of material into lungs
Esophageal trauma, esophagitis
Gastric irritation

PROCEDURE 9-4

Anal Sac Palpation and Expression

PURPOSE

To palpate and assess the anal sacs, as well as to express their contents

INDICATIONS

1. Anal sacs should be palpated as part of a routine physical examination in dogs, and if they are full they should be emptied.
2. Dogs with full or inflamed anal sacs will often "scoot" across the floor or lick at their anal region. These behaviors suggest that the anal sacs should be evaluated.
3. A mass (neoplastic or abscess) may occur in association with the anal sacs.

CONTRAINDICATIONS AND WARNINGS

None

EQUIPMENT

- Latex glove
- Lubricating jelly
- Gauze sponges

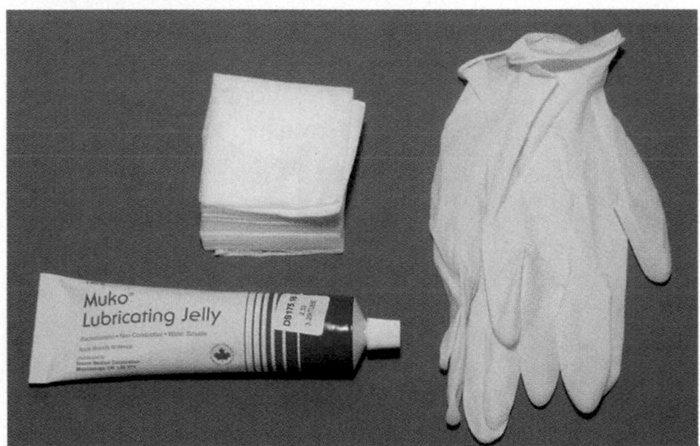

Equipment required for anal sac palpation and expression.

POSITIONING AND RESTRAINT

The animal should be restrained in a standing position on a table and should be supported under the abdomen by the assistant, to prevent sitting and minimize movement.

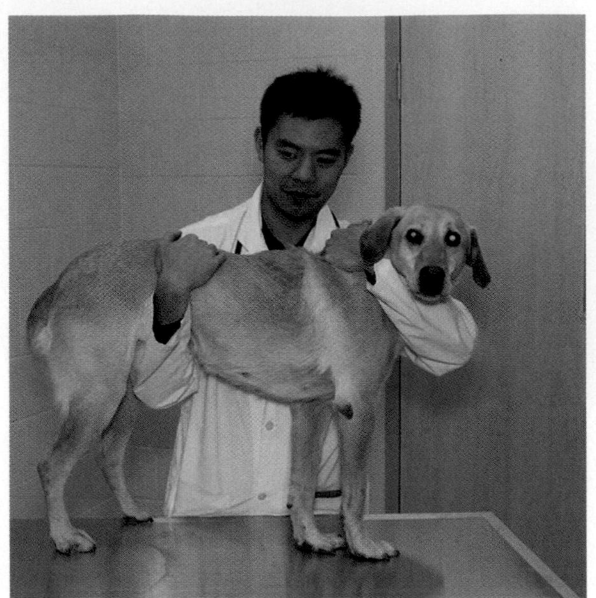

Restraint of a dog for anal sac palpation.

SPECIAL ANATOMY

The anal sacs are located at 5 and 7 o'clock relative to the anus.

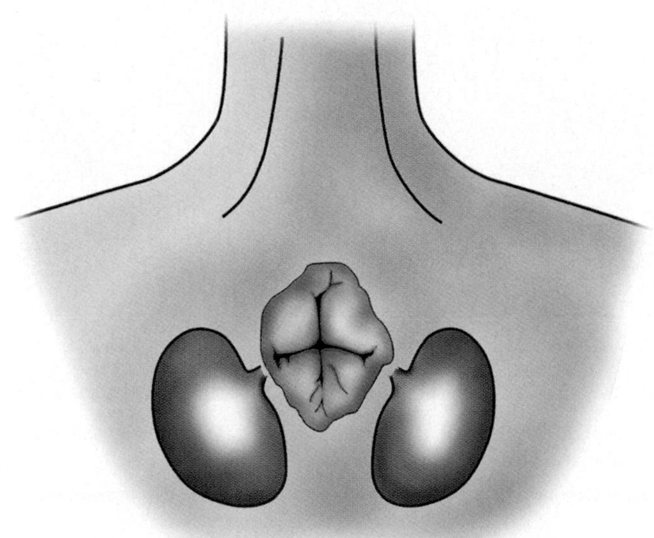

The anal sacs are located at 5 and 7 o'clock relative to the anus.

TECHNIQUE

1. Insert a gloved and lubricated index finger into the rectum and palpate the anal region and rectum for any abnormalities.

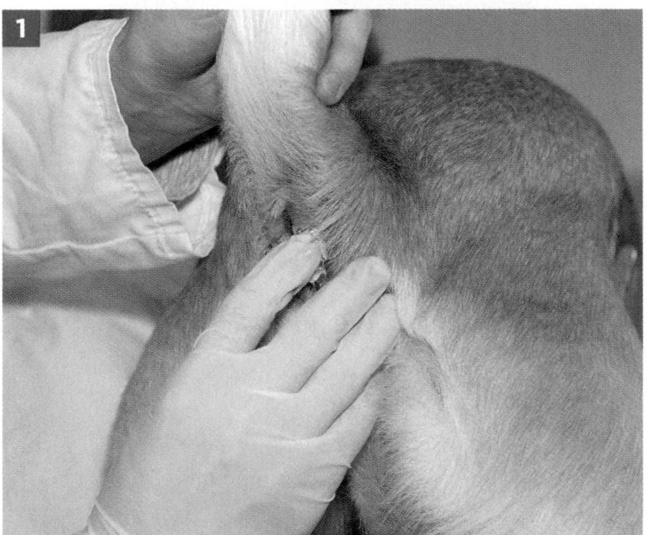

Inserting a gloved and lubricated index finger into the rectum.

2. Identify the anal sacs at 5 and 7 o'clock and palpate each one between the index finger inside the rectum and the thumb in the perineal region.

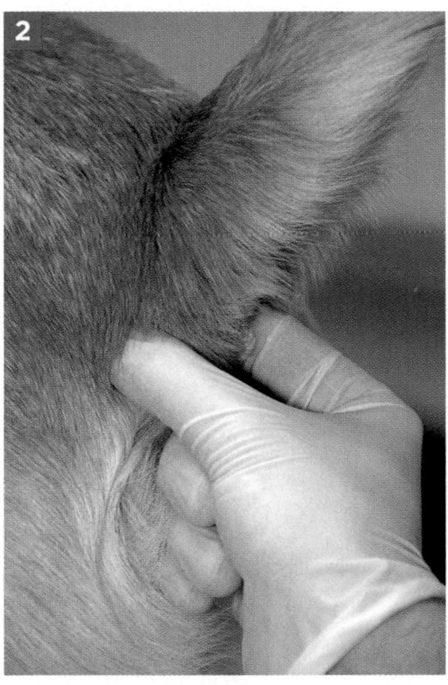

Palpating the anal sac between the index finger inside the rectum and the thumb in the perineal region.

3. If the anal sacs are to be expressed, place a gauze sponge or other absorbent material over the anal sac opening at the anorectal margin and gently but firmly squeeze the anal sac from the ventral surface toward the anal sac opening until it is empty

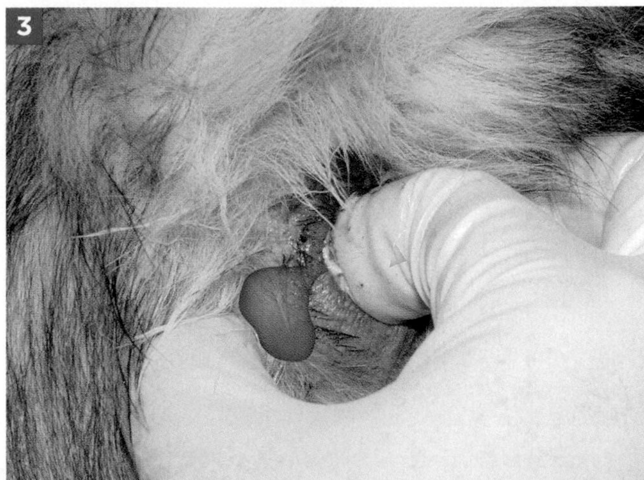

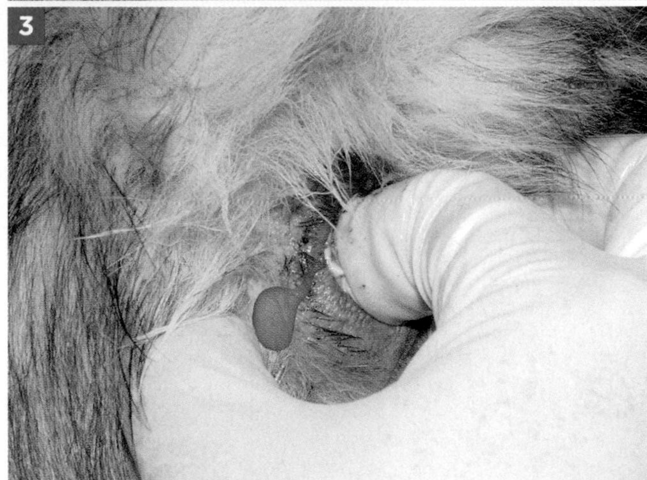

Squeezing the anal sac gently but firmly from the ventral surface toward the anal sac opening to express its contents.

PROCEDURE 9-4 Anal Sac Palpation and Expression—cont'd

4. Normal anal sac contents can vattry in color and consistency. Most often the secretions are yellow, gray, or brown.

Normal anal sac contents are typically yellow, gray, or brown.

5. Palpate the empty anal sac for any thickenings or masses.

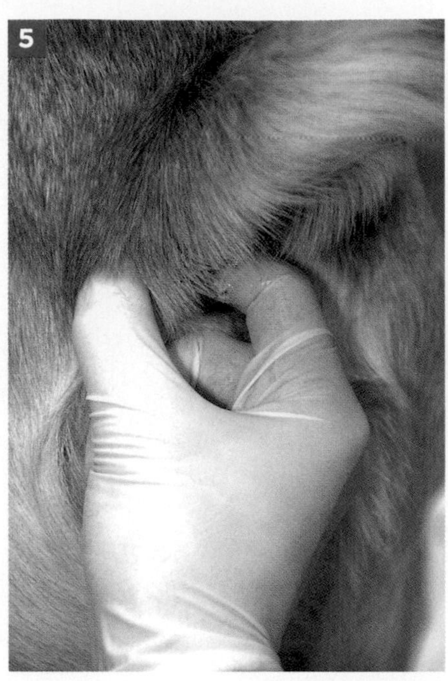

Palpating the anal sac for thickenings or masses once it is empty.

PROCEDURE 9-5

Percutaneous Transabdominal Liver Biopsy

PURPOSE

To obtain a sample of liver tissue for histologic analysis

INDICATIONS

1. Animals with liver dysfunction, hepatic enlargement, and ultrasound evidence of diffuse, uniform hepatic parenchymal disease when obtaining a wedge biopsy by exploratory or laparoscopy is not an option
2. Percutaneous biopsy of discrete or focal liver masses can also be attempted using ultrasound guidance.

CONTRAINDICATIONS AND WARNINGS

1. Hemostatic abnormalities are common in patients with liver failure. Before percutaneous biopsy, a platelet count, coagulation profile, and bleeding time should be evaluated and any abnormalities addressed (e.g., fresh plasma, vitamin K).
2. Vascular liver tumors like hemangiosarcoma often bleed excessively when biopsied.
3. Animals with posthepatic obstruction and dilated bile ducts should not be biopsied percutaneously. Surgical exploration is recommended to diagnose and relieve their obstruction. Percutaneous biopsy in these patients might lead to bile peritonitis.
4. Hepatic cysts or abscesses should not be biopsied percutaneously using this technique. Surgical exploratory or ultrasound guided drainage is recommended.
5. Animals with surgically correctable disease such as posthepatic obstruction or portosystemic shunt should have exploratory surgery rather than a percutaneous biopsy.
6. Percutaneous biopsies are less invasive and less expensive than surgery or laparoscopy, but the results obtained do not always correlate well with the results obtained with larger tissue samples. Diffuse liver disorders such as lipidosis and lymphoma are most reliably diagnosed, whereas inflammatory, vascular, and fibrotic disorders are difficult to diagnose.

EQUIPMENT

- Tru-Cut needle (preferably 14-gauge) (for needle technique see Box 9-1, page 136)
- #11 scalpel blade
- Lidocaine blocking solution (2% lidocaine mixed 9:1 with 8.4% sodium bicarbonate)
- Sterile gloves

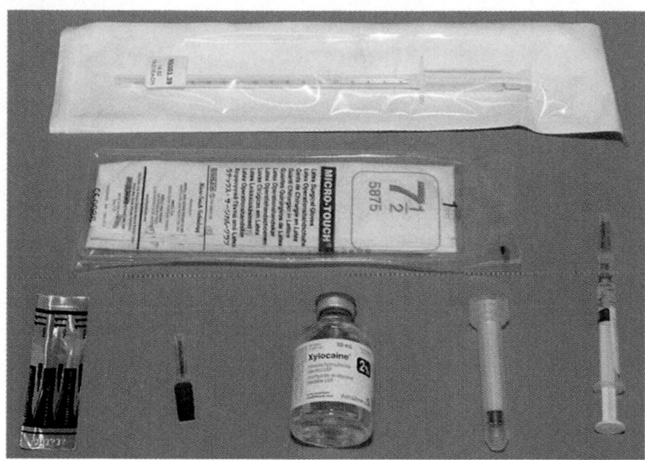

Equipment required for percutaneous liver biopsy.

POSITIONING AND RESTRAINT

1. Light sedation and local anesthesia will be adequate in most patients.
2. Lidocaine blocking solution (2% lidocaine mixed 9:1 with 8.4% sodium bicarbonate) can be used to block the skin and subcutaneous tissues. The addition of bicarbonate decreases the sting of injection and speeds the local analgesic effect of the lidocaine.
3. If performing a liver biopsy under ultrasound guidance, any position in which the liver and gallbladder can be easily visualized is acceptable.
4. When performing a blind percutaneous liver biopsy it is important to use patient positioning to maximize exposure of the liver for biopsy and to minimize the chance of gallbladder puncture. The animal should be placed in dorsal recumbency with the chest higher than the abdomen and the entire body tilted to the right.

SPECIAL ANATOMY

1. The gallbladder is located on the right side of the liver, and is often distended in patients with liver disease associated with cholestasis or anorexia. Care should be taken to prevent puncture of the gallbladder during liver biopsy. The animal is placed in dorsal recumbency and tilted to the right, whereas the biopsies are obtained from the left lobes of the liver.
2. The liver does not normally protrude past the costal arch. When the liver is enlarged, percutaneous biopsy is relatively simple. When the liver is small or normal sized the patient should be tilted with the chest higher than the abdomen so that the liver will fall caudally beyond the costal arch.

PROCEDURE 9-5 Percutaneous Transabdominal Liver Biopsy—cont'd

BOX 9-1

Needle Technique

Before proceeding, it is important to become familiar with the operation of a Tru-Cut needle.

1. The needle is advanced, in the closed position to the liver and through the liver capsule.

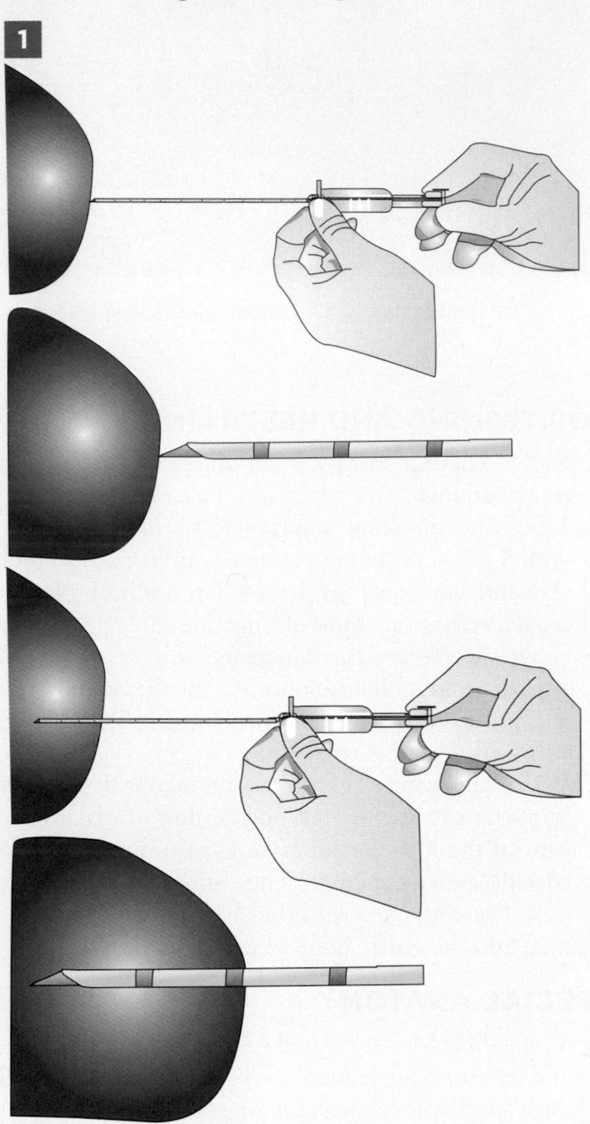

2. The inner obturator is then advanced into the liver.

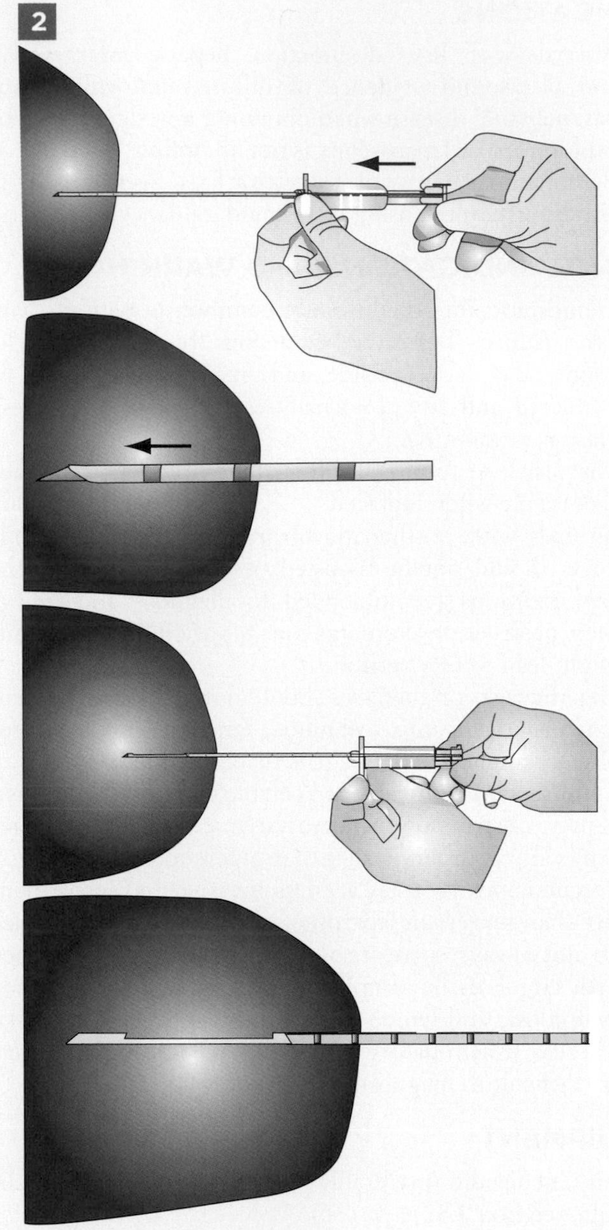

BOX 9-1

Needle Technique—cont'd

3. While holding the inner obturator steady in the advanced position, the outer cannula is advanced over the inner obturator, cutting a core of liver tissue.

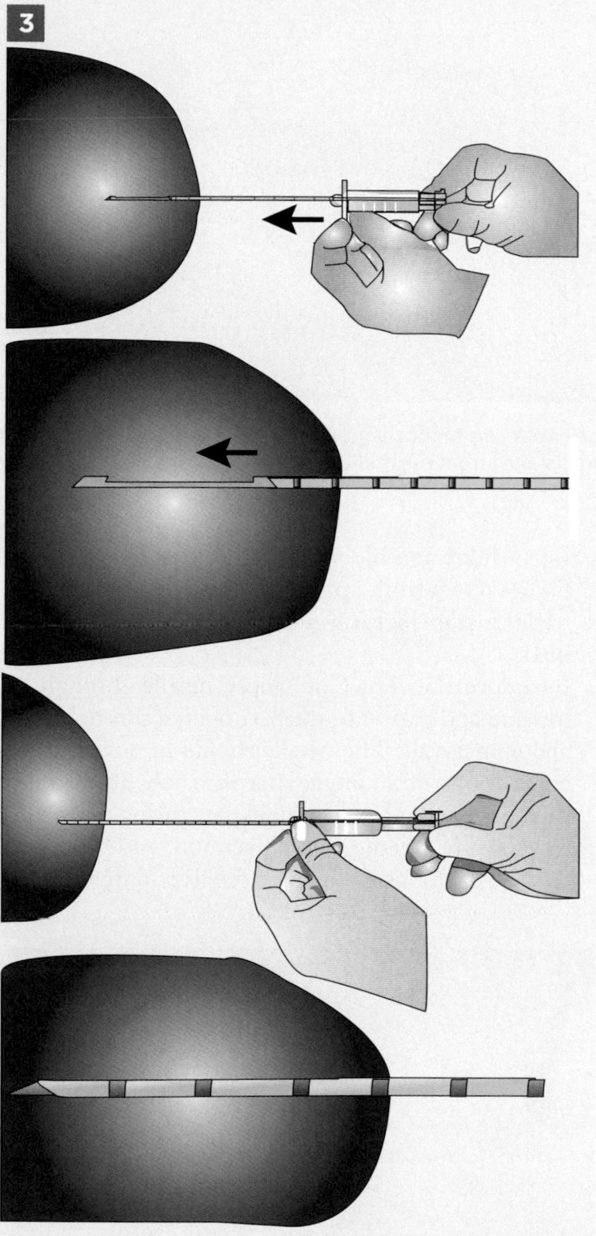

4. The needle is then withdrawn from the liver and the skin.

5. The inner obturator is advanced to expose the biopsy.

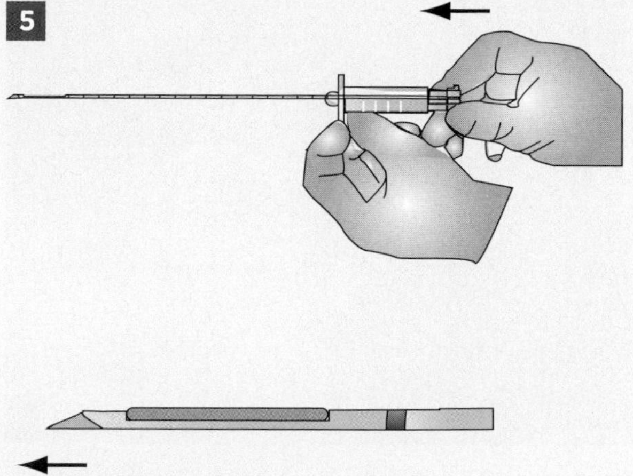

6. A small-gauge needle is used to tease the piece of liver off the biopsy needle.

PROCEDURE 9-5 Percutaneous Transabdominal Liver Biopsy—cont'd

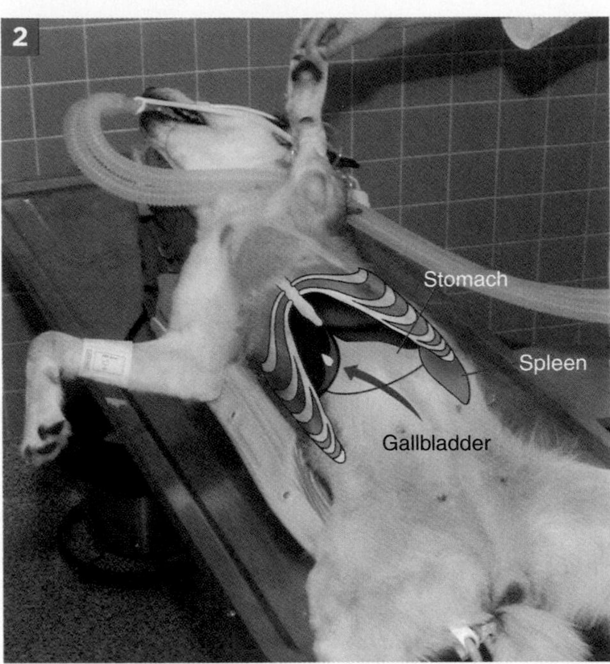

Tilting the body to the right and raising the thorax relative to the abdomen maximizes exposure of the liver and decreases the chance of gallbladder puncture when the liver biopsy is taken from the left side.

TECHNIQUE

1. Sedate the animal as required so it remains immobile during the procedure.
2. Place the patient in dorsal recumbency on a tilted or padded table with the chest higher than the abdomen, and tilt the entire body toward the right side of table surface at 30 to 45 degrees. Clip and prep the region. Wear gloves and use aseptic technique.

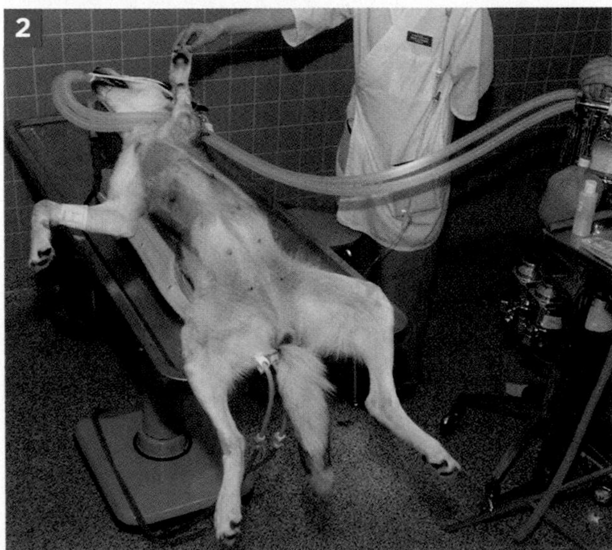

This dog is positioned properly for percutaneous liver biopsy.

3. Identify the tip of the xiphoid. The entrance site for the needle is at the level of the xiphoid, half the distance from the midline to the left costal arch at that level.

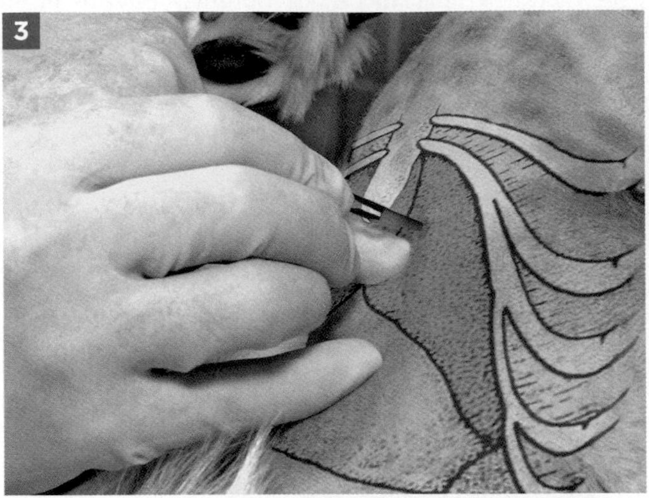

The entrance site for the needle is at the level of the xiphoid, half the distance from the midline to the left costal arch at that level.

4. Inject lidocaine blocking solution to block the skin and tissues down to the peritoneum at this site.
5. Make a stab incision at this site using the #11 scalpel blade
6. Introduce the Tru-Cut biopsy needle through the stab incision and then into the peritoneum through the ventral abdominal wall. The needle should be advanced cranially and dorsally at an angle approximately 30 degrees left of the midsagittal plane (to avoid puncturing the gallbladder).
7. Advance the needle to the liver and, with the needle still in the closed position, enter the liver parenchyma.

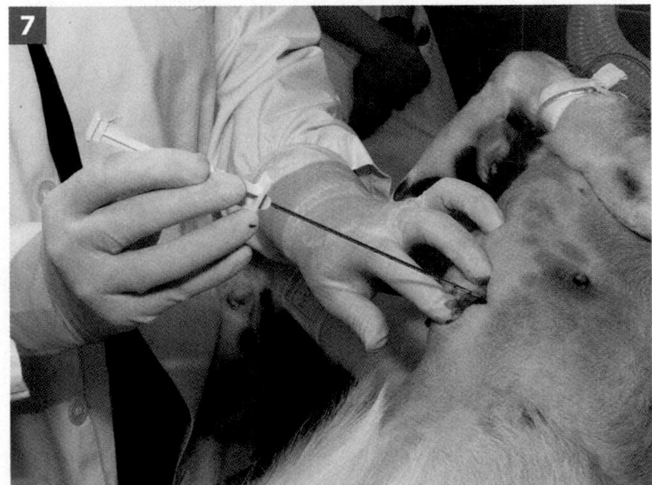

The needle is advanced to the liver and inserted into the liver parenchyma with the needle still in the closed position.

8. Push the inner obturator into the liver.

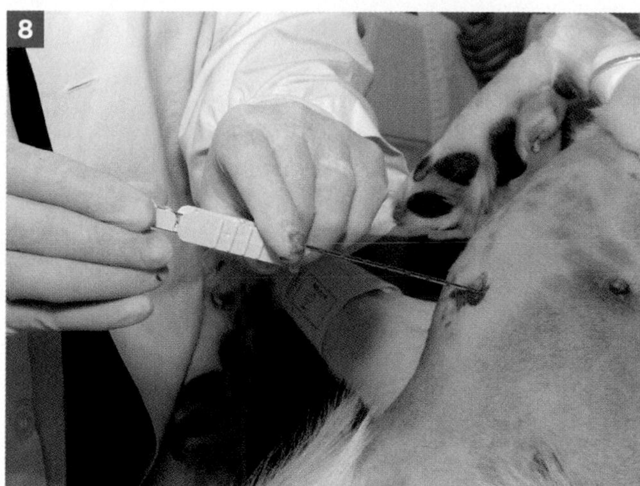

Advancing the inner obturator into the liver.

9. Advance the outer cannula over the inner obturator, cutting a core of liver tissue.

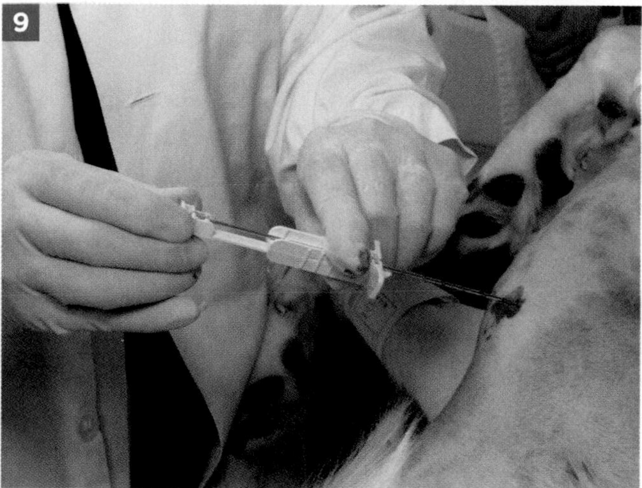

Advancing the outer cannula over the inner obturator.

10. Withdraw the entire apparatus. Push the inner obturator forward to reveal the biopsy. Use a small-gauge needle to tease the piece of liver off of the biopsy needle.

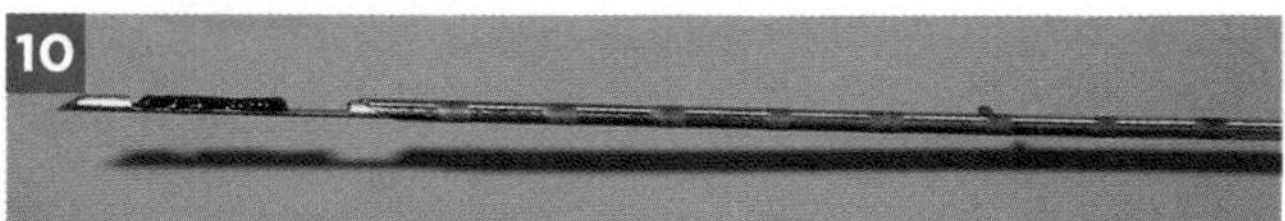

Pushing the inner obturator forward to reveal the biopsy.

POTENTIAL COMPLICATIONS

Hemorrhage
Laceration of viscera
Puncture of gallbladder or bile peritonitis
Pneumothorax if needle is advanced through diaphragm into lung

Caution: The diagnostic accuracy of blindly obtained percutaneous liver biopsies is significantly lower than biopsies obtained under visualization during exploratory laparotomy or laparoscopy.

PROCEDURE 9-6

Fine-Needle Aspiration Biopsy of the Liver

In some patients with diffuse liver disease, fine-needle aspiration of the liver provides sufficient diagnostic information so that tissue biopsy may be delayed or avoided. This technique is most effective for confirming a suspected diagnosis of hepatic lipidosis or hepatic lymphoma when done blindly, and may be useful in the diagnosis of other hepatic neoplasms when performed with ultrasound guidance.

EQUIPMENT

- 1½- or 2½-inch, 22-gauge spinal needle with a stylet

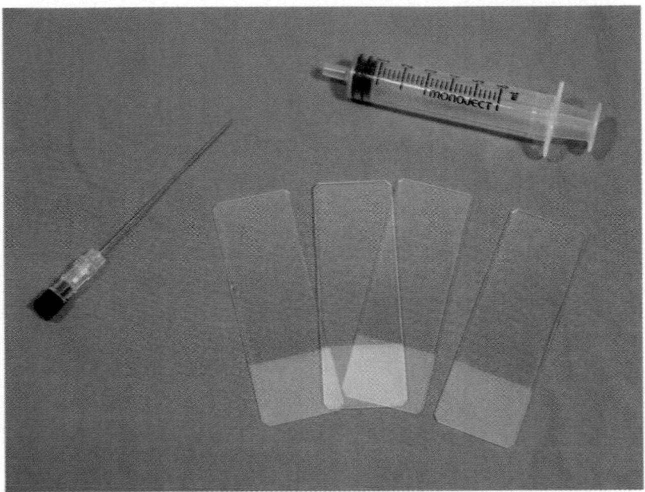

Equipment required for fine-needle aspiration of the liver.

TECHNIQUE

1. Sedate the animal as required to have it remain immobile during the procedure.
2. Place the animal in dorsal recumbency with the chest higher than the abdomen and the entire body tilted to the right to maximize the exposure of the liver and decrease the risk of gallbladder puncture.

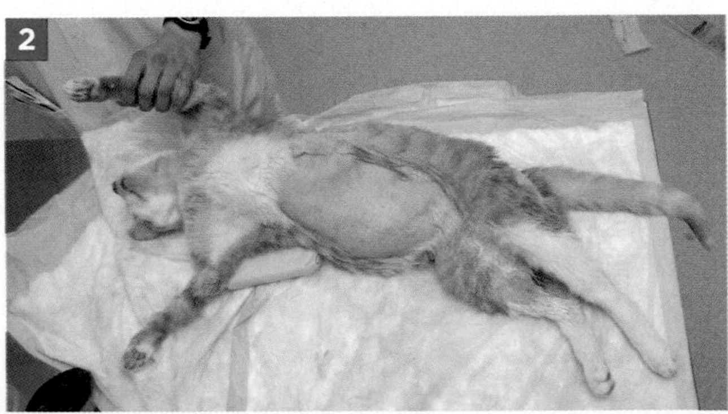

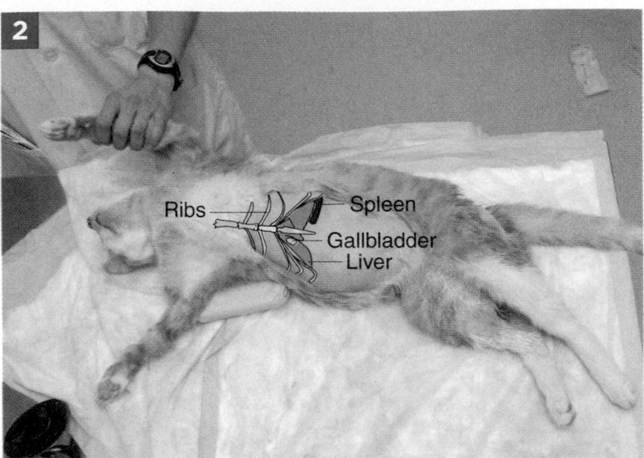

This cat is positioned properly to maximize the exposure of the liver and decrease the risk of gallbladder puncture.

3. Clip and prep the anterior ventral abdomen. Wear gloves and use aseptic technique.
4. Use ultrasound guidance or the positioning and landmark techniques described as follows to advance the needle to the desired region within the liver parenchyma.
5. When there is diffuse or extensive multifocal disease, "blind" aspirates can be obtained using similar landmarks as used for percutaneous liver biopsy. The entrance site for the needle is at the level of the xiphoid, half the distance from the midline to the left costal arch at that level. Advance the needle craniodorsally at an angle approximately 30 degrees left of the midsagittal plane (to avoid the gallbladder).

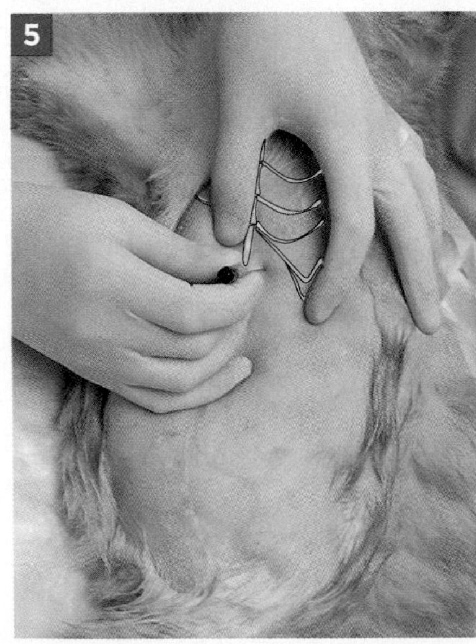

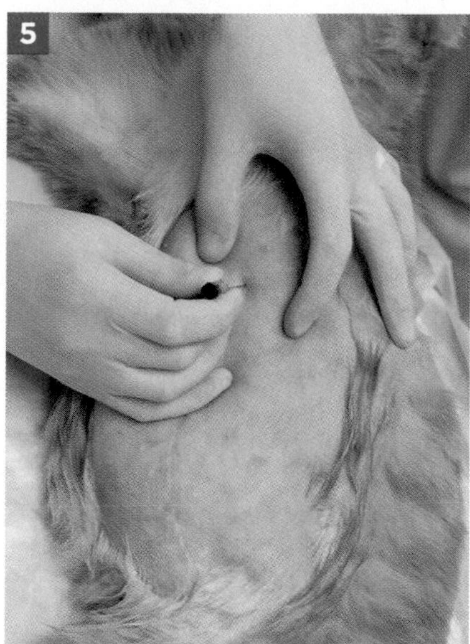

The entrance site for the needle is at the level of the xiphoid, half the distance from the midline to the left costal arch at that level.

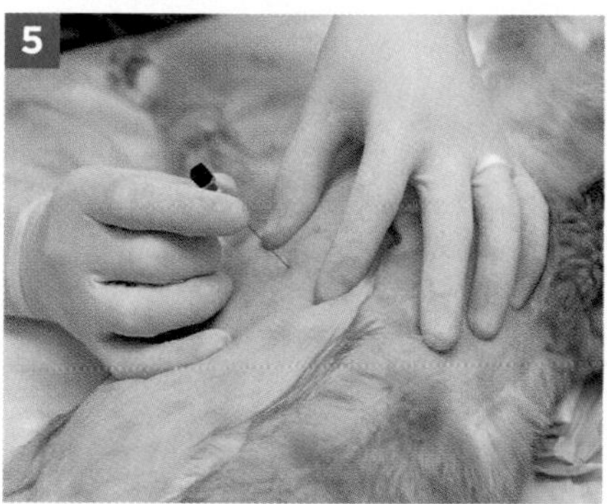

The biopsy needle is advanced into the liver craniodorsally at an angle approximately 30 degrees left of the midsagittal plane (to avoid the gallbladder).

6. Remove the stylet.

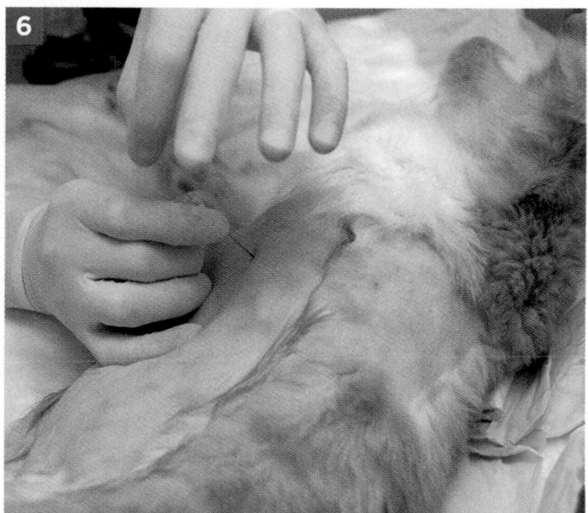

The needle stylet is removed.

7. Holding the needle by the hub, advance the needle several times into the liver while twisting the needle. This forces cells into the needle.

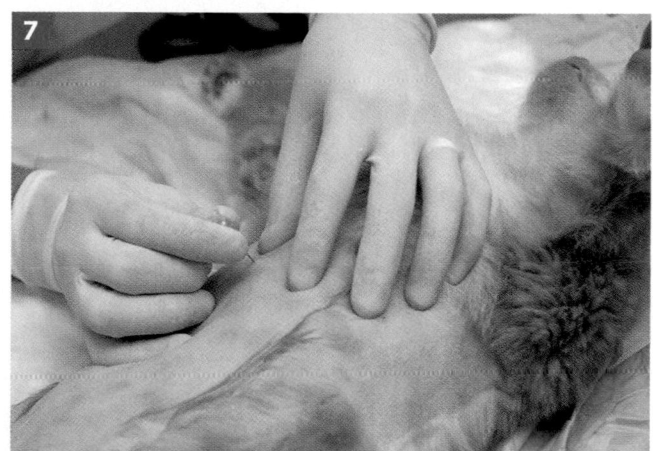

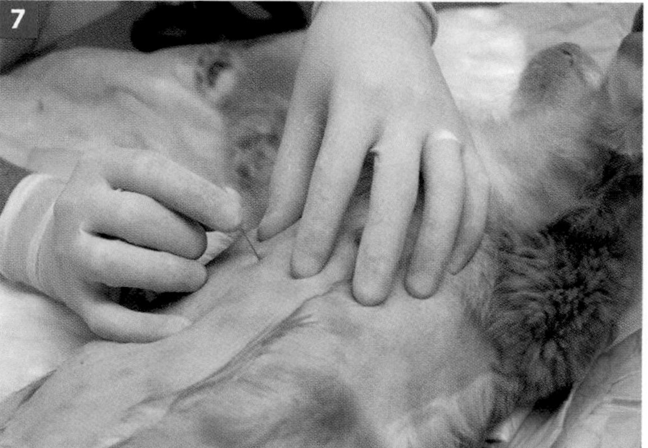

PROCEDURE 9-6 Fine-Needle Aspiration Biopsy of the Liver—cont'd

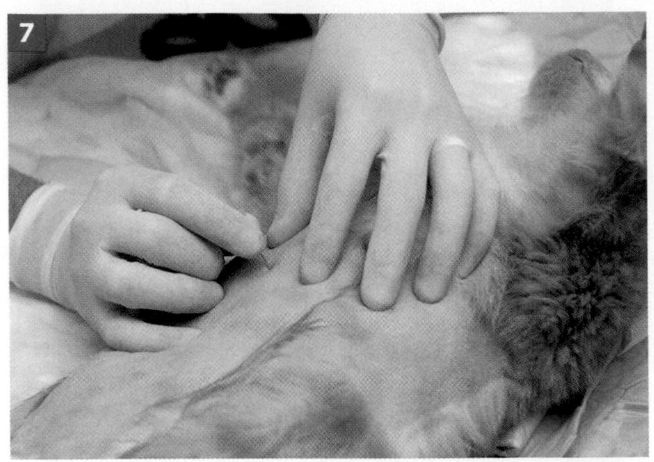

Advancing the needle several times into the liver while twisting, to force cells into the needle.

8. Remove the needle from the abdomen.
9. Attach a syringe with 2 to 3 mL of air inside.
10. Squirt the sample onto a glass microscope slide.
11. Smear gently and stain for cytologic evaluation.

POTENTIAL COMPLICATIONS

Complications are minimized by the use of a small-gauge needle.

Hemorrhage and puncture of gallbladder, and bile peritonitis are still potential complications.

Warning: The diagnostic accuracy of this technique is low, except in patients with diffuse hepatic lymphoma or cats with primary hepatic lipidosis.

PROCEDURE 9-7
Abdominocentesis

PURPOSE

To collect a sample of peritoneal fluid for analysis

INDICATIONS

The presence of an abdominal effusion

CONTRAINDICATIONS AND WARNINGS

1. Care must be taken to avoid perforation or laceration of enlarged abdominal organs.
2. Whenever possible, abdominal radiographs should be performed prior to performing abdominocentesis because air may enter the peritoneal cavity during this procedure and be mistaken for spontaneous pneumoperitoneum.
3. It is common for abdominocentesis to be negative if only a small volume of effusion (<6 mL/kg) is present.

EQUIPMENT

- 14- to 22-gauge butterfly catheter or 1{1/2}-inch needle with extension tubing
- Syringe
- Tubes

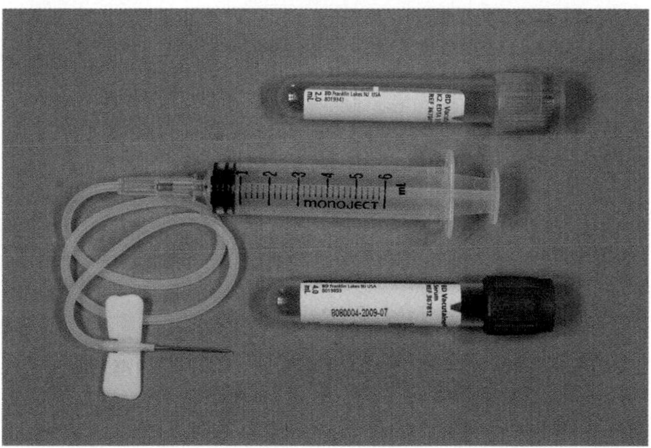

Equipment required for abdominocentesis.

POSITIONING AND RESTRAINT

The animal should be restrained in lateral recumbency or should be standing. No sedation is usually required.

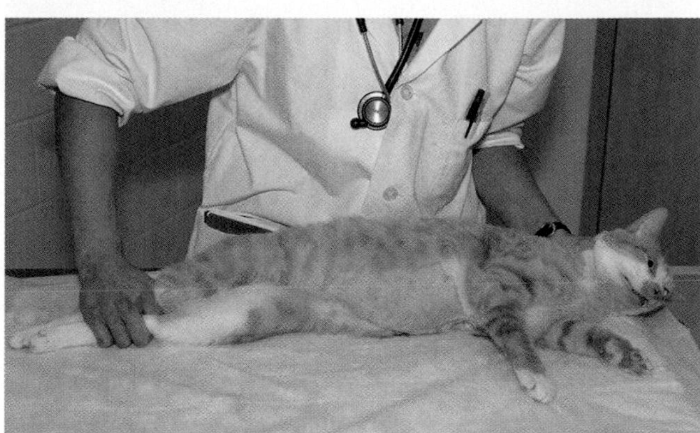

A cat restrained in lateral recumbency for abdominocentesis.

SPECIAL ANATOMY

In an animal with a large volume of effusion, the ideal site is slightly caudal to the umbilicus on midline.

TECHNIQUE

1. Clip the ventral midline and clean with a disinfectant scrub.
2. Attach the butterfly catheter or needle with extension tubing to the syringe, and slowly introduce the needle into the peritoneal cavity on midline 2 to 3 cm caudal to the umbilicus.

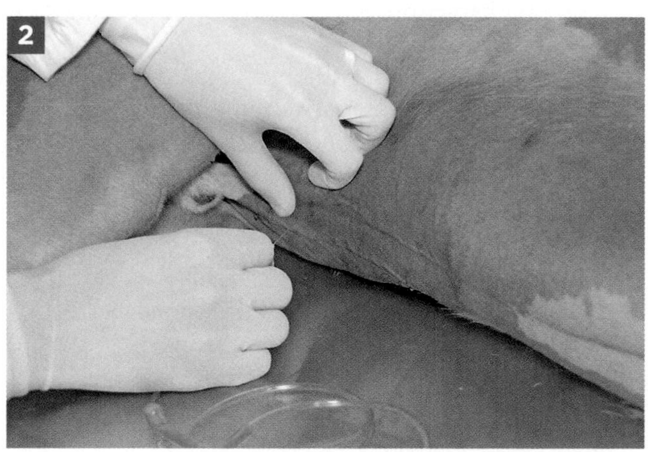

PROCEDURE 9-7 Abdominocentesis—cont'd

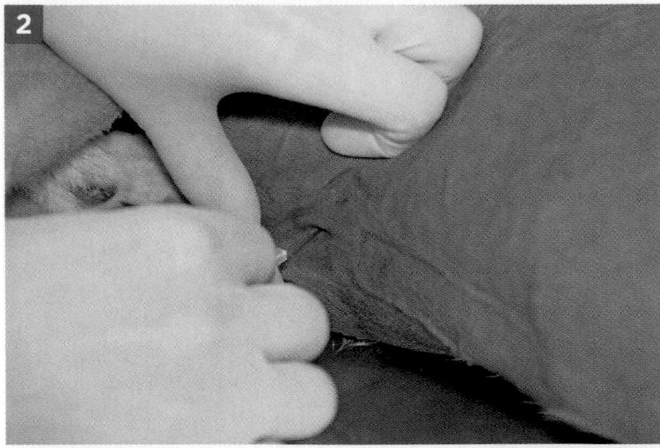

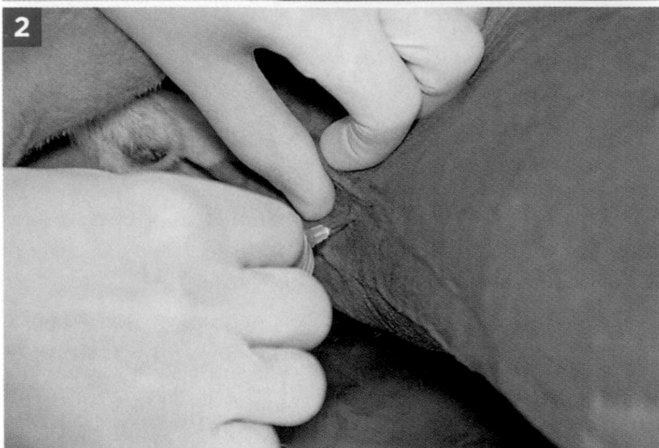

A needle is slowly introduced into the peritoneal cavity on midline 2 to 3 cm caudal to the umbilicus for abdominocentesis.

3. Apply gentle suction on the syringe as the needle enters the abdominal cavity.
4. If no fluid is obtained, withdraw the needle slightly and redirect or change the animal's position.
5. If still no fluid is obtained, remove the syringe from the needle and rotate the needle 360 degrees along its axis to clear the tip and redirect the needle.
6. Collect fluid directly into a syringe and submit for cytologic analysis and, when warranted, for biochemical and microbial analysis.

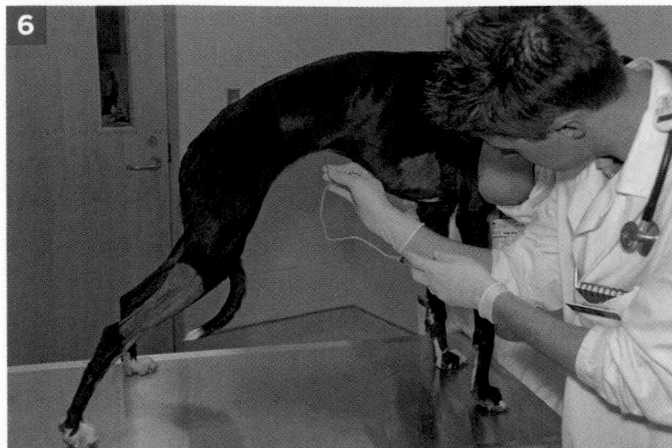

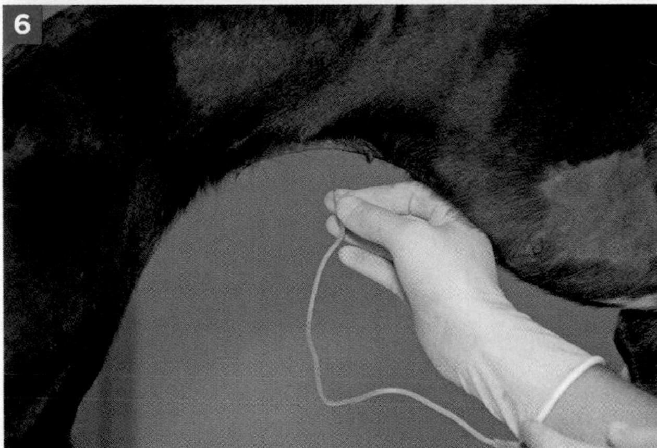

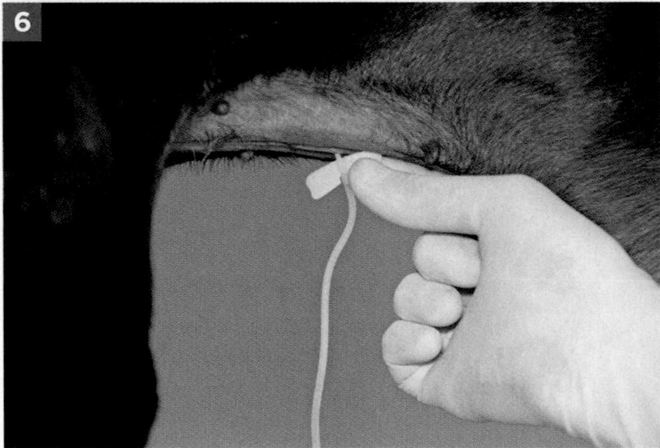

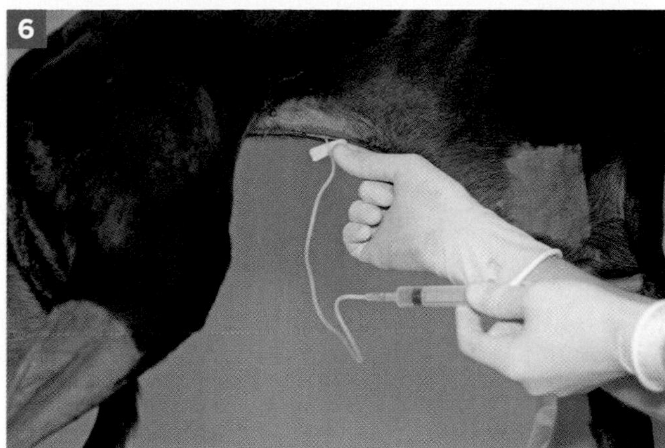

Abdominocentesis in a standing dog.

RESULTS

This figure shows the cytology of an abdominal effusion from a dog with septic peritonitis caused by dehiscence of a full-thickness intestinal biopsy site.

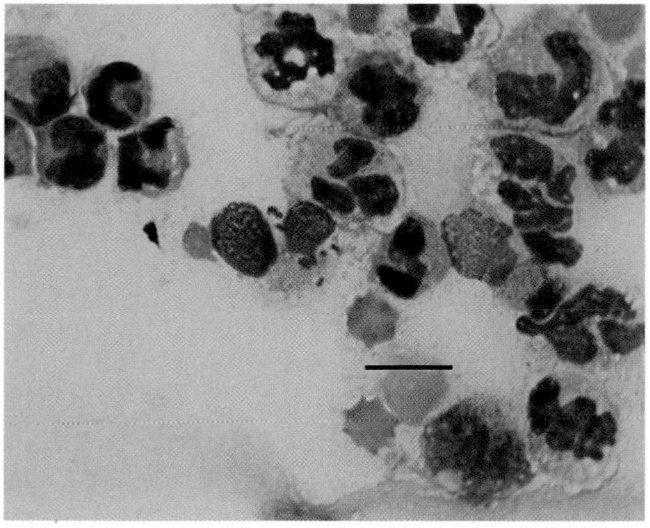

Abdominal effusion from a 6-year-old Bulldog with septic peritonitis following dehiscence of a full-thickness intestinal biopsy site. Large numbers of degenerate neutrophils are present, some of which have engulfed bacteria of different species. **(Courtesy Dr. Marion Jackson, University of Saskatchewan.)**

These figures show the gross and microscopic appearance of a viscous, yellow abdominal effusion from a cat with the wet form of feline infectious peritonitis.

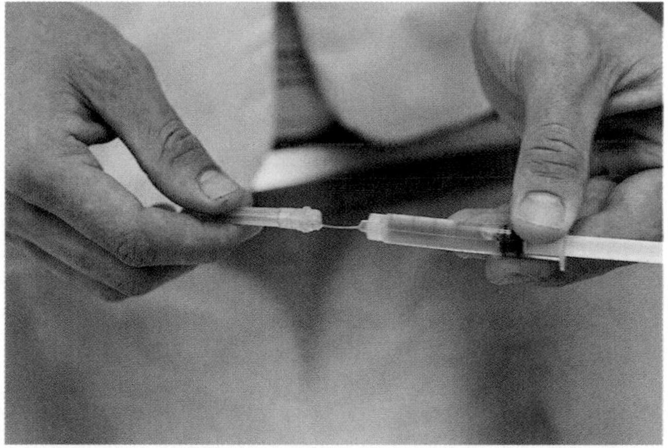

Viscous, yellow abdominal effusion collected from a cat. The total protein content of this fluid was 65 g/L.

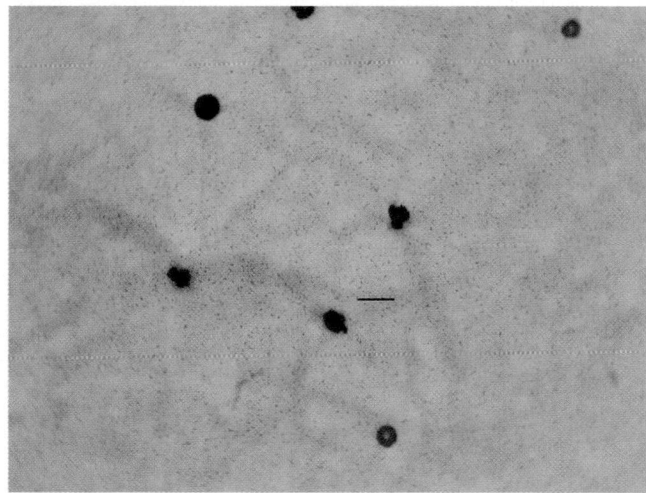

Cellularity of the fluid is high, with most cells (85%) nondegenerate neutrophils as well as some macrophages and occasional lymphocytes. The basophilic stippling in the background suggests a high protein content. This nonseptic pyogranulomatous exudate is typical of the effusion found in cats with the wet form of feline infectious peritonitis. **(Courtesy Dr. Marion Jackson, University of Saskatchewan.)**

PROCEDURE 9-8

Diagnostic Peritoneal Lavage (DPL)

PURPOSE

To collect a washing of the peritoneal cavity for diagnostic evaluation

INDICATIONS

1. The presence of a small volume of abdominal effusion that cannot be sampled by abdominocentesis
2. Animals with unexplained acute abdominal pain together with a fever or inflammatory leukogram
3. Animals with suspected postoperative intestinal surgical dehiscence
4. Animals suffering blunt or penetrating trauma, when rupture of a hollow viscous is suspected

CONTRAINDICATIONS AND WARNINGS

Fluid collected by DPL must be interpreted with caution because dilution of total cell count and chemical analytes can occur.

EQUIPMENT

- 14-gauge 2½- to 3½-inch over-the-needle catheter
- Warm (37° C) isotonic crystalloid solution (Normosol-R, lactated Ringer's, or 0.9% saline)
- IV fluid administration set; rapid infusion IV pressure bag
- 3-mL syringe, 14- to 22-gauge butterfly catheter or 1½-inch needle with extension tubing for fluid collection
- Tubes
- Sterile gloves

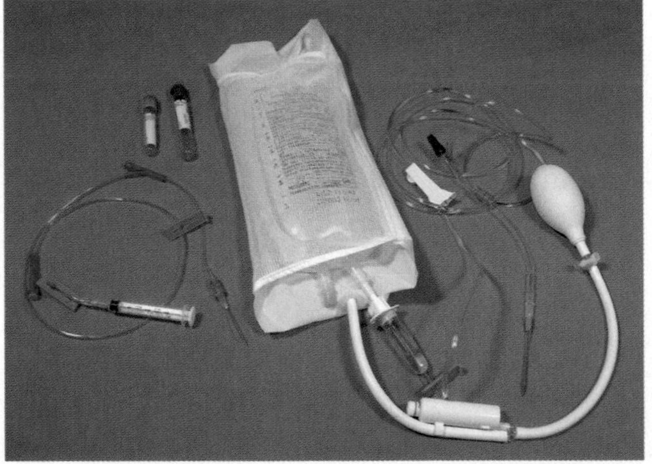

Equipment required for diagnostic peritoneal lavage.

POSITIONING AND RESTRAINT

Restrain the animal in lateral recumbency

TECHNIQUE

1. Clip the ventral abdomen in a 10 × 10–cm square centered on the umbilicus and aseptically prepare the clipped region.
2. Wearing sterile gloves, insert the over-the-needle catheter into the abdominal cavity 2 cm caudal and 2 cm to the right of the umbilicus.
3. Once the needle has penetrated the abdominal wall, advance the catheter slowly with a gentle twisting motion to prevent inadvertent puncture of any abdominal organs.
4. Withdraw the needle, and collect and analyze any fluid that can be retrieved from the catheter.
5. Instill 20 mL/kg of warmed saline into the abdominal cavity over a period of 5 minutes.
6. Remove the catheter and roll the animal from side to side, or allow the animal to walk while the abdomen is massaged to distribute the fluid.
7. Lay the animal in lateral recumbency, and aseptically prepare the abdomen as previously described.
8. Perform abdominocentesis to remove at least 1 mL of the lavage fluid for analysis.

SAMPLE ANALYSIS

1. Degenerate neutrophils with bacteria, vegetable fibers, or a white blood cell count more than 2000/mL suggest septic peritonitis, requiring surgery.
2. Pink fluid indicates intraabdominal hemorrhage, with a packed cell volume (PVC) greater than 4% suggesting significant hemorrhage.
3. Further analysis of lavage fluid may reveal increased bilirubin or bile crystals indicating biliary tree rupture, increased creatinine, and potassium compared with serum suggesting urinary tract rupture, or nonseptic inflammation and high amylase levels compared with serum suggesting acute pancreatitis.

Urinary System Techniques

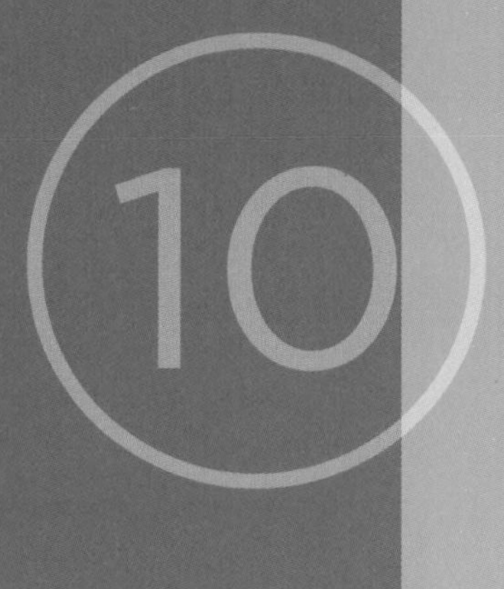

PROCEDURE 10-1

Urine Collection by Cystocentesis

PURPOSE

To collect urine directly from the bladder

INDICATIONS

1. To obtain a urine sample not contaminated by bacteria, cells, and debris from the lower urinary tract
2. To aid localization of hematuria, pyuria, and bacteruria

CONTRAINDICATIONS

1. Bleeding disorders
2. Potential pyometra or prostatic abscess that could be inadvertently ruptured by this technique
3. Bladder cancer that may be seeded to the peritoneum by this technique
4. Animals with urinary outflow obstruction, or animals likely to have urinary outflow obstruction before the hole created in the bladder by this technique has a chance to heal

EQUIPMENT

- 22-gauge needle, 1 inch or 1½ inches
- 6-mL syringe
- Alcohol

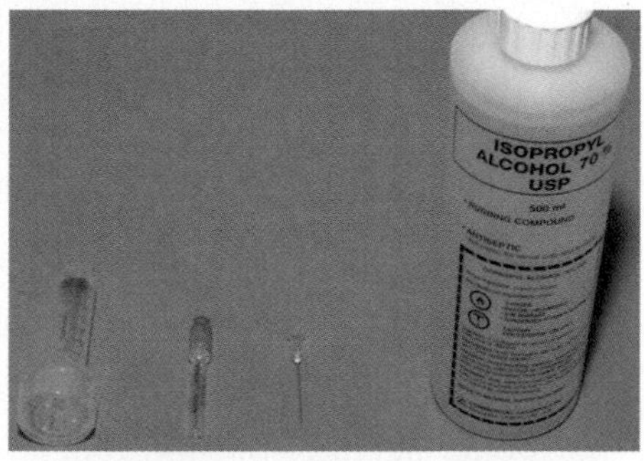

Equipment required for cystocentesis.

TECHNIQUE

1. Restrain the patient in dorsal recumbency.
2. Palpate the bladder, if possible, to assess size and location, and clean the skin surface with alcohol.

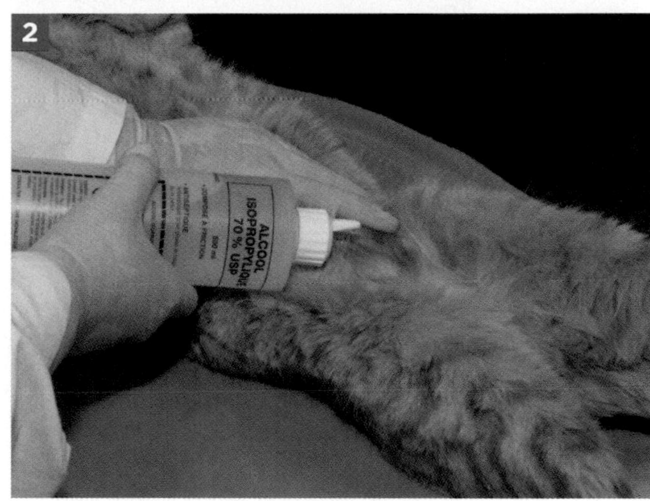

Cleaning the skin surface with alcohol.

PROCEDURE 10-1 Urine Collection by Cystocentesis—cont'd

3. Localize and immobilize the urinary bladder if possible. Do not apply excessive digital pressure before, during, or following cystocentesis.

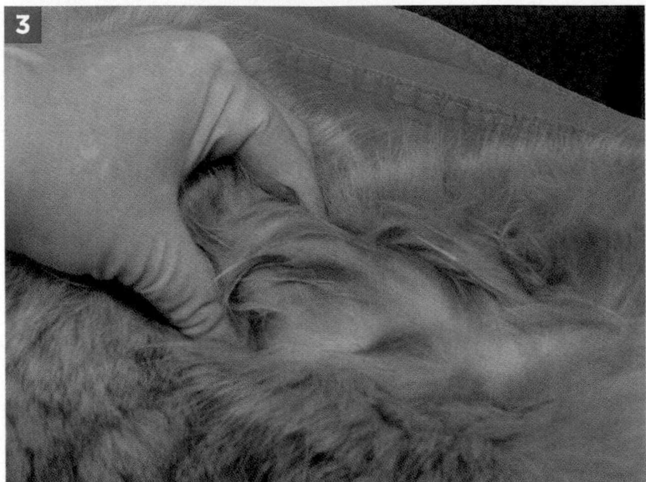

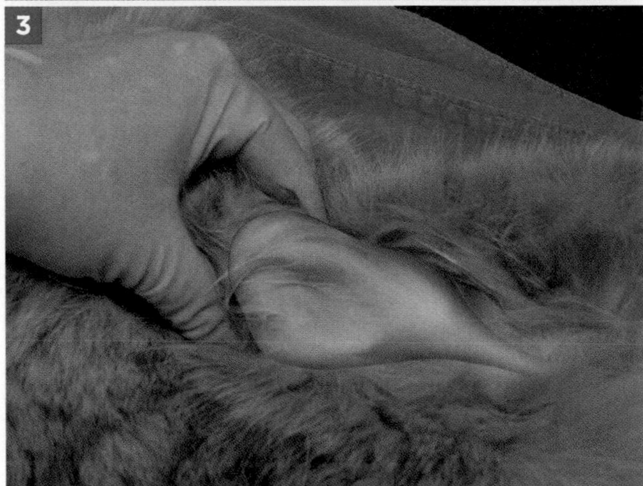

Locating and immobilizing the urinary bladder by gentle palpation.

4. Attach the needle to the syringe.
5. Advance the needle through the ventral abdominal wall to the bladder, taking care to insert the needle through the bladder wall at an oblique angle directed dorsocaudally, so that as the bladder shrinks, the needle tip remains within the bladder lumen. Apply suction.

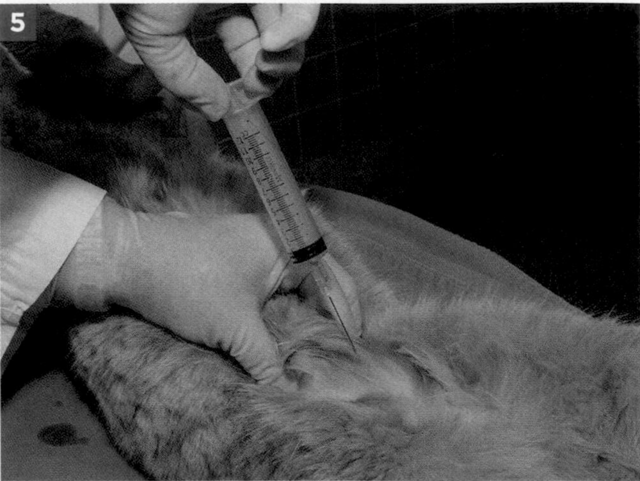

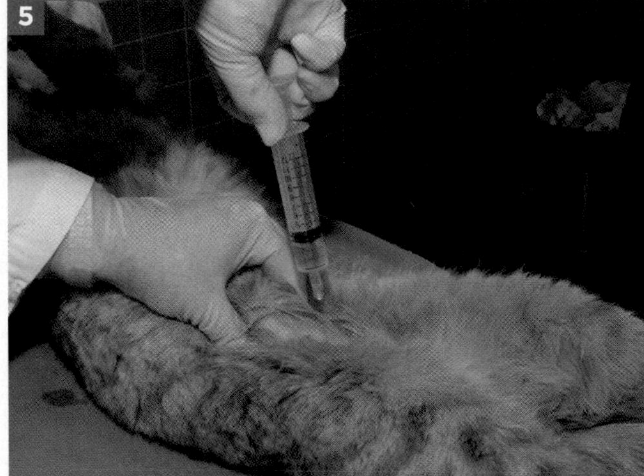

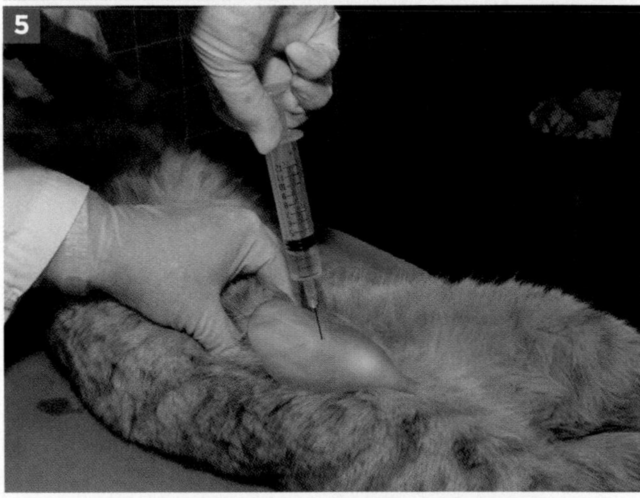

Directing the needle dorsocaudally during cystocentesis.

6. Release all suction once the sample has been obtained to minimize the chance of sample contamination.
7. Withdraw the needle from the abdomen.
8. Change the needle and place the urine sample in a tube.

ALTERNATE TECHNIQUE: BLIND CYSTOCENTESIS

If the bladder cannot be palpated because the patient is tense or obese, attempt a blind cystocentesis. This is usually successful if the bladder is moderately full.

1. Restrain the patient in dorsal recumbency.

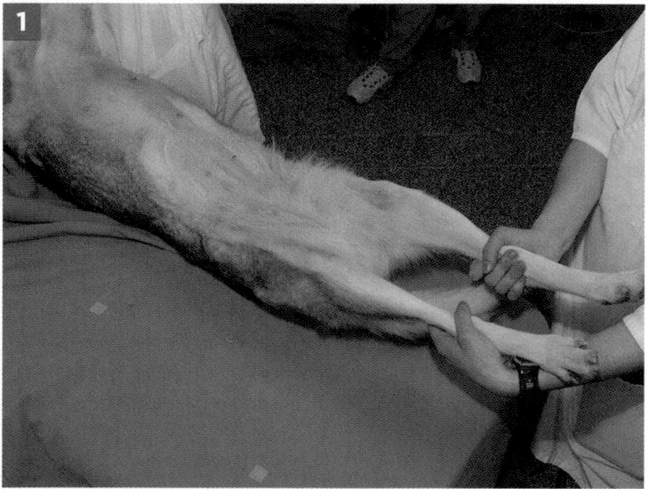

Restraint in dorsal recumbency for blind cystocentesis.

2. Apply alcohol liberally to the caudal abdomen.

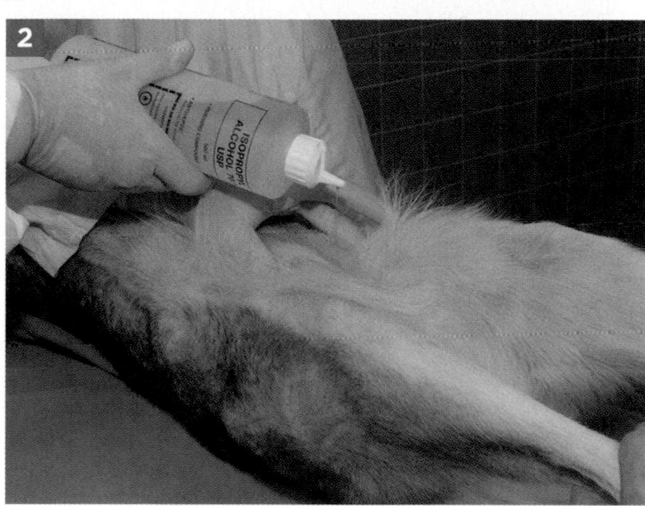

Applying alcohol liberally to the caudal abdomen.

3. Apply some pressure to the abdomen to push the abdominal contents caudally and estimate the location of the bladder. In females, the cystocentesis needle should usually enter the abdomen where the alcohol pools. In male dogs, the needle should be inserted lateral to the penis, approximately halfway between the tip of the prepuce and the scrotum.
4. Attach the needle to the syringe.
5. Advance the needle through the ventral abdominal wall to the bladder, taking care to insert the needle through the bladder wall at an oblique angle directed dorsocaudally, so that as the bladder shrinks, the needle tip remains within the bladder lumen. Apply suction.

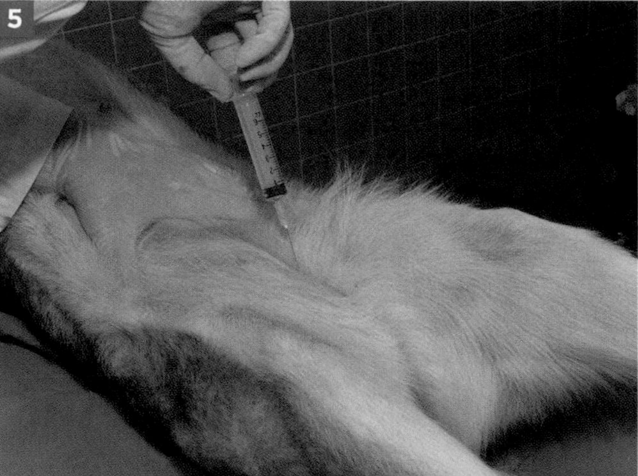

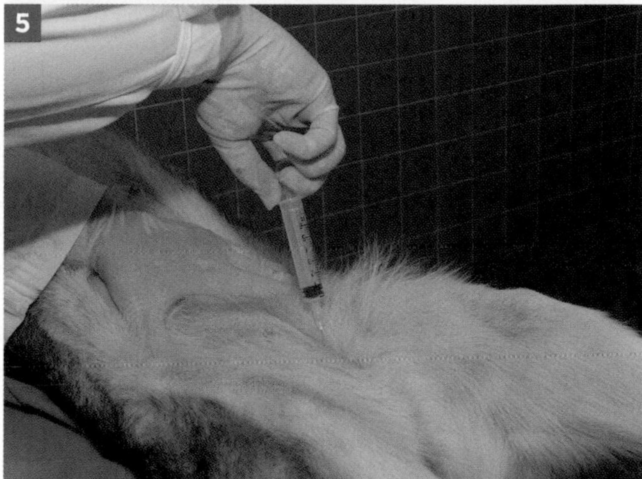

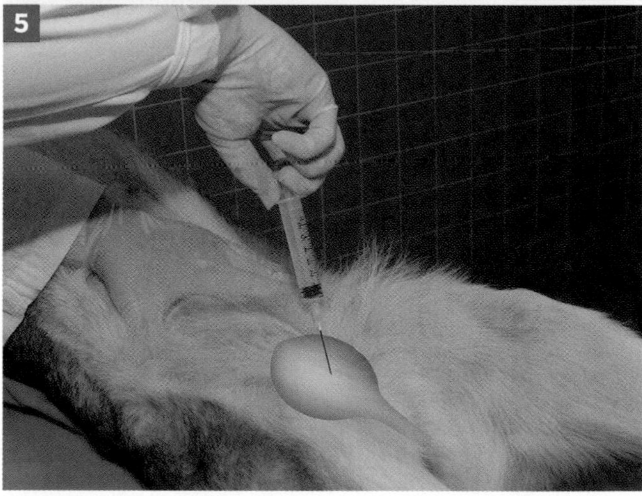

The needle is directed dorsocaudally so that as the bladder shrinks, the needle tip remains within the bladder lumen.

6. Release all suction once the sample has been obtained to minimize the chance of sample contamination.
7. Withdraw the needle from the abdomen.
8. Change the needle and place the urine sample in a tube.

PROCEDURE 10-2

Urinary Catheterization: Male Cat

PURPOSE

To provide access to the urinary bladder to collect urine, relieve urinary obstruction, or instill substances

INDICATIONS

1. Collection of urine for urinalysis or culture
2. Collection of accurately timed volumes of urine for renal function studies
3. Monitoring urinary output
4. Instilling radiographic contrast material
5. Evaluation of the urethral lumen for calculi, masses, or strictures
6. Collection of a urine sample for cytologic evaluation when bladder neoplasia is suspected
7. To relieve structural or functional urethral obstruction

POTENTIAL COMPLICATIONS

1. Trauma to the urethra or bladder
2. Introduction of infection

EQUIPMENT

- Sterile gloves
- Sterile lubricant
- Sterile flush fluid (saline)
- An appropriate urinary catheter

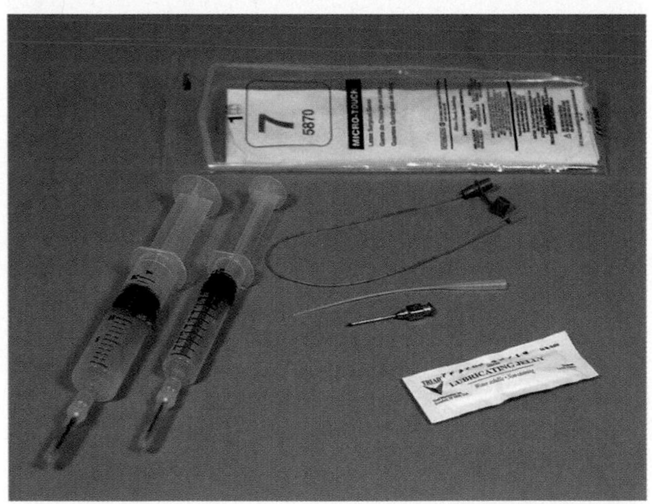

Equipment required to pass a urinary catheter in a male cat.

URINARY CATHETERS USED

1. An open-ended tomcat catheter, which is a 3½ French polypropylene catheter, is typically used to relieve urethral obstruction in cats. This catheter has an open end, allowing flushing during catheterization to resolve urethral blockage and aid passage. This stiff catheter is not recommended for use as an indwelling catheter because it causes bladder trauma and urethral irritation.

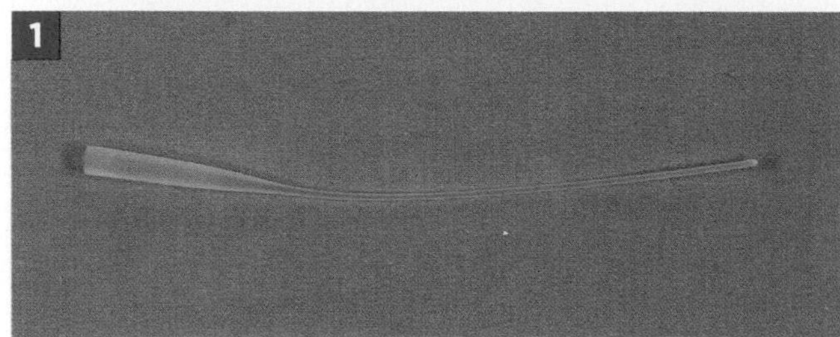

Open-ended tomcat catheter.

2. A soft infant feeding tube, consisting of 3½ or 5 French polyethylene tubing, is most often used as an indwelling catheter following relief of urethral obstruction. This catheter may also be used to collect a urine sample from a cat without urethral obstruction.

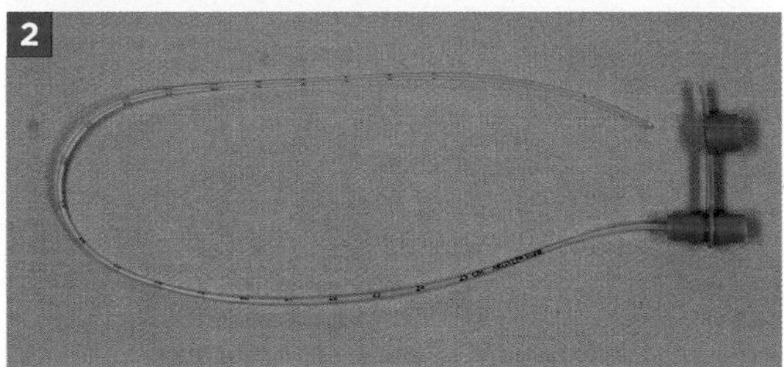

Soft polyethylene infant feeding tube.

3. An open-ended olive-tip metal catheter can be used to relieve urethral obstruction. This catheter is stiff to allow passage, has a central lumen to allow flushing, and has a rounded atraumatic tip. This catheter is short, however, and will not reach the bladder lumen.

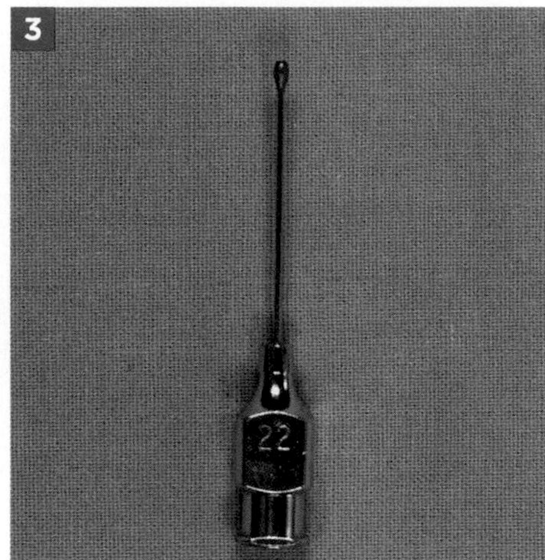

Open-ended olive tip metal catheter.

TECHNIQUE

1. Sedate the cat if necessary.
2. Restrain the cat in lateral or dorsal recumbency.

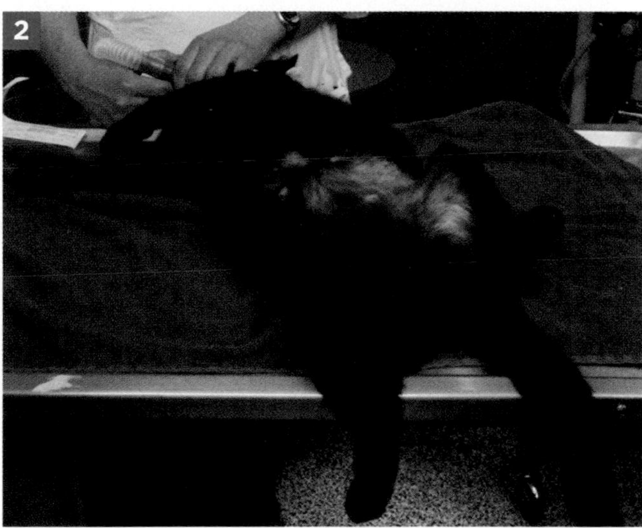

Cat restrained in dorsal recumbency for urethral catheterization.

3. Extrude the penis by pushing the penis caudally while grasping the prepuce and pulling the prepuce forward.
4. Once the penis is extruded, maintain this and hold the penis by tightly pinching the prepuce around the base of the penis.

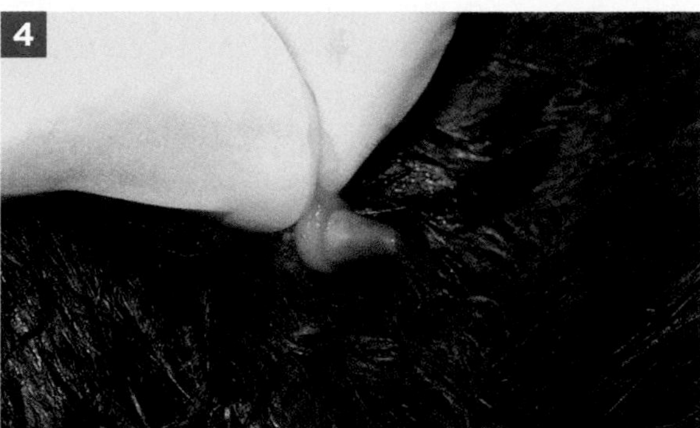

Maintaining the penis extruded by tightly pinching the prepuce around the base of the penis.

5. Gently wash the end of the penis with antiseptic solution and rinse with saline.
6. Pull the penis straight back caudally so that the long axis of the penile urethra is parallel to the vertebral column, reducing the natural curvature of the urethra and simplifying passage of the catheter.

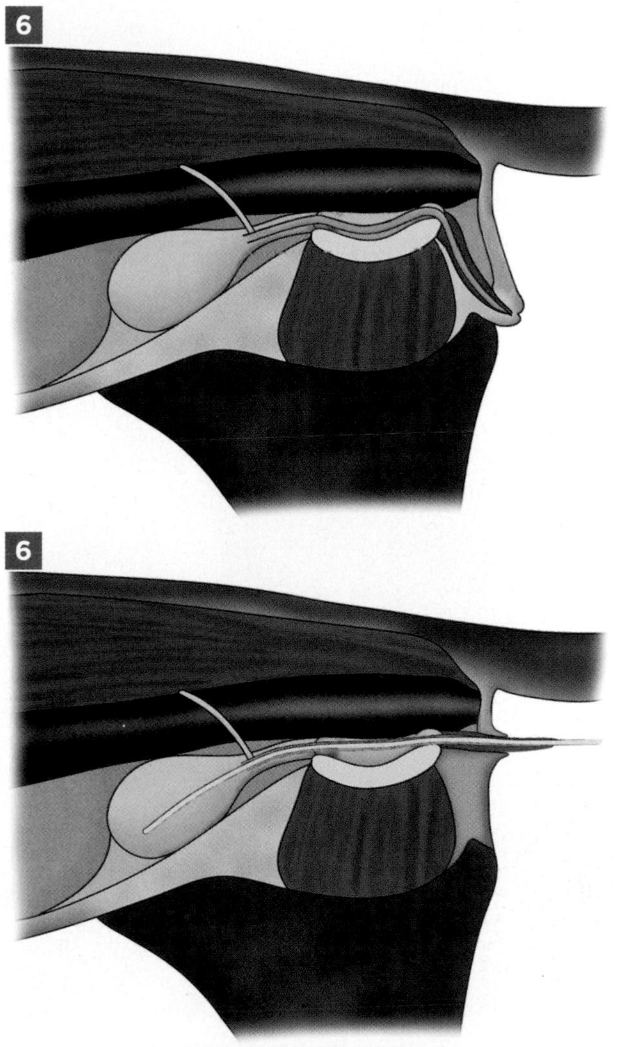

Pulling the extruded penis straight back caudally reduces the natural curvature of the urethra and simplifies passage of a urinary catheter.

PROCEDURE 10-2 Urinary Catheterization: Male Cat—cont'd

7. Lubricate the tip of the catheter with sterile aqueous lubricant

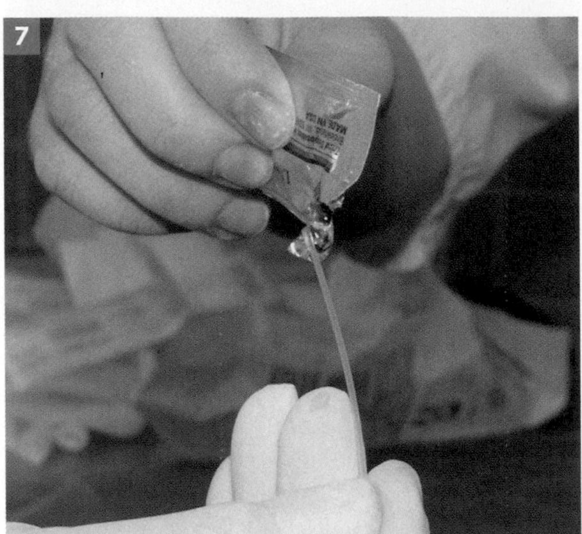

Lubricating the tip of a tomcat urinary catheter.

8. Gently insert the tip of the catheter into the external urethral orifice and advance it into the lumen of the bladder.

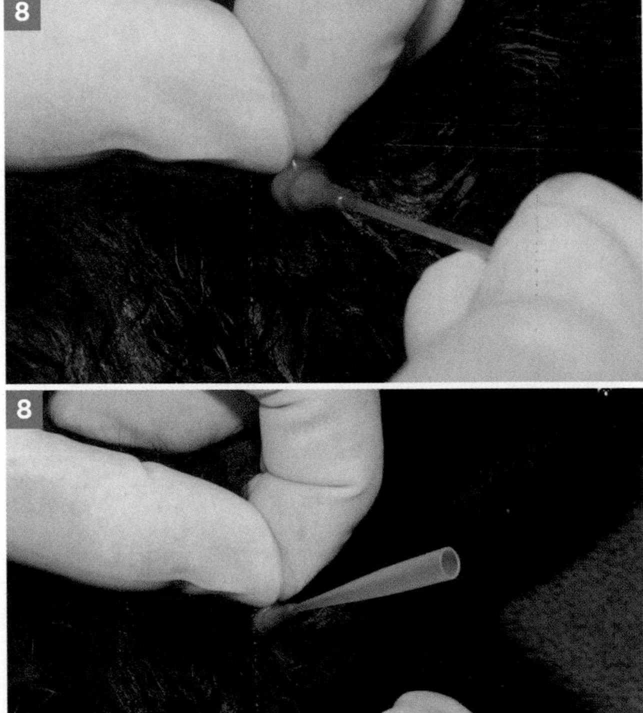

Inserting the catheter tip into the external urethral orifice and advancing it into the bladder lumen.

9. If resistance is met, the catheter can be flushed during advancement with sterile saline—be aware that this will alter test results on the urine obtained.

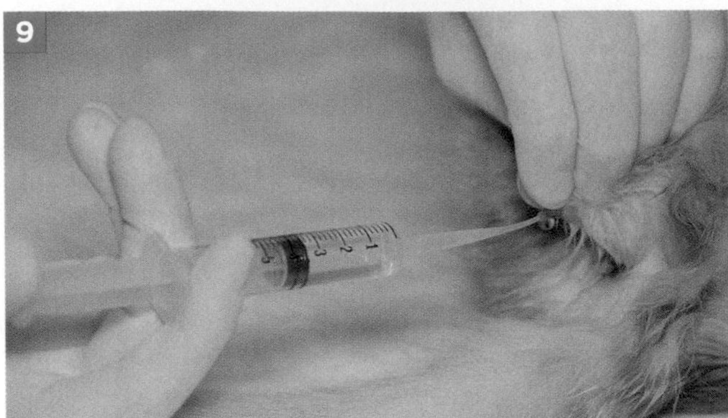

Flushing can help relieve a urethral obstruction and facilitate catheter advancement.

PROCEDURE 10-3

Urinary Catheterization: Male Dog

PURPOSE

To provide access to the urinary bladder to collect urine, relieve urinary obstruction, or instill substances

INDICATIONS

1. Collection of urine for urinalysis or culture
2. Collection of accurately timed volumes of urine for renal function studies
3. Monitoring urinary output
4. Instilling radiographic contrast material
5. Evaluation of the urethral lumen for calculi, masses, or strictures
6. Collection of a urine sample for cytologic evaluation when bladder neoplasia is suspected
7. To relieve structural or functional urethral obstruction

EQUIPMENT

- Sterile gloves
- Sterile lubricant
- An appropriate urinary catheter

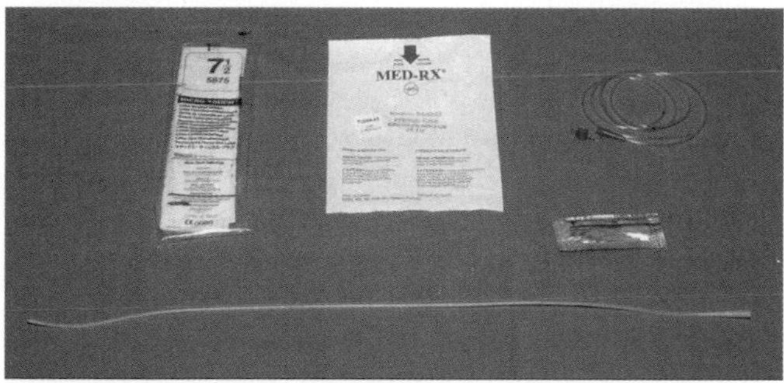

Equipment required to pass a urinary catheter in a male dog.

URINARY CATHETERS USED

1. A 4 to 10 French (depending on size of dog) stiff polypropylene catheter may be used for a single urine collection or for relief of urethral obstruction. This stiff catheter is not recommended for use as an indwelling catheter because it causes bladder trauma and urethral irritation.

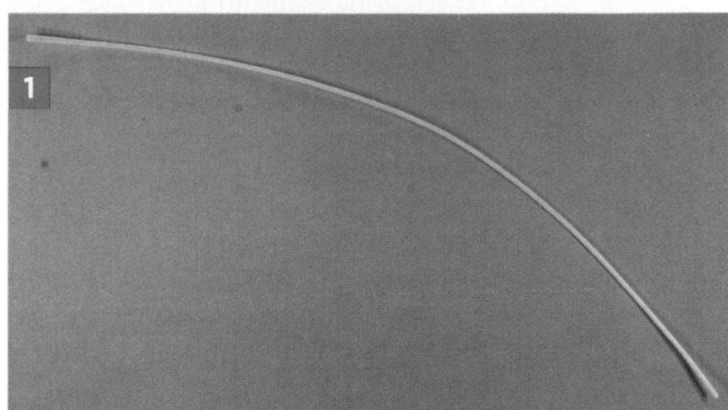

Stiff polypropylene catheter.

2. A 4 to 10 French soft infant feeding tube made of polyethylene tubing can be used to collect a urine sample or as an indwelling catheter.

TECHNIQUE

1. Restrain the dog in lateral or dorsal recumbency.
2. Estimate the length of catheter to be inserted by holding the catheter next to the dog.

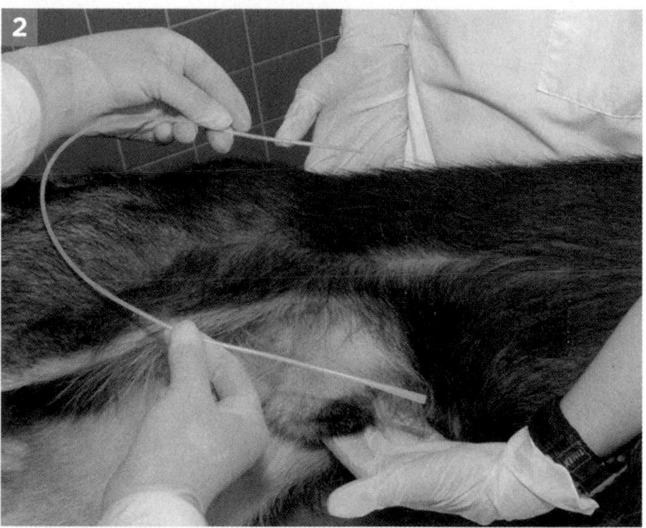

Estimating the length of catheter to be inserted in a dog.

PROCEDURE 10-3 Urinary Catheterization: Male Dog—cont'd

3. Extrude the penis by pushing the penis cranially from the base while pushing the prepuce caudally off the penis. Maintain penile extrusion by continuing to push cranially on the base of the penis and caudally on the prepuce.

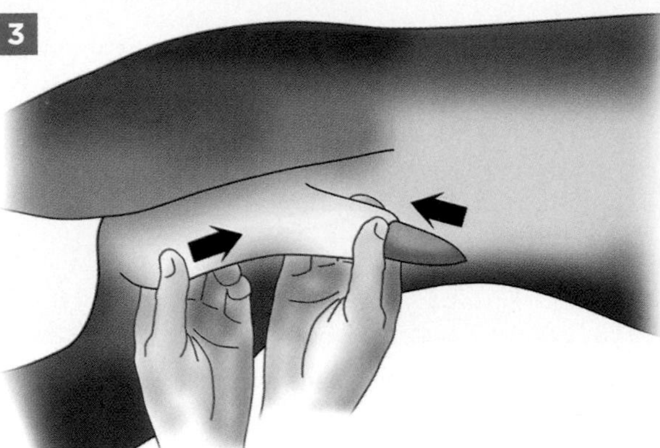

Extruding the penis.

4. Gently wash the end of the penis with antiseptic solution and rinse with saline.

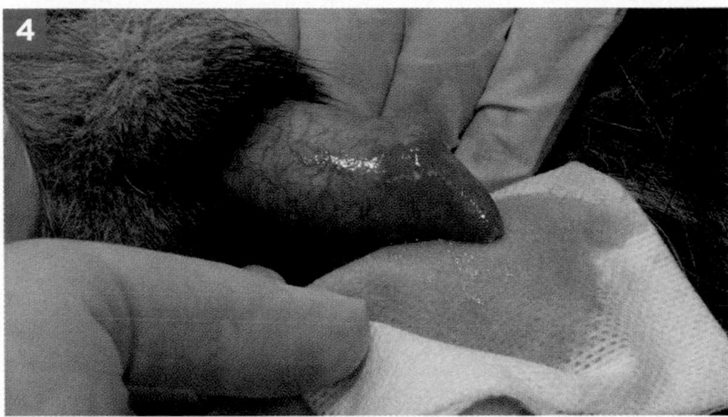

Washing the end of the penis with antiseptic solution.

5. Lubricate the tip of the catheter with sterile aqueous lubricant.

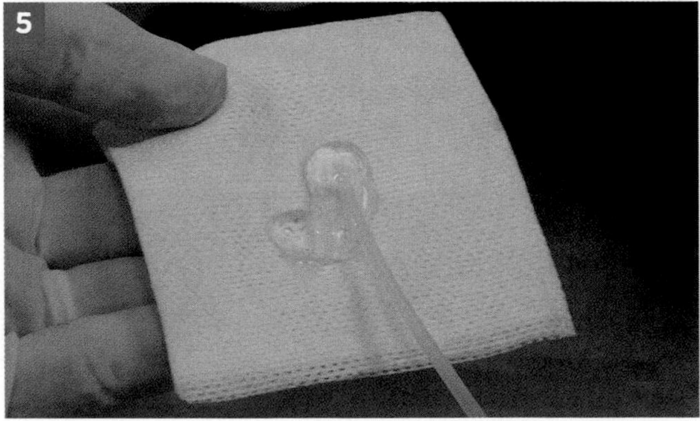

Lubricating the tip of the catheter.

6. Gently insert the tip of the catheter into the external urethral orifice and advance it into the lumen of the bladder, being careful not to advance too far.

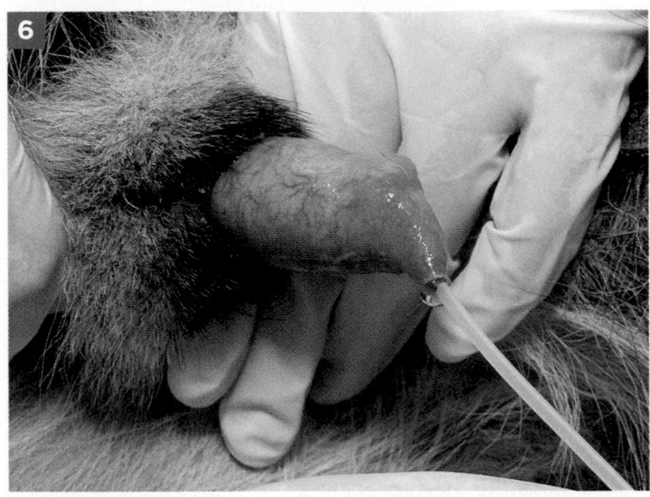

Inserting the tip of the catheter into the external urethral orifice.

7. Collect and discard the first 5 to 6 mL of urine, then collect a sample for urinalysis and culture.

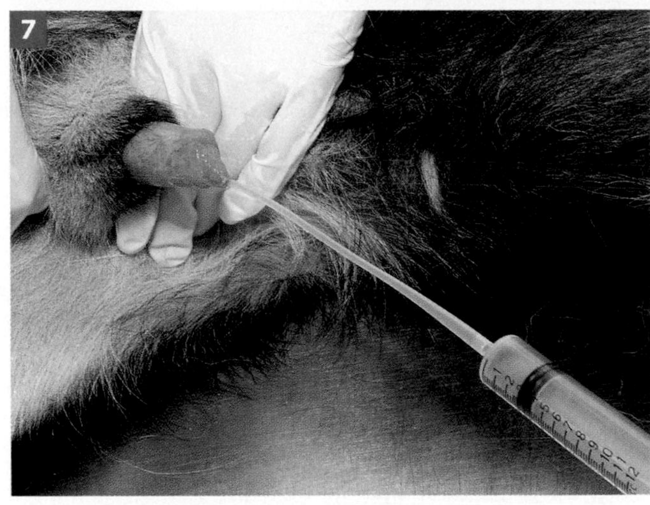

Collecting urine through a urinary catheter.

PROCEDURE 10-4
Urinary Catheterization: Female Dog

EQUIPMENT

- Speculum
- Sterile gloves
- Sterile lubricant
- An appropriate catheter

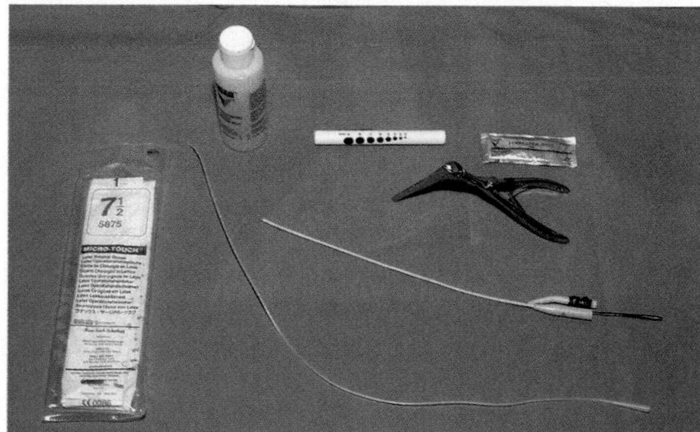

Equipment required to catheterize a female dog.

URINARY CATHETERS USED

1. A 4 to 10 French (depending on size of dog) stiff polypropylene catheter may be used for a single urine collection or for relief of urethral obstruction This stiff catheter is not recommended for use as an indwelling catheter because it causes bladder trauma and urethral irritation.

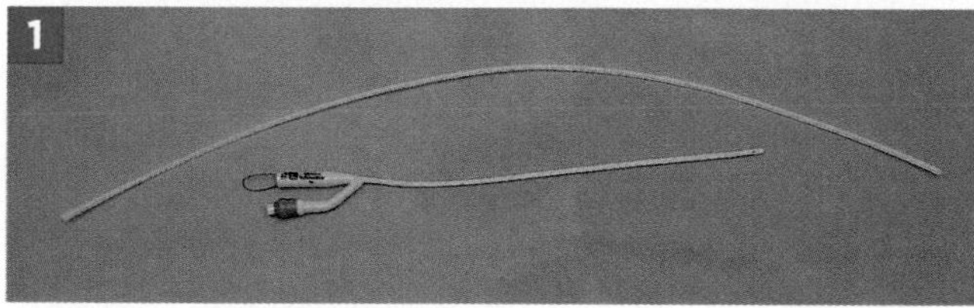

Urinary catheters used in female dogs include a stiff polypropylene catheter and a Foley catheter.

2. A 3 to 10 French Foley with a self-retaining inflatable balloon can be inserted to use as an indwelling catheter. A wire stylet can be used to add rigidity during catheter placement.

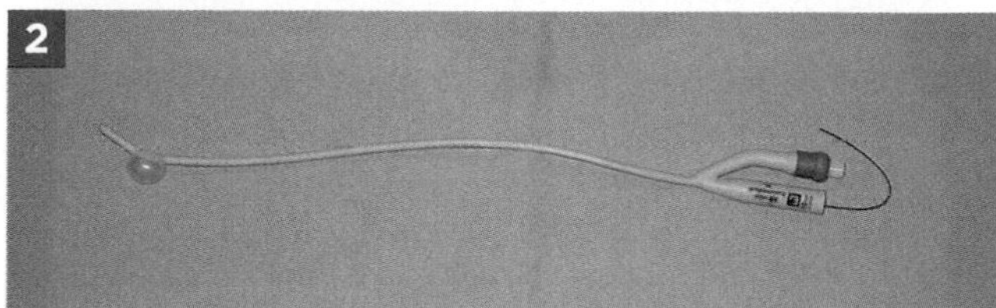

A Foley catheter with a self-retaining inflatable balloon and a wire stylet.

SPECIAL ANATOMY

1. The external urethral orifice lies within a tubercle on the ventral floor of the vagina.
2. When passing the speculum and the catheter, it is important to insert them near the dorsal commissure of the vulva to avoid the sensitive clitoral fossa.
3. The caudal portion of the vagina is the vestibule, which is angled steeply dorsocranial until just past the urethral tubercle.

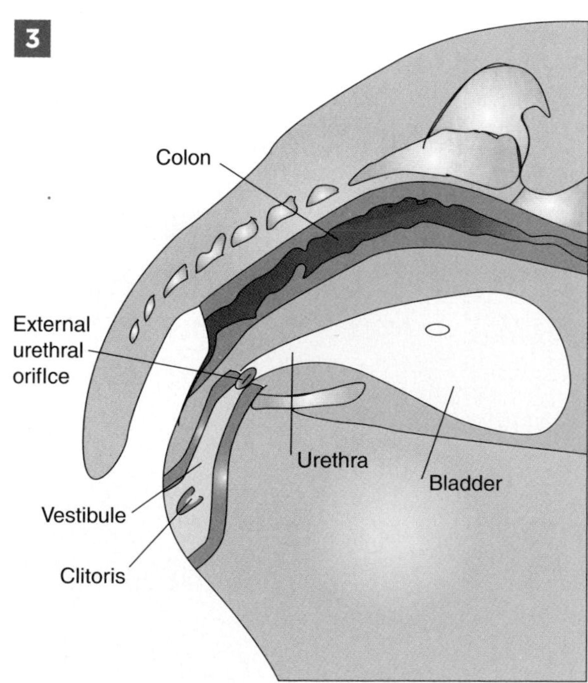

The caudal portion of the vagina is the vestibule, which is angled steeply dorsocranially until just past the urethral tubercle.

PROCEDURE 10-4 Urinary Catheterization: Female Dog—cont'd

4. In the mature small to medium-sized female dog, the external urethral orifice is located on the ventral floor of the vagina, 3 to 5 cm cranial to the ventral commissure of the vulva.

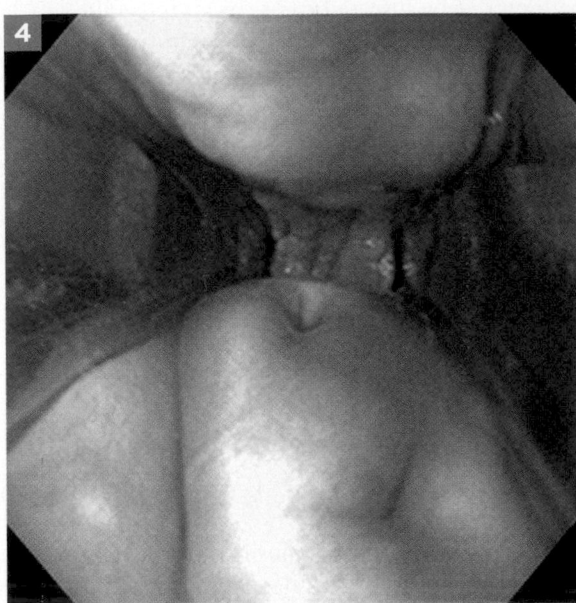

The external urethral orifice is located on the ventral floor of the vagina.

TECHNIQUE: VISUALIZING URETHRAL ORIFICE

1. Sedate the dog if necessary.
2. Restrain the dog standing or else in sternal recumbency with feet off the end of the table.

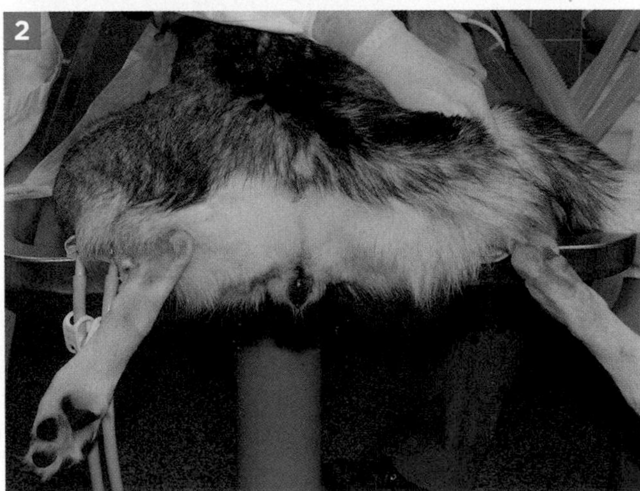

Restraint for urinary catheterization.

3. Cleanse the perivulvar skin and vulva with antiseptic solution and rinse with saline.

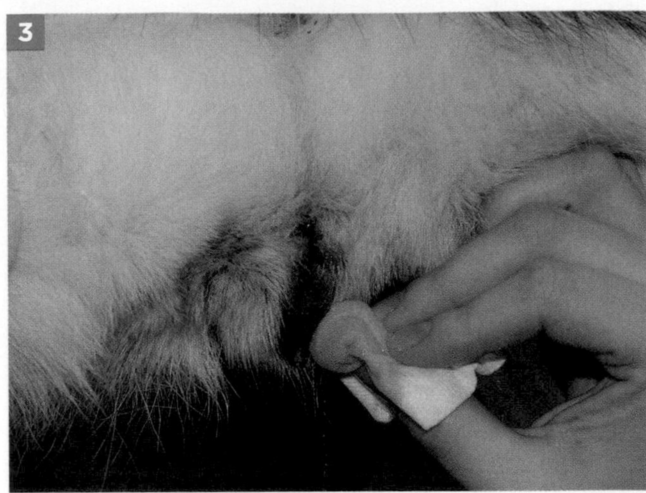

The perivulvar skin and vulva are cleaned with antiseptic solution and rinsed.

4. Flush the vestibule with sterile saline injected through a syringe.

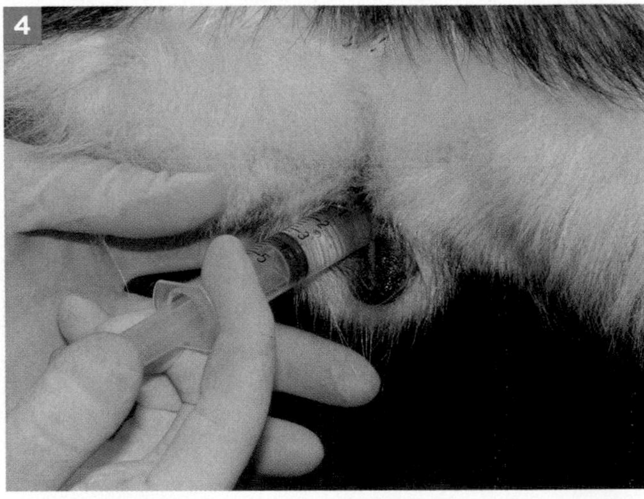

The vagina and vestibule are flushed with sterile saline injected through a syringe.

5. Use a speculum and light source to visualize the tubercle and the external urethral orifice. The speculum must be directly quite dorsally initially after insertion through the vulvar lips to avoid the clitoral fossa. Spread the wings of the speculum to distend the vaginal lumen.

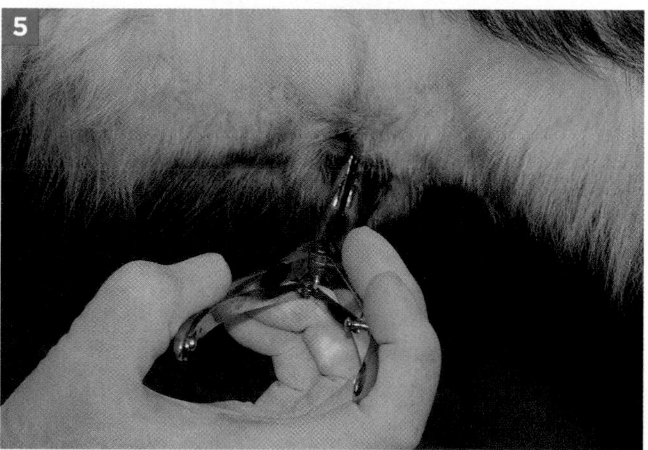

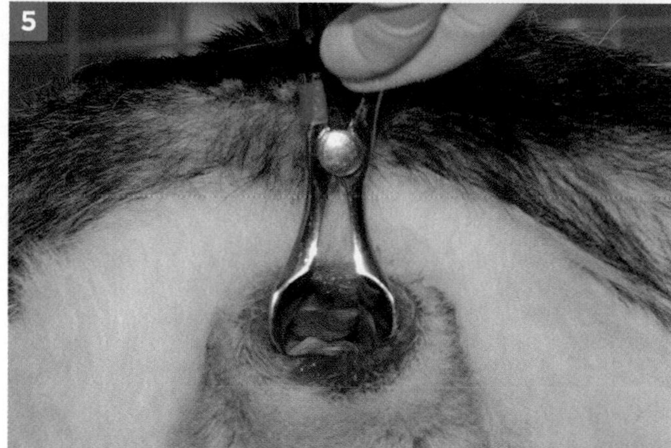

A speculum is directed dorsally after insertion through the vulvar lips, and once inserted the wings are spread to visualize the vestibule and vagina.

6. Visualize the urethral orifice, located on a small tubercle on the ventral floor of the vagina.

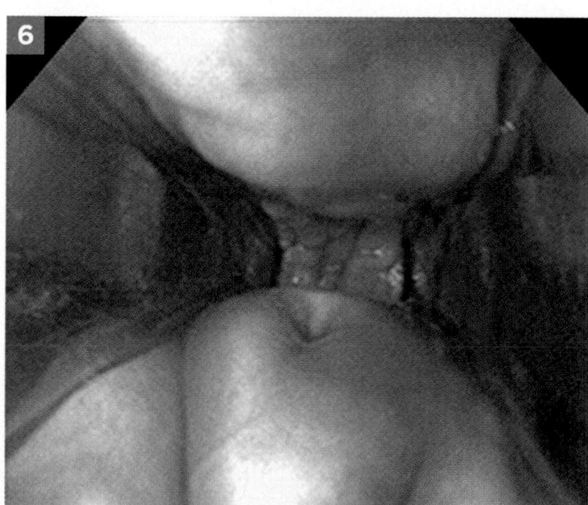

The urethral orifice is located on a small tubercle on the ventral floor of the vagina.

7. Lubricate the tip of the catheter with sterile aqueous lubricant.

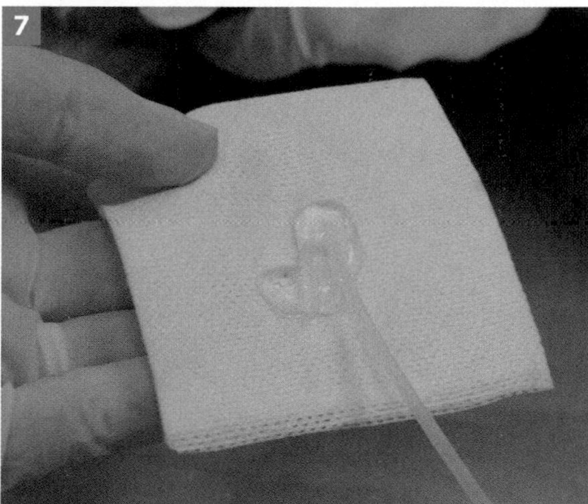

Lubricating the tip of the catheter with sterile aqueous lubricant.

8. Gently insert the tip of the catheter into the external urethral orifice and advance it into the lumen of the bladder, being careful not too advance too far.

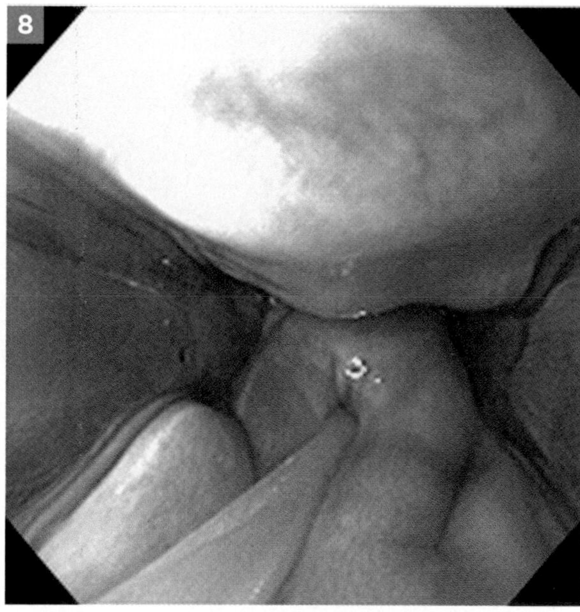

The catheter is inserted into the external urethral orifice and advanced into the lumen of the bladder.

PROCEDURE 10-4 Urinary Catheterization: Female Dog—cont'd

TECHNIQUE: BLIND DIGITAL APPROACH

In large female dogs the catheter can sometimes be guided into the urethra digitally.

1. Restrain the dog in the standing or sternal position and sedate if necessary.
2. Cleanse the perivulvar skin and vulva with antiseptic solution and rinse with saline.
3. Flush the vestibule with sterile saline injected through a syringe.
4. Wearing sterile gloves, lubricate the index finger and insert it into the vagina. In some dogs the external urethral orifice is palpable.
5. Insert a lubricated sterile catheter through the dorsal commissure of the vulva to avoid the clitoral fossa.
6. Guide the catheter under the index finger, along the ventral floor of the vagina.
7. Although the external urethral orifice cannot always be palpated, entry of the catheter into the urethra can be confirmed when the catheter disappears into the floor of the vagina.

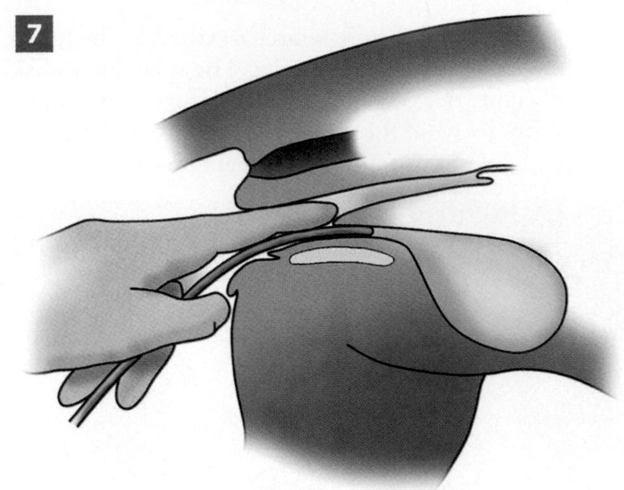

Using the blind digital approach to urinary catheterization, a catheter is inserted and guided under the index finger along the ventral floor of the vagina until it disappears into the urethral orifice on the floor of the vagina.

PROCEDURE 10-5

Prostatic Wash

PURPOSE

To collect a sample of cells and fluid from the prostate gland

INDICATIONS

1. Suspected prostatic disease based on recurrent urinary tract infections, stranguria, or spontaneous urethral bleeding (dripping blood)
2. Palpable abnormalities of the prostate including enlargement, asymmetry, irregularity, or painfulness
3. Collection of prostatic fluid and cells for cytology and culture in a dog with possible prostatitis or infertility

CONTRAINDICATIONS AND WARNINGS

1. When inflammation is present, prostatic epithelial cells may become dysplastic and exhibit some criteria of malignancy. If inflammation can be resolved (as by treating a bacterial infection), cytology should be reassessed.
2. Although evaluation of an ejaculate may have a higher diagnostic yield than a prostatic wash, an ejaculate may be impossible to collect in a dog that is sick, in pain, or neutered.
3. Other methods for evaluating the prostate may include radiographs, ultrasound, and fine-needle aspiration.

EQUIPMENT

- 5 to 10 French (depending on size of dog) stiff polypropylene catheter 28 inches long
- Sterile saline
- Syringes
- Gloves
- Lubricant

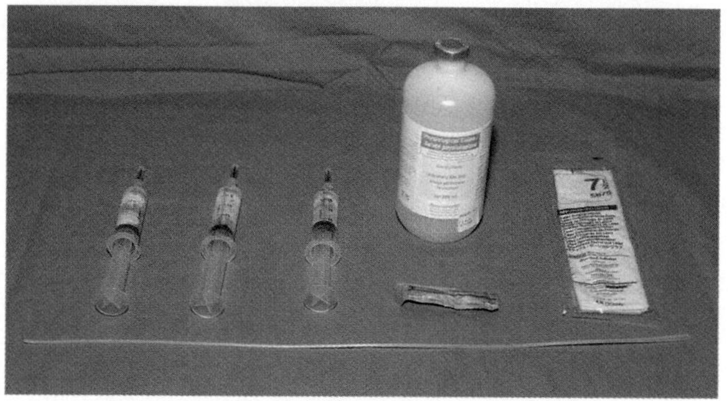

Equipment required to perform a prostatic wash.

SPECIAL ANATOMY

The normal prostate is a bilobed structure surrounding the urethra just caudal to the trigone of the bladder. In most dogs it is palpable per rectum, but when it enlarges it may move forward, out of reach.

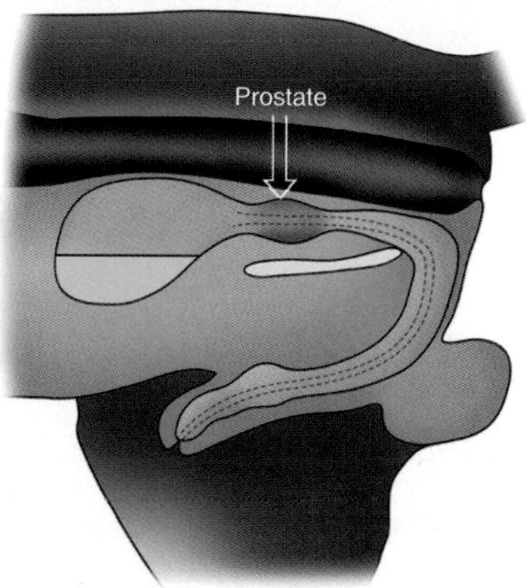

The prostate is a bilobed structure surrounding the urethra just caudal to the trigone of the bladder.

TECHNIQUE

1. Sedate the dog if necessary. This is advised if the dog is in severe pain or very large, making palpation of the prostate difficult.
2. Pass a urethral catheter into the bladder.

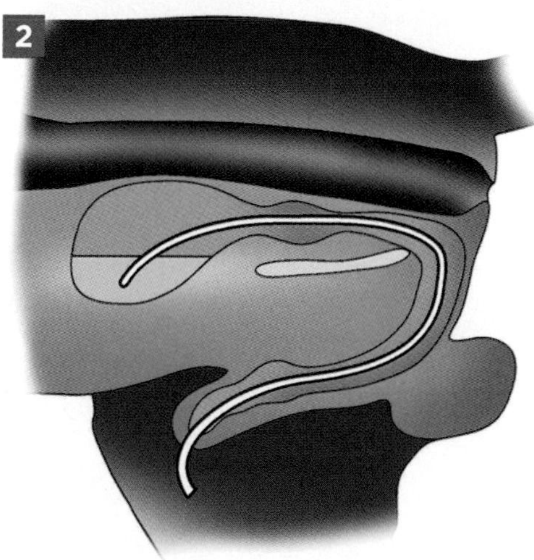

Passing a urethral catheter into the bladder.

PROCEDURE 10-5 Prostatic Wash—cont'd

3. Empty the bladder.

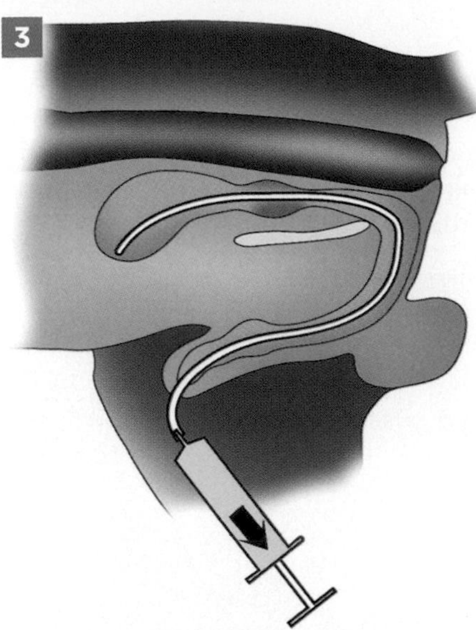

Emptying the bladder.

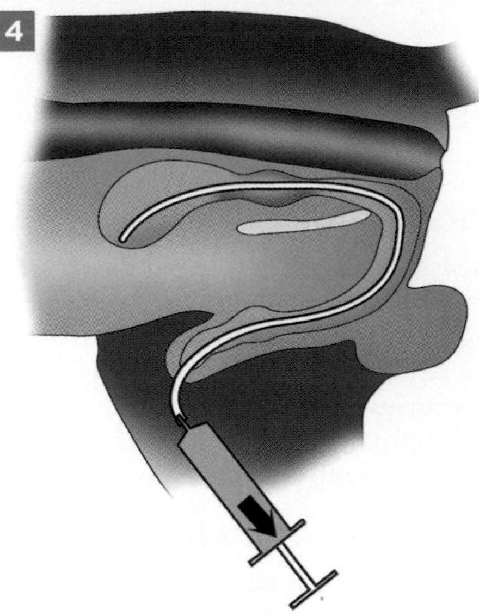

The bladder is flushed and emptied repeatedly until the flush comes back clear.

4. Flush the bladder with sterile saline, and empty it repeatedly until the flush comes back clear.

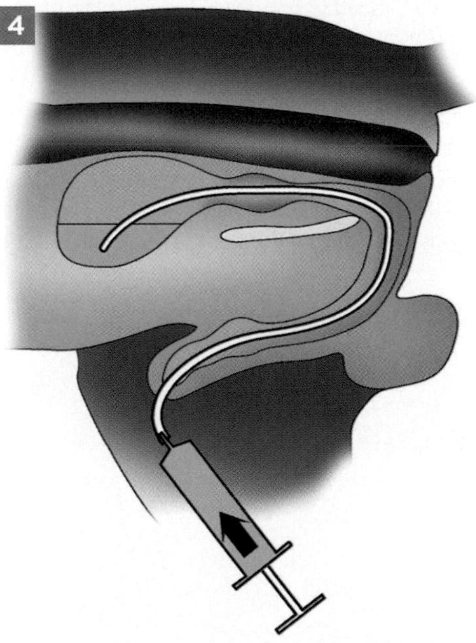

5. Perform a rectal palpation and pull the urethral catheter back until the tip can be felt in the urethra just caudal to the prostate.

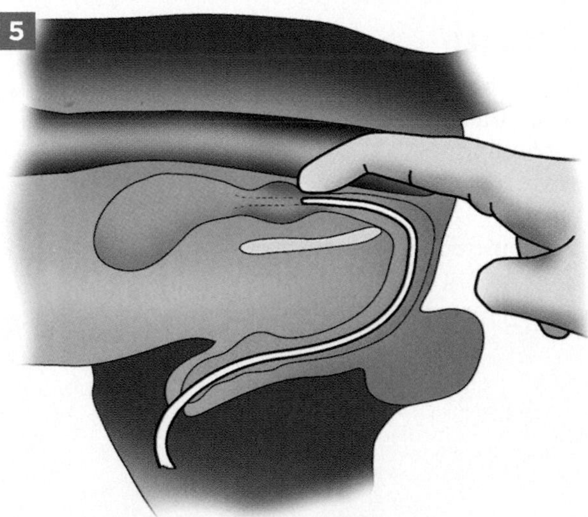

Withdraw the urethral catheter until the tip can be felt in the urethra just caudal to the prostate.

6. Massage the prostate rectally for 1 minute.

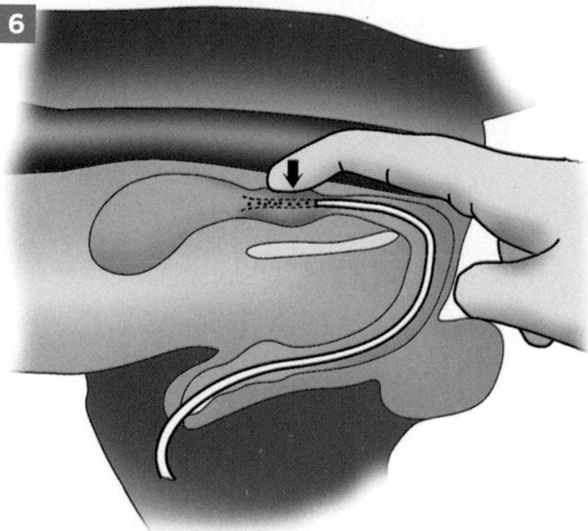

The prostate is massaged rectally for 1 minute.

7. Inject 5 to 10 mL of saline slowly through the catheter while the external urethral orifice is gently occluded around the catheter (to prevent leakage of fluid).

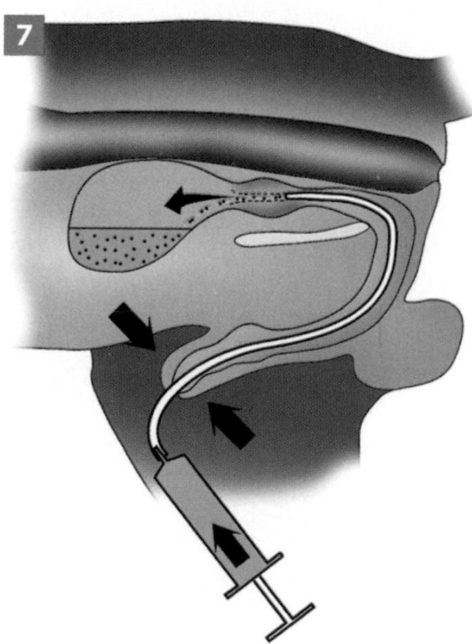

Saline is injected slowly through the catheter into the bladder while the external urethral orifice is gently occluded around the catheter.

8. Advance the catheter into the bladder and aspirate the fluid.

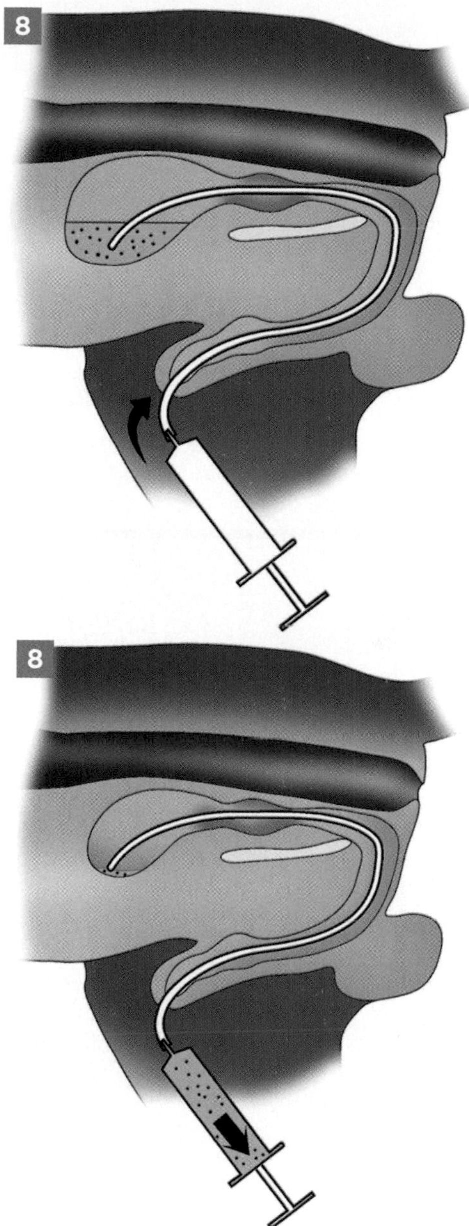

The catheter is advanced into the bladder and the prostatic wash fluid is aspirated.

9. Submit the fluid for cytology and culture.

PROCEDURE 10-5 Prostatic Wash—cont'd

RESULTS

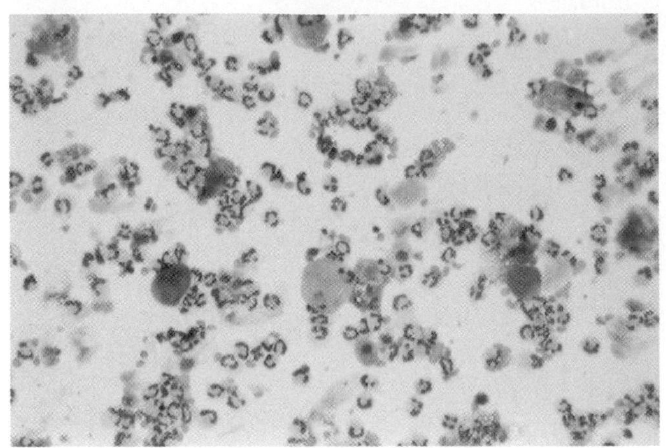

Prostatic wash cytology revealing septic inflammation due to prostatitis. **(Courtesy Dr. Sherry Myers, Prairie Diagnostic Services, Saskatoon, Saskatchewan.)**

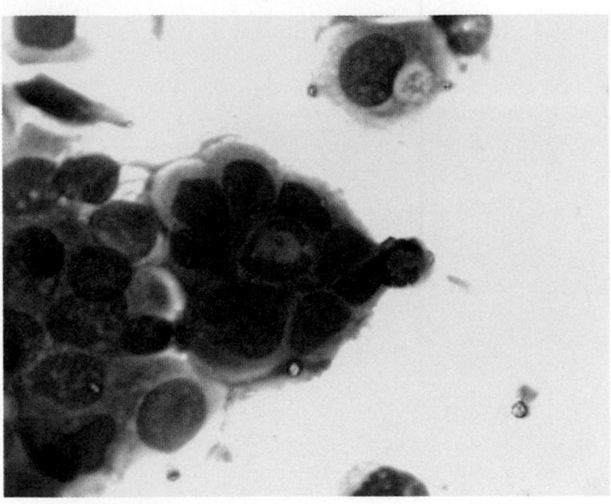

Prostatic wash cytology with no inflammation but many abnormal epithelial cells indicating prostatic carcinoma.

11 Vaginal Cytology

PROCEDURE 11-1 Obtaining Vaginal Samples

PURPOSE

To obtain samples from the vagina for cytologic evaluation

INDICATIONS

1. To determine whether a bitch with a hemorrhagic vulvar discharge is "in heat"
2. To assess the degree of estrogen influence in a breeding bitch during a heat cycle
3. To determine the first day of diestrus for timing parturition
4. To differentiate between mucoid, septic, and nonseptic vulvar discharges

CONTRAINDICATIONS AND CONCERNS

1. Vaginal cytology can determine the degree of estrogen influence, but does not predict ovulation date.
2. Poor technique can result in vaginal swabs that are not representative of true superficial vaginal cytology.

SPECIAL ANATOMY

1. The caudal portion of the vagina is the vestibule, which extends from the vulvar labia to the cingulum, a narrowing just anterior to the urethral papilla. The vestibule is angled steeply dorsocranial.

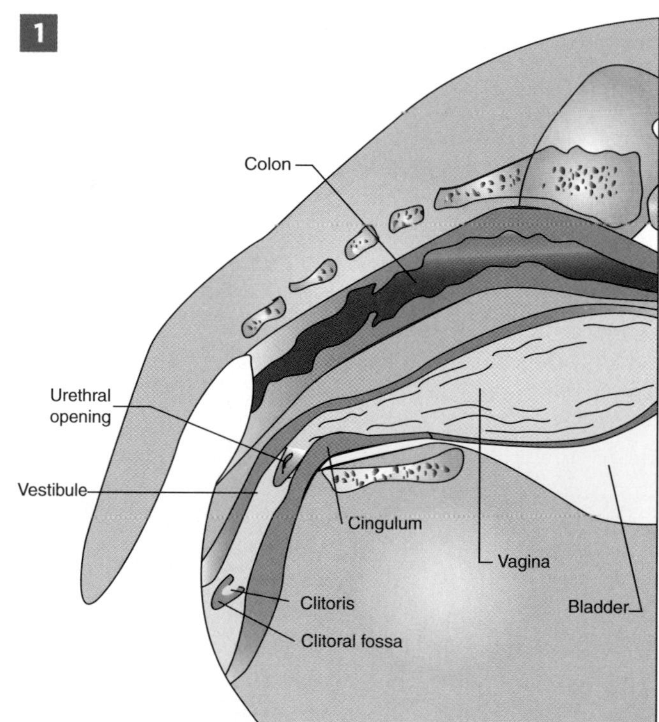

PROCEDURE 11-1 Obtaining Vaginal Samples—cont'd

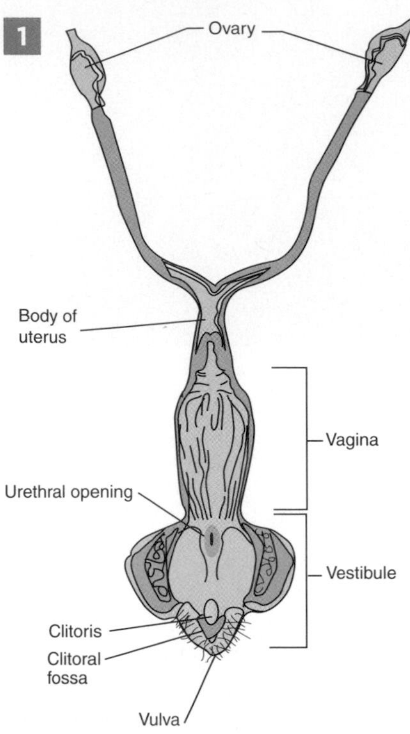

Anatomy of the caudal portion of the reproductive tract in a bitch.

2. When the vulvar lips (labia) are parted, the clitoris can be visualized within the ventral commissure of the vulvar lips. When passing swabs or a scope, it is important to begin their insertion near the dorsal vulvar commissure to avoid the sensitive clitoral fossa.

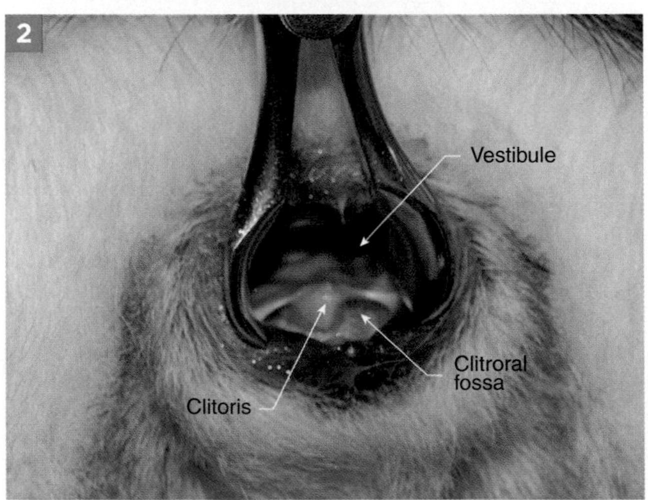

Anatomy of the clitoral fossa and clitoris.

3. The urethral tubercle is located on the ventral wall (floor) of the anterior vestibule.

EQUIPMENT

- Cotton-tipped swabs
- Otoscope cone
- Glass microscope slides
- Syringe with saline

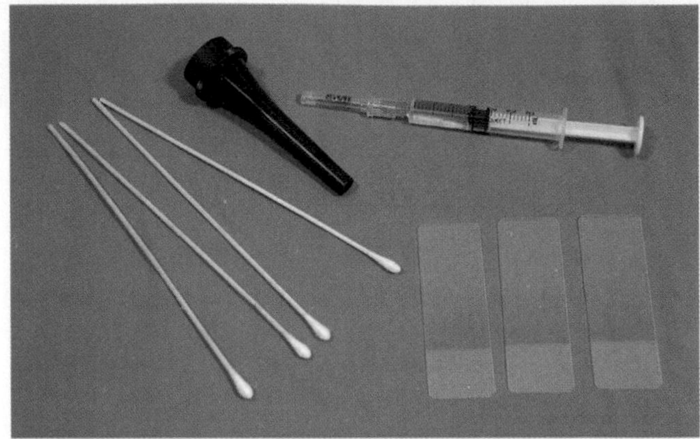

Equipment needed to make vaginal cytology slides from a bitch.

TECHNIQUE

1. Moisten a cotton-tipped swab with saline.

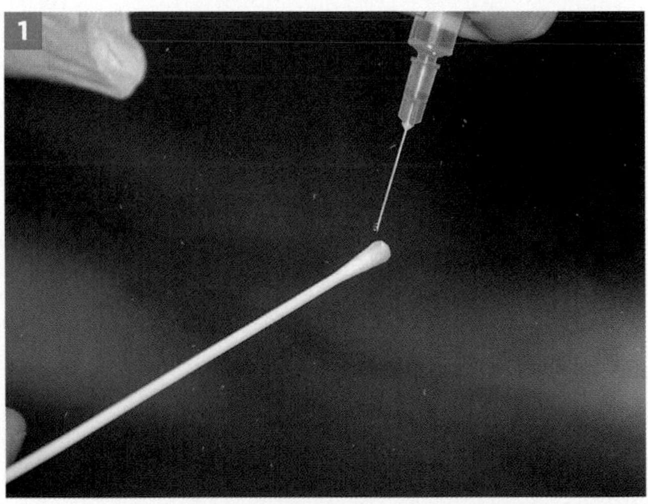

Moistening a cotton-tipped swab with saline.

2. Gently part the vulvar lips and insert the swab at the dorsal commissure of the vulva.

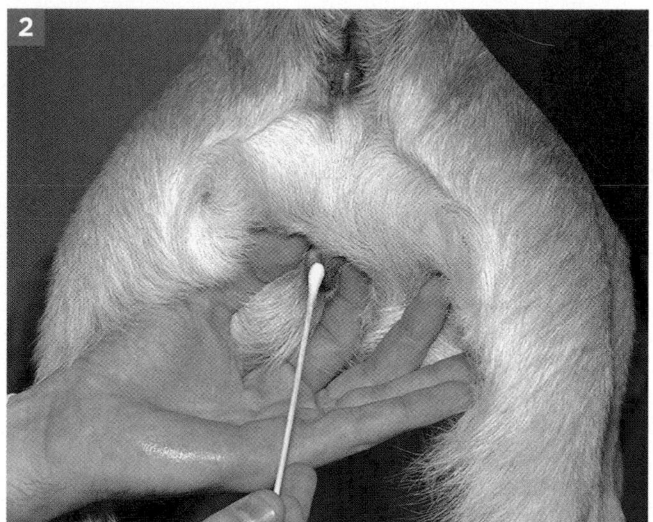

Inserting the swab at the dorsal commissure of the vulva.

3. Advance the swab dorsally and angle slightly cranially until the swab goes over the ischial arch, then advance slightly cranially.

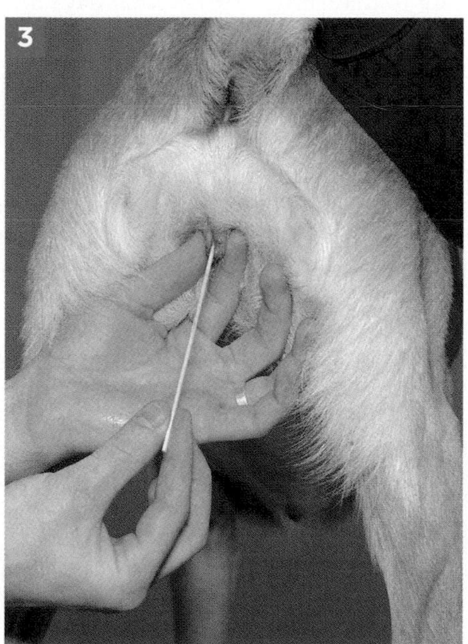

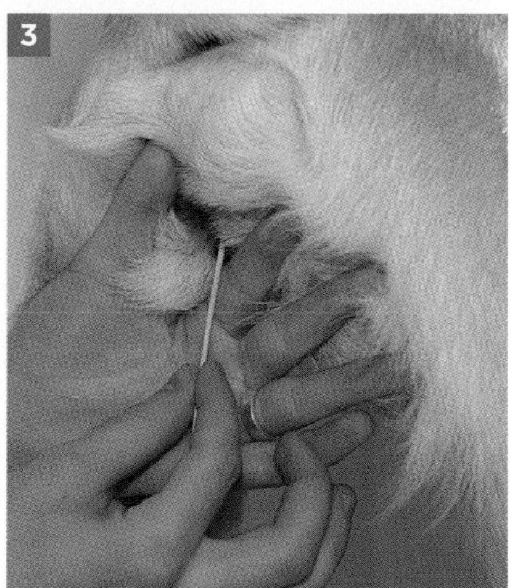

The swab is advanced craniodorsally until the swab goes over the ischial arch, then it is advanced slightly cranially.

4. Alternative technique: If the dog is large enough, pass an otoscope cone up through the vestibule into the vagina and use the otoscope cone as a speculum. Pass the cotton swab up through the speculum so that it comes into contact with the dorsal wall of the posterior vagina. The advantage to using a speculum is that you sample cells only from the vagina and not from the vestibule. Cells in the vagina are more responsive to changing hormone levels than cells in the vestibule.

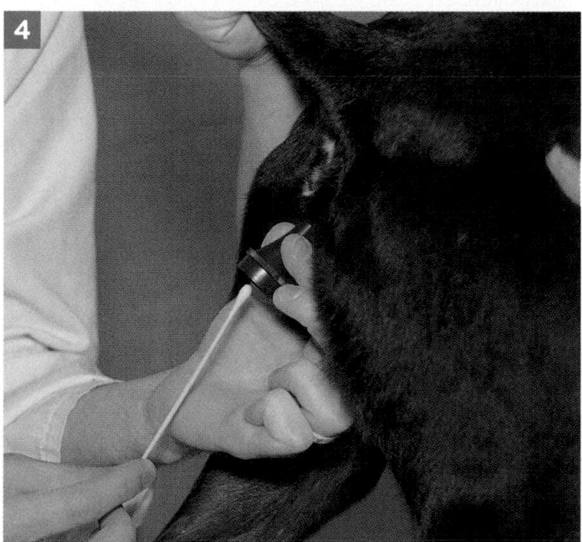

PROCEDURE 11-1 Obtaining Vaginal Samples—cont'd

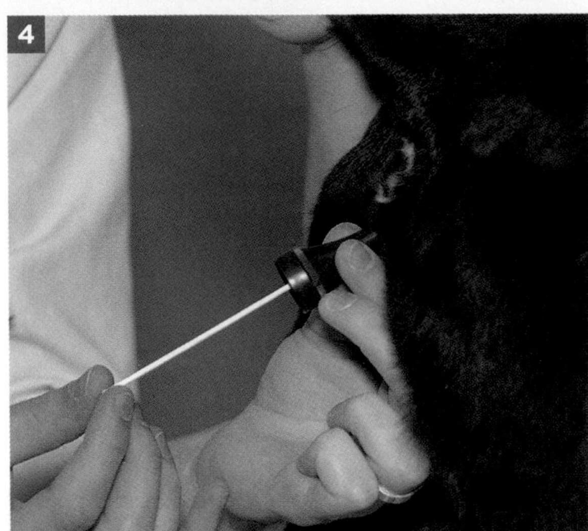

4

An otoscope cone can be used as a speculum for vaginal cytology swab collection, bypassing the vestibule.

5. Gently roll the swab against the dorsal vaginal surface, then pull it straight out.
6. Roll the swab on a glass slide, allow to air dry, and stain with Diff-Quik or Wright-Giemsa stain.

COMPLICATIONS

None

RESULTS

1. Vaginal cytology normally varies with the stage of the estrus cycle and the degree of estrogen influence.
   - A. During proestrus there are small, round parabasal cells with large darkly stained nuclei as well as slightly larger intermediate cells and red blood cells.

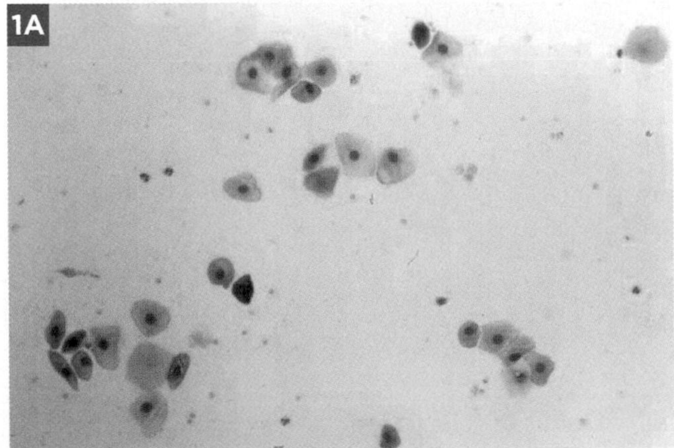

1A

Vaginal smear from a bitch in proestrus contains red blood cells, parabasal cells, and intermediate cells. **(Courtesy Dr. Klaas Post, University of Saskatchewan.)**

   - B. During estrus the proportion of superficial mature cornified cells increases. Superficial cells are polygonal, with a small round nucleus that becomes pyknotic over time. Eventually the cells become anuclear.

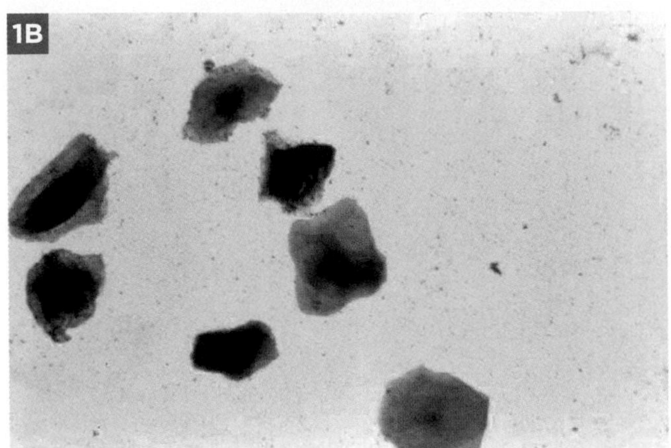

1B

Vaginal cytology during estrus consists primarily of superficial mature cornified epithelial cells. **(Courtesy Dr. Klaas Post, University of Saskatchewan.)**

2. Vaginal cornification of 50% to 60% has been recommended as the best time to begin sequential progesterone testing to determine the optimal days for breeding.
3. At the onset of diestrus there is an abrupt transition of vaginal cytology from estrus (80% to 100% superficial mature cornified cells) to diestrus (80% to 100% parabasal and intermediate cells plus neutrophils). Onset of cytologic diestrus is usually 6 days following ovulation, suggesting that it is too late to breed during the current cycle. Parturition, if a bitch becomes pregnant, typically occurs 58 (±1) days after the first day of cytologic diestrus.

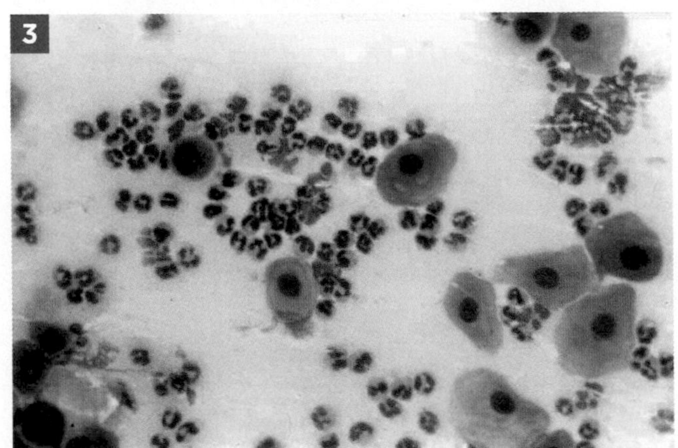

3

Diestrus is characterized by an abrupt transition of vaginal cytology to predominantly parabasal and intermediate cells plus neutrophils. **(Courtesy Dr. Klaas Post, University of Saskatchewan.)**

4. When vaginal cytology performed in a spayed female dog that is showing signs of estrus (bloody discharge, attractive to males) demonstrates estrogen influence (cornified cells), this suggests that an ovarian remnant may be present.

Bone Marrow Collection

12

PROCEDURE 12-1

Bone Marrow Aspiration

PURPOSE

To collect bone marrow for evaluation

INDICATIONS

1. Persistent or unexplained pancytopenia, neutropenia, or thrombocytopenia
2. Nonregenerative anemia
3. Investigation of atypical cells seen in the peripheral blood
4. Diagnosis or staging of neoplastic disease (especially lymphoma, plasma cell myeloma, histiocytic neoplasia, and mast cell neoplasia)
5. Investigation of patients with hypercalcemia or hyperglobulinemia
6. Evaluation of iron stores
7. Diagnosis of specific infectious diseases such as leishmania, ehrlichiosis, histoplasmosis, and cytauxzoonosis

CONTRAINDICATIONS AND COMPLICATIONS

1. None. Even patients with severe thrombocytopenia or severe coagulopathy are unlikely to bleed excessively from this procedure.
2. It is important to submit a current complete blood count (CBC) and blood smear to facilitate interpretation of bone marrow cytology.

RESTRAINT

1. Sedation combined with local anesthesia will be adequate in most cases.
2. Lidocaine blocking solution (2% lidocaine mixed 9:1 with 8.4% sodium bicarbonate) can be used to block the skin, subcutaneous tissues, and periosteum. The addition of bicarbonate decreases the sting of injection and speeds the local analgesic effect of the lidocaine.
3. Firm restraint may be required during the actual bone marrow aspiration because disruption of endosteal nerves causes some discomfort.

EQUIPMENT

Illinois bone marrow biopsy needle (15- to 18-gauge, 1 to 1½ inches). For bone marrow aspiration, a specialized needle with an inner stylet is used. The stylet is useful to prevent occlusion of the needle with a core of bone. Often these needles have a mechanism for locking the stylet in place during insertion, and they may have a cap that fits over the proximal end to maintain sterility and facilitate handling.

- Sterile gloves
- Lidocaine blocking solution
- #11 scalpel blade
- 12-mL syringe

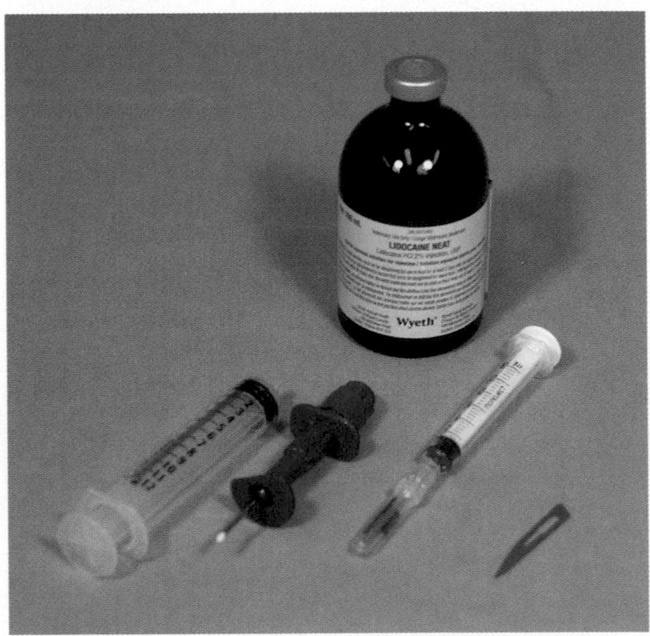

The equipment required for bone marrow aspiration.

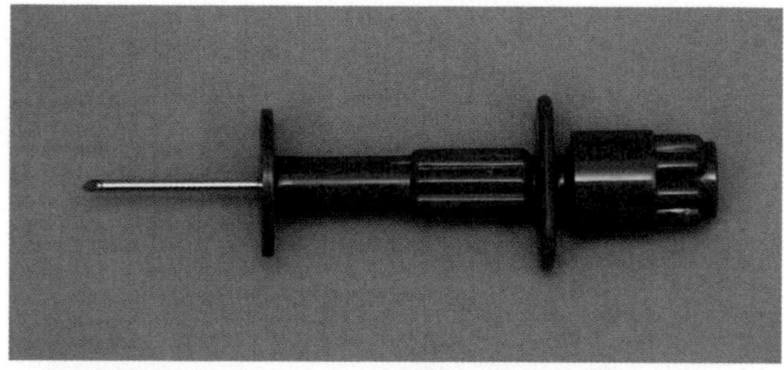

An Illinois bone marrow needle used for bone marrow aspiration.

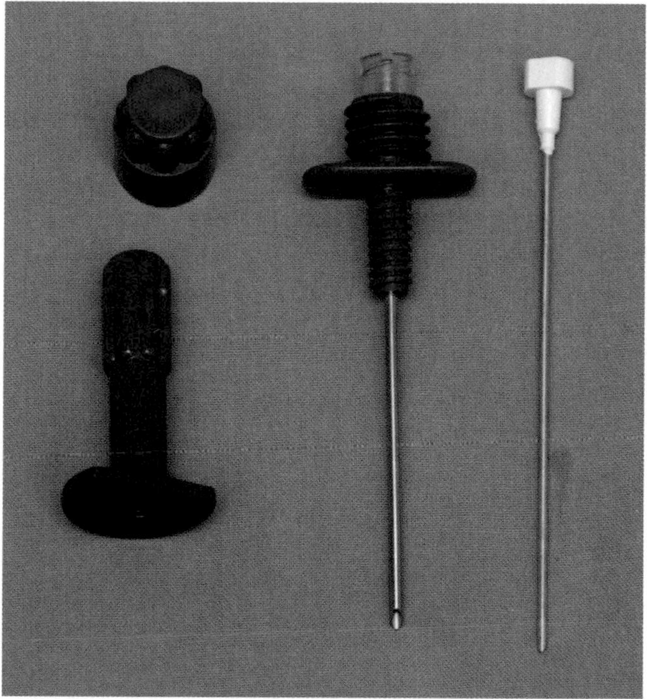

Components of an Illinois bone marrow needle include a needle, a stylet, a depth guard, and a screw-on cap.

SPECIAL ANATOMY

Sites selected for bone marrow biopsy should be easily and safely accessed and should normally contain active (red) marrow. The preferred sites in dogs and cats include the proximal femur, the proximal humerus, and the iliac crest of the pelvis. Anatomic landmarks are described under each of the following procedures.

TECHNIQUE: PROXIMAL FEMUR—TROCHANTERIC FOSSA APPROACH

1. With this approach, the needle enters the marrow cavity of the proximal femur through the trochanteric fossa, just medial to the greater trochanter and is directed down the shaft of the femur toward the stifle.

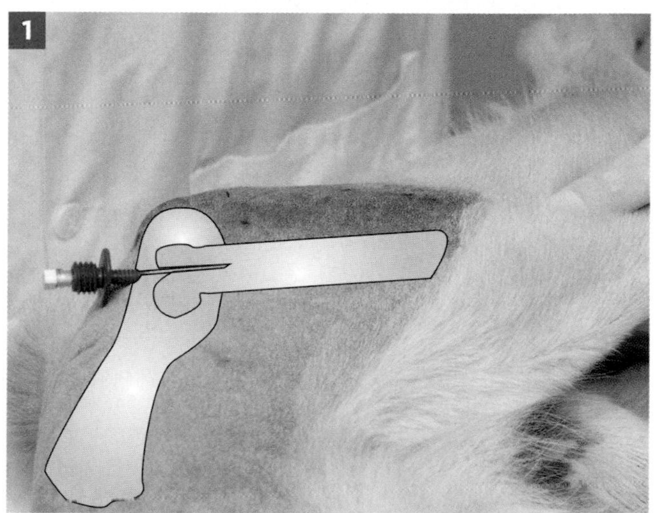

Anatomic overlay showing the position of a bone marrow needle properly inserted in the trochanteric fossa of the femur.

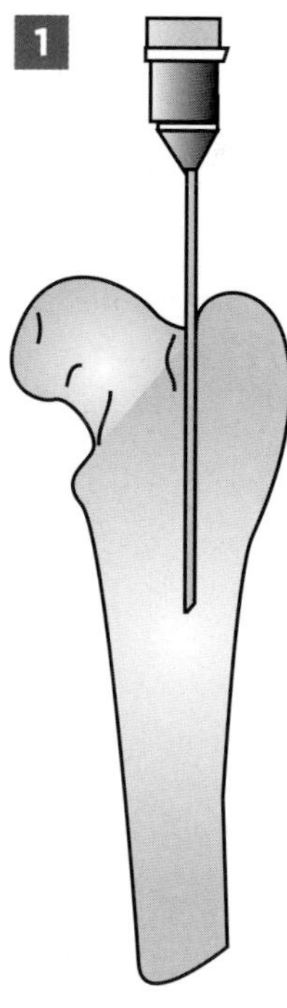

Anatomic drawing of the proximal femur with a bone marrow needle inserted in the trochanteric fossa.

PROCEDURE 12-1 Bone Marrow Aspiration—cont'd

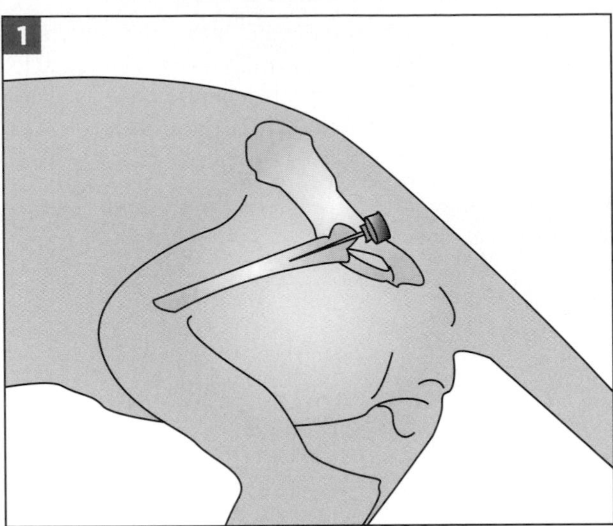

Anatomic drawing of the pelvis and femur, showing proper placement of a bone marrow needle in the trochanteric fossa.

2. Restrain the patient in lateral recumbency.
3. Clip and surgically prep the region. Bone marrow aspiration should be performed as a sterile procedure.
4. Inject lidocaine blocking solution to block the skin and underlying tissues down to the bone.

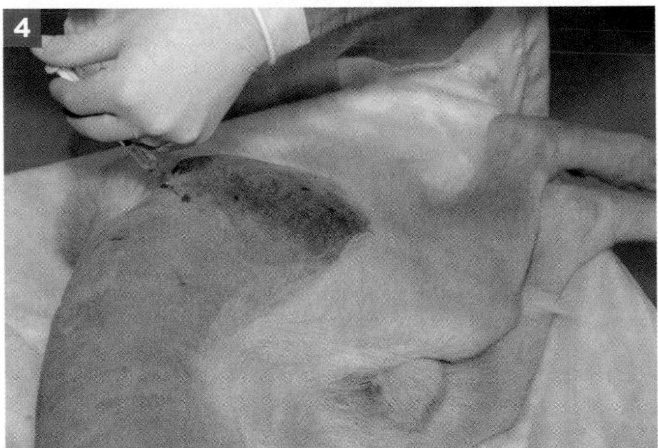

Injecting lidocaine blocking solution to block the skin and underlying tissues down to the bone.

5. Palpate the greater trochanter. The tip of the needle should be positioned just medial to this prominence.

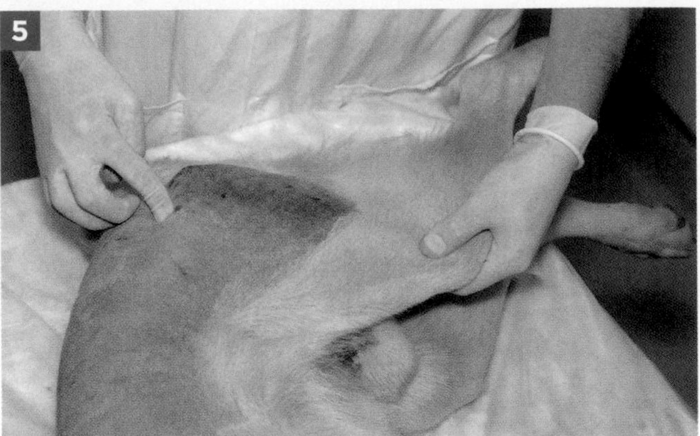

Palpating the greater trochanter.

6. Stabilize the femur by grasping the stifle and applying slight internal (medial) rotation.
7. Use a scalpel blade (#11) to make a stab incision in the skin.

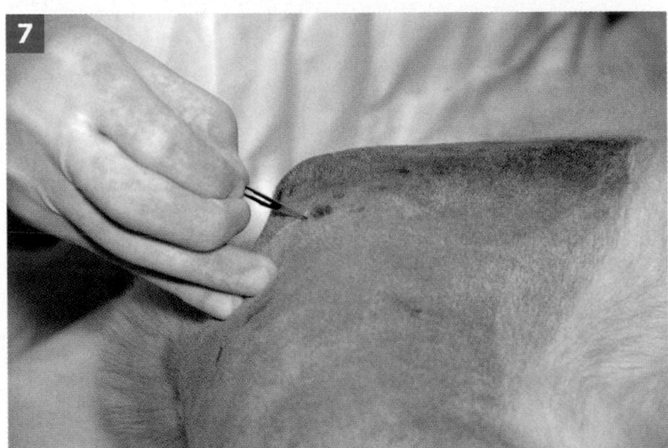

Making a stab incision in the skin using a #11 scalpel blade.

8. Make sure the stylet is properly seated in the needle and (if available) the cap is screwed on the needle. Hold the needle using a modified pencil grip with the proximal end of the needle firmly against the palm or the first metacarpophalangeal joint. Insert the needle through the hole in the skin and advance it toward the bone until the cortex is encountered.

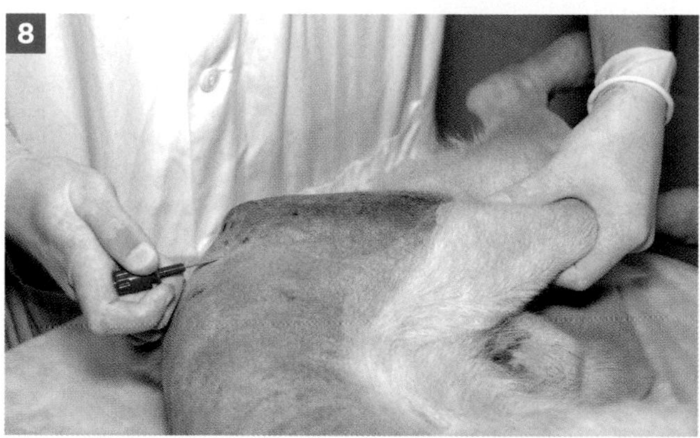

Inserting the needle to the bone, just medial to the greater trochanter.

9. Using a rotating motion, apply pressure and advance the needle forcefully by rotation into the marrow cavity down the shaft of the femur.

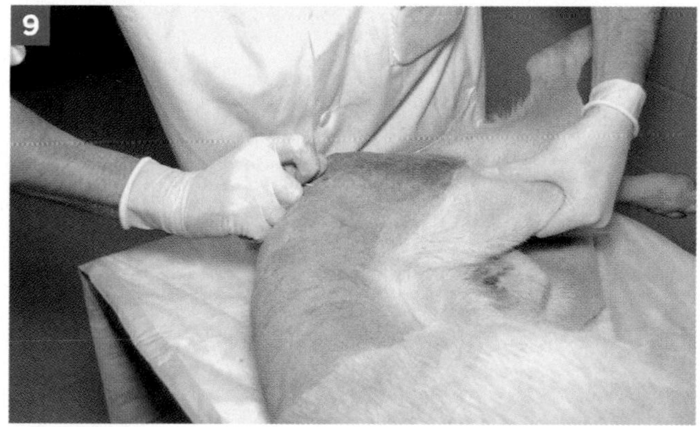

Using pressure and a rotating motion, the needle is advanced down the shaft of the femur into the marrow cavity.

10. The needle entry and insertion should maintain the shaft of the needle parallel to the center of the femoral shaft, with the tip in the center of the marrow cavity directed toward the stifle. It is important to remember that the sciatic nerve is located caudal to the femur and can be injured if the needle slips caudal to the femur.
11. Advance the needle until it is seated firmly in the bone. Once the needle is well seated, it will move with the femur.

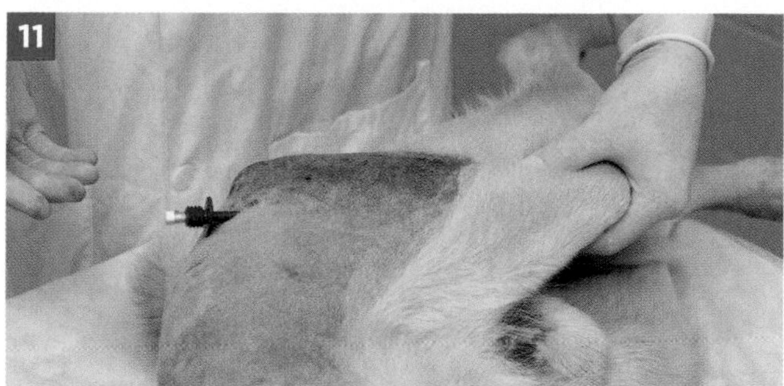

Seating the bone marrow needle firmly in the bone.

12. Remove the stylet and attach a 12-mL syringe.

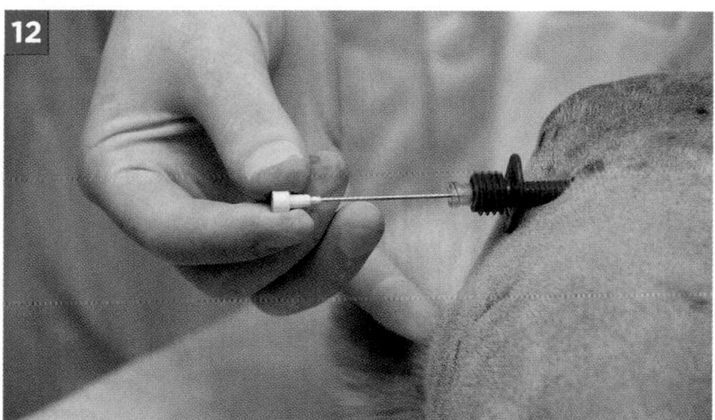

Removing the stylet.

13. Withdraw the syringe plunger, applying full negative pressure (6 to 8 mL) rapidly and vigorously until blood enters the hub of the needle.

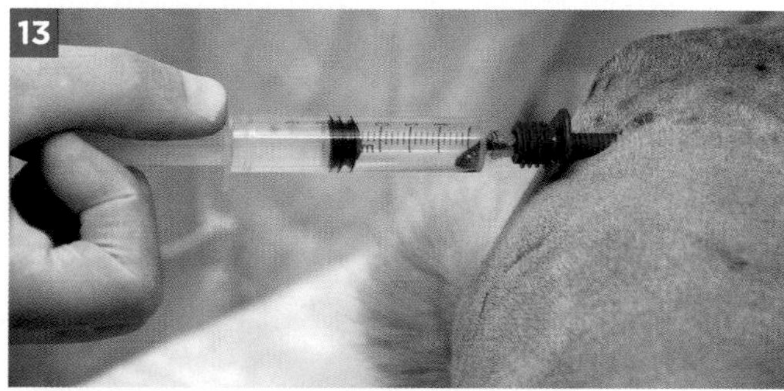

Aspirating vigorously until blood enters the hub of the needle.

14. As soon as blood is seen in the needle hub, discontinue suction to minimize hemodilution of the sample.
15. Quickly disconnect the syringe from the needle and prepare slides for examination as outlined following.

PROCEDURE 12-1 Bone Marrow Aspiration—cont'd

TECHNIQUE: PROXIMAL FEMUR—LATERAL APPROACH

1. With this approach, the needle directly enters the marrow cavity of the proximal femur from the lateral aspect. This method is most useful in cats and very small dogs.

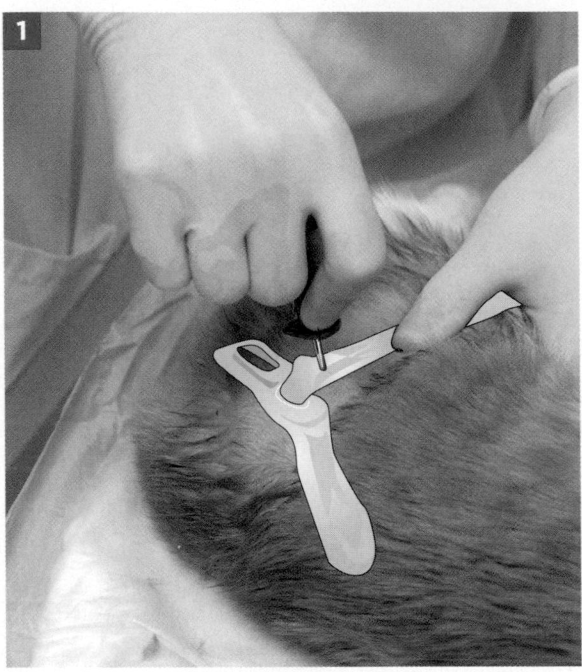

Anatomic overlay showing the position of a bone marrow needle properly inserted in the proximal femur through a lateral approach.

2. Restrain the patient in lateral recumbency.

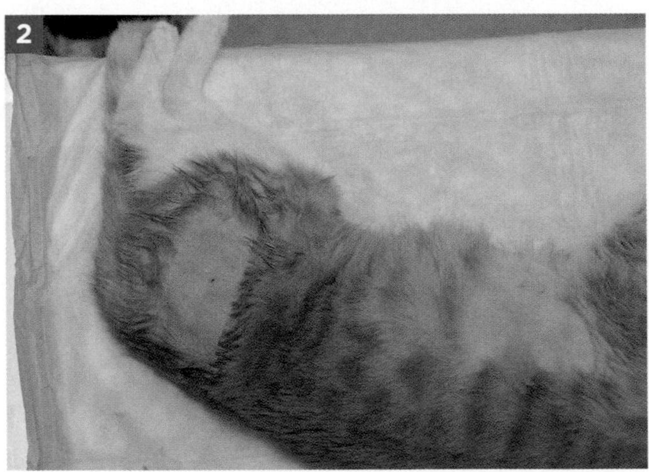

The animal is restrained in lateral recumbency.

3. Clip and surgically prep the region.
4. Inject lidocaine blocking solution to block the skin and underlying tissues down to the bone.

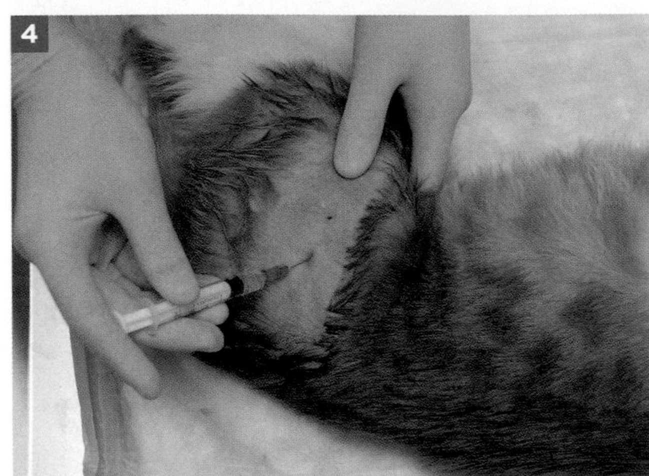

Lidocaine blocking solution is injected to block the skin and underlying tissues.

5. Use a scalpel blade (#11) to make a stab incision in the skin.

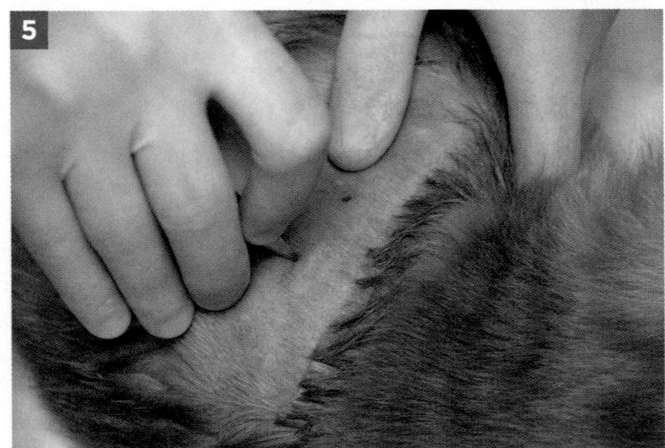

A #11 scalpel blade is used to make a stab incision in the skin.

6. Stabilize the femur by firmly grasping the stifle.

7. Using a modified pencil grip, insert the needle through the hole in the skin and advance it straight in, perpendicular to the proximal femur, until the cortex is encountered.

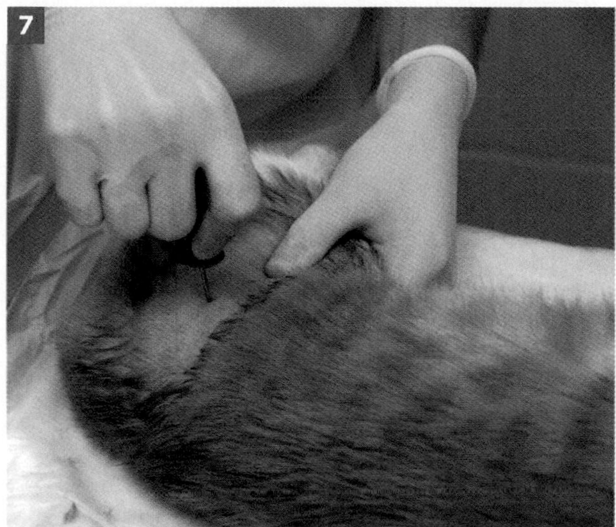

The needle is advanced straight in, perpendicular to the proximal femur.

8. Using a rotating motion, apply pressure and advance the needle forcefully by rotation through the cortex into the marrow cavity. There will usually be a palpable loss of resistance when the marrow cavity is entered.

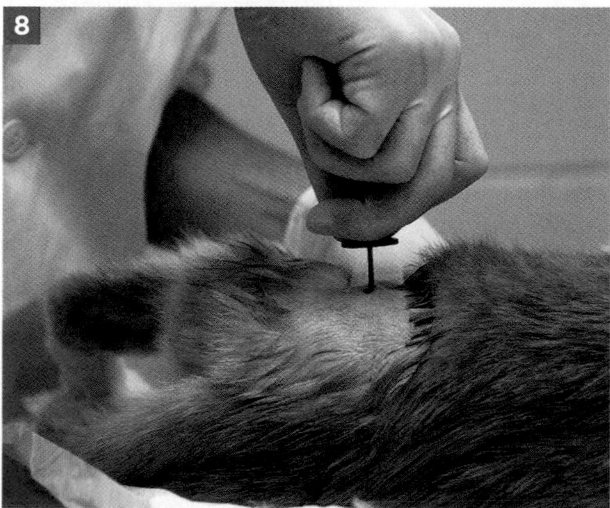

The needle is advanced forcefully by rotation through the cortex into the marrow cavity.

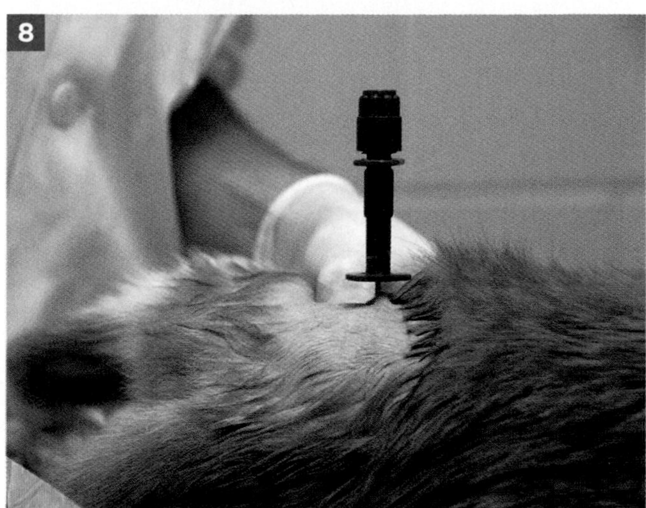

Bone marrow needle in place.

9. Remove the stylet and attach a 12-mL syringe.

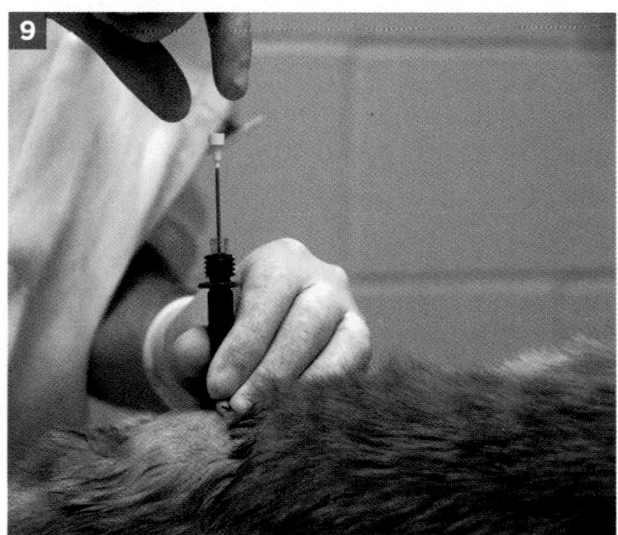

The stylet is removed.

PROCEDURE 12-1 Bone Marrow Aspiration—cont'd

10. Withdraw the syringe plunger, applying full negative pressure (6 to 8 mL) rapidly and vigorously until blood enters the hub of the needle.

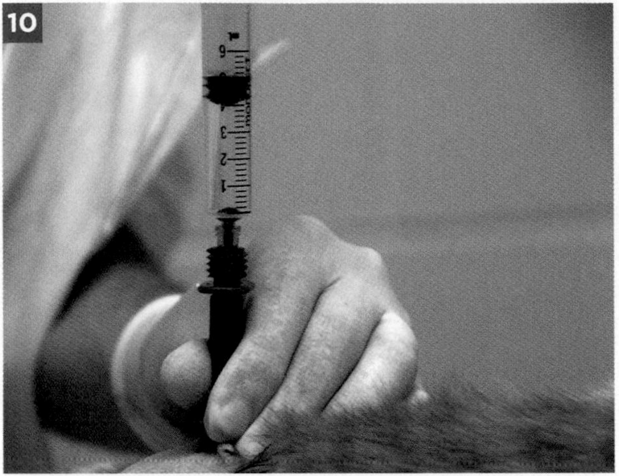

Full negative pressure is applied repeatedly until blood enters the hub of the needle.

11. As soon as blood is seen in the needle hub, discontinue suction to minimize hemodilution of the sample.

12. Quickly disconnect the syringe from the needle, and prepare slides for examination as outlined following.

TECHNIQUE: PROXIMAL HUMERUS—LATERAL APPROACH

1. With this approach, the needle directly enters the marrow cavity of the proximal humerus from the craniolateral aspect.

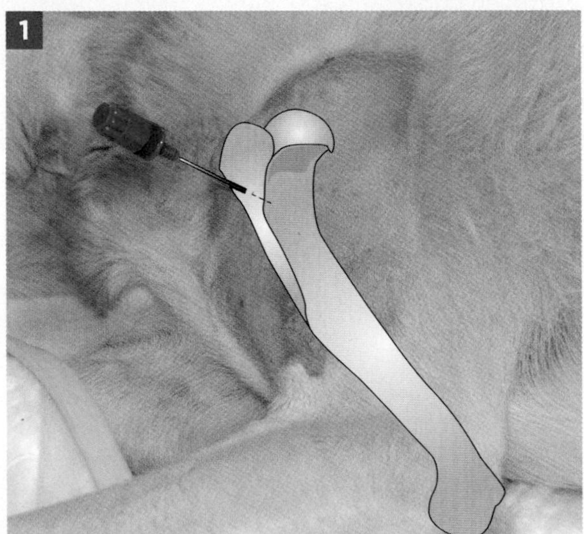

Anatomic overlay showing a bone marrow needle properly inserted in the proximal humerus through a lateral approach.

2. Restrain the patient in lateral recumbency.

3. Clip and surgically prep the skin lateral to the shoulder and proximal humerus.

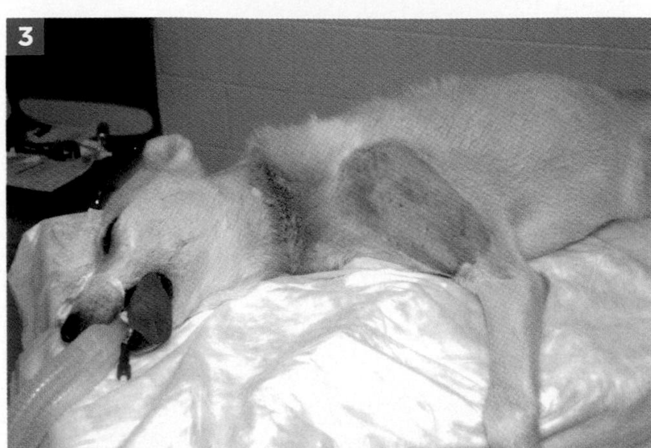

The animal is positioned properly, and the region is clipped and surgically prepped.

4. The site of entry into the bone is the flattened area on the craniolateral side of the proximal humerus, just distal to the greater tubercle. This site can be identified by palpating down the spine of the scapula—the first bony prominence palpated is the acromion and the next is the greater tubercle of the humerus.

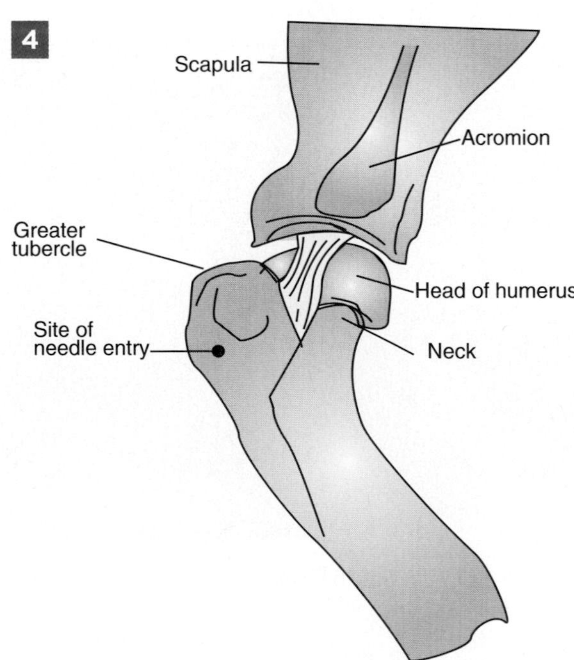

The humerus showing anatomic landmarks.

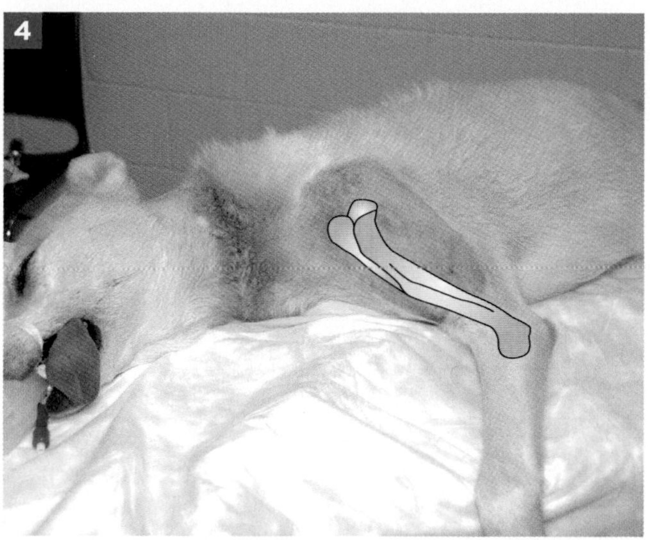

The site of entry into the bone is the flattened area on the craniolateral side of the proximal humerus, just distal to the greater tubercle.

5. Inject lidocaine blocking solution to block the skin and underlying tissues down to the bone.

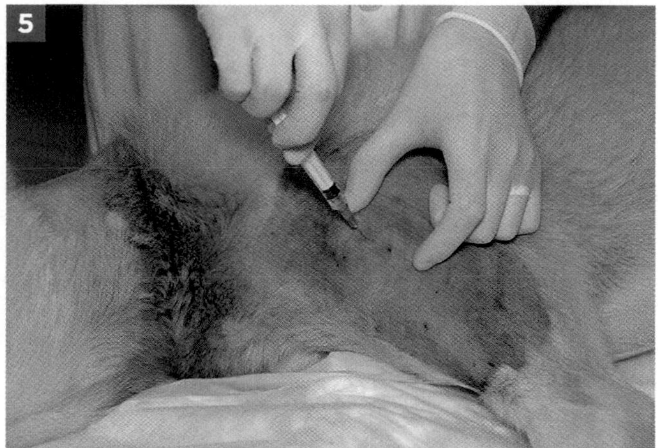

Lidocaine blocking solution is injected to block the skin and underlying tissues down to the bone.

6. Use a scalpel blade (#11) to make a stab incision in the skin.

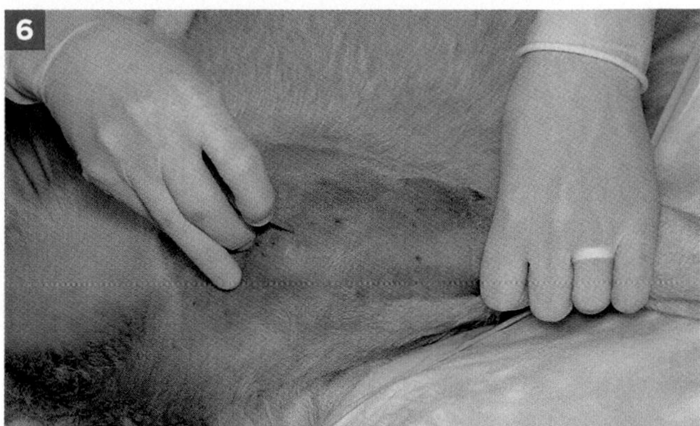

A stab incision is made in the skin.

7. Grasp the elbow to stabilize the limb and maintain the humerus in a standing dog position while being able to counter the pressure applied to the proximal humerus.

8. The needle is inserted just distal to the greater tubercle, perpendicular to the long axis of the humerus, and advanced forcefully by rotation laterally to medially until it is seated firmly in the bone. There may be a palpable loss of resistance when the marrow cavity is entered. Penetration of the medial cortex should be avoided because this could result in entry into the bicipital bursa that communicates with the scapulohumeral joint on the medial side of the limb.

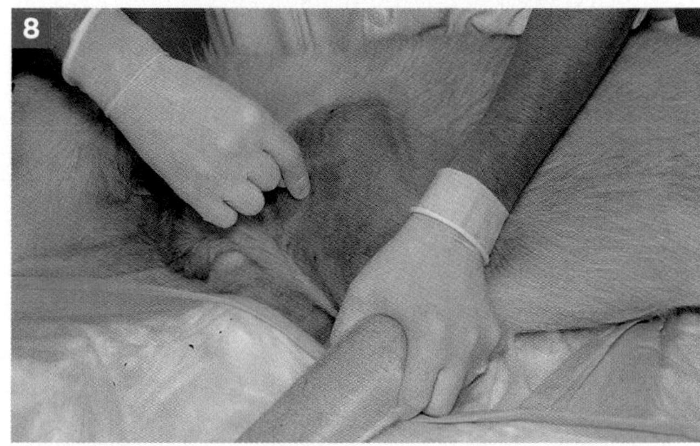

The needle is inserted just distal to the greater tubercle, perpendicular to the long axis of the humerus, and advanced forcefully by rotation laterally to medially.

PROCEDURE 12-1 Bone Marrow Aspiration—cont'd

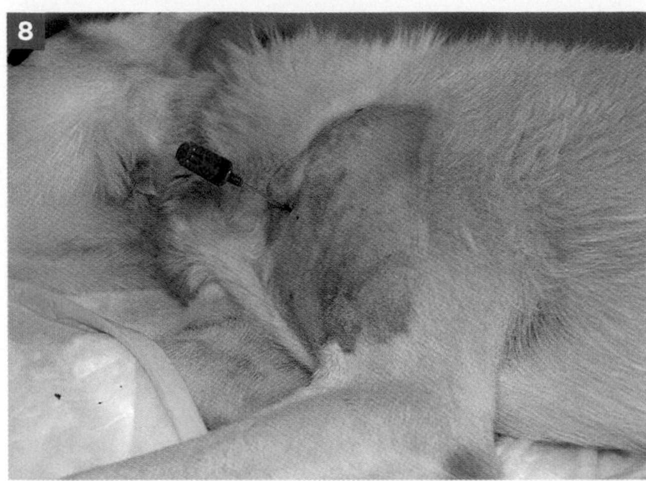

When the marrow cavity is entered there is a loss of resistance, but the needle is firmly seated in the bone.

9. Remove the stylet and attach a 12-mL syringe.
10. Withdraw the syringe plunger, applying full negative pressure (6 to 8 mL) rapidly and vigorously until blood enters the hub of the needle.

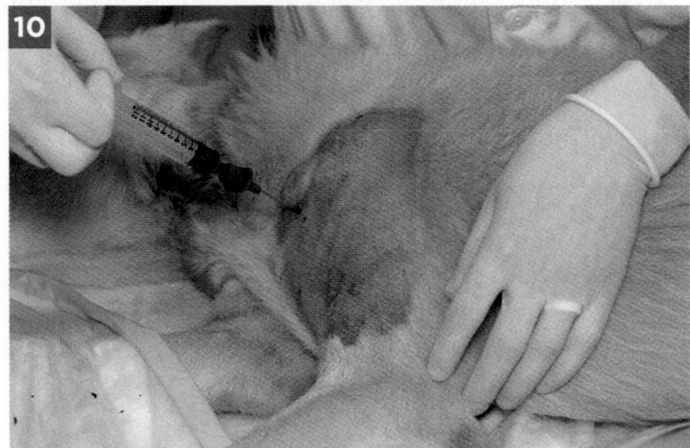

Full negative pressure is applied rapidly and vigorously on the syringe until blood enters the hub of the needle.

11. As soon as blood is seen in the needle hub, discontinue suction to minimize hemodilution of the sample.
12. Quickly disconnect the syringe from the needle and prepare slides for examination as outlined following.

TECHNIQUE: PROXIMAL HUMERUS—ANGLE APPROACH

1. This alternate approach to collecting bone marrow from the proximal humerus has the same site of entry as the lateral approach, but directs the needle toward the elbow, thus sampling the marrow cavity of the humerus 2 to 4 cm further distal.

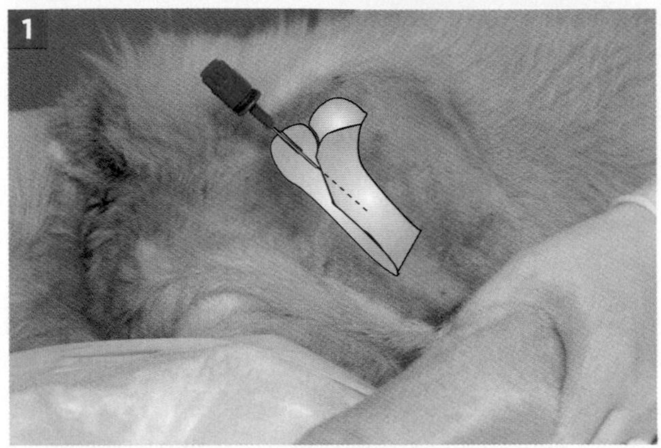

Anatomic overlay showing a bone marrow needle properly inserted in the proximal humerus through the angle approach.

2. Restrain the patient in lateral recumbency. Grasp the elbow to stabilize the limb and maintain the humerus in a standing dog position while being able to counter the pressure applied to the proximal humerus.
3. Clip and surgically prep the skin lateral to the shoulder and proximal humerus.
4. The site of entry into the bone will be the same as for the lateral approach——the flattened area on the craniolateral side of the proximal humerus, just distal to the greater tubercle.

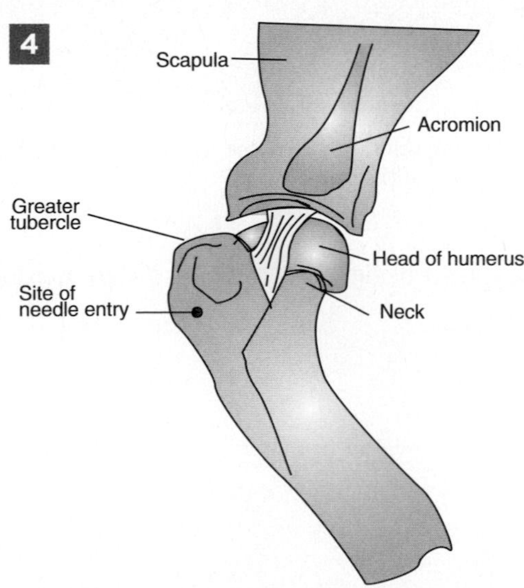

The humerus showing anatomic landmarks.

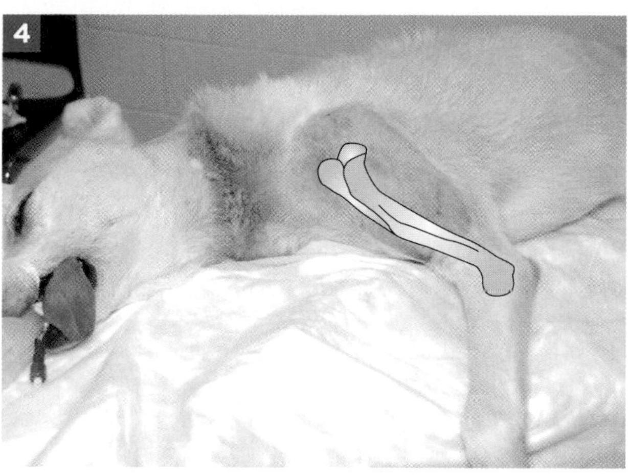

The site of entry into the bone is the flattened area on the craniolateral side of the proximal humerus, just distal to the greater tubercle.

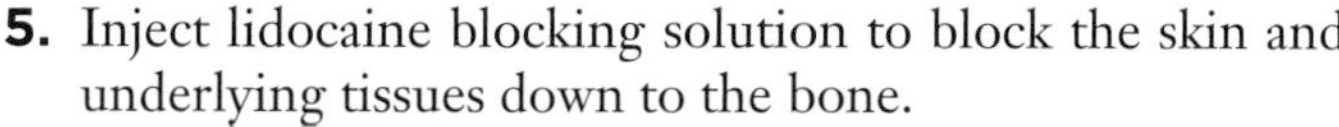

5. Inject lidocaine blocking solution to block the skin and underlying tissues down to the bone.
6. Use a scalpel blade (#11) to make a stab incision in the skin
7. The needle is inserted just distal to the greater tubercle, and the needle tip is directed distally toward the elbow, at an angle 45 degrees from the long axis of the humerus. It is important to maintain control of the needle as it is being seated into the bone because the needle may slide down the surface of the bone instead of penetrating the cortex, resulting in damage to adjacent soft tissues.

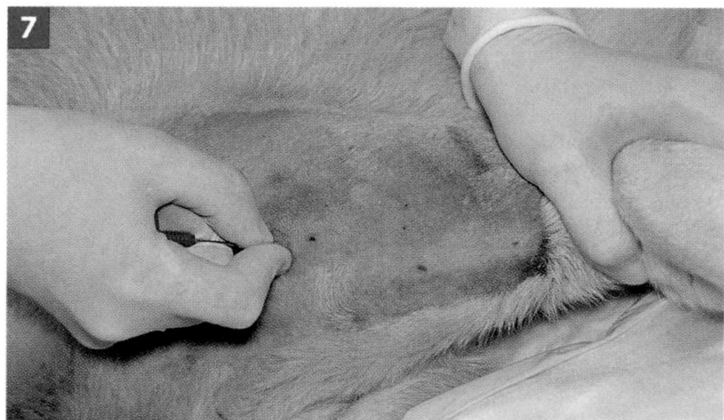

The needle is inserted just distal to the greater tubercle, and the needle tip is directed distally toward the elbow.

8. Once the cortex has been penetrated, the needle is advanced forcefully by rotation until it is firmly seated within the medullary cavity.

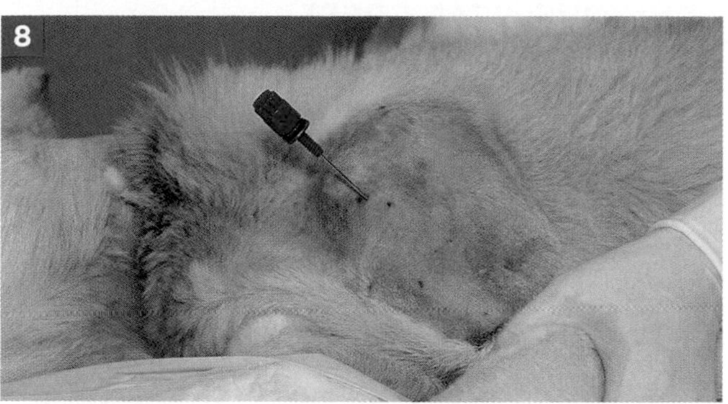

The properly placed needle is firmly seated within the medullary cavity.

9. Remove the stylet and attach a 12-mL syringe.

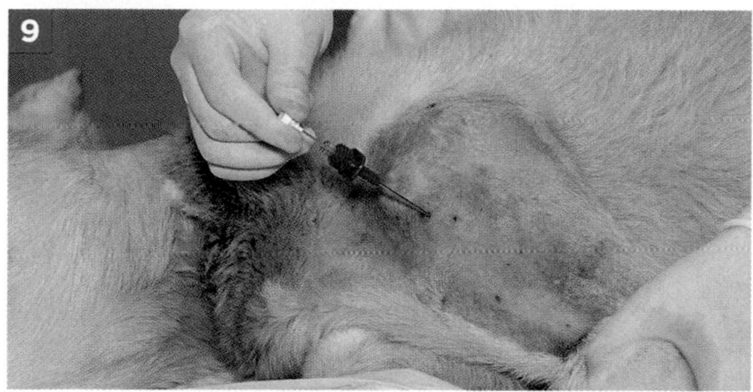

The stylet is removed.

10. Withdraw the syringe plunger, applying full negative pressure (6 to 8 mL) rapidly and vigorously until blood enters the hub of the needle.

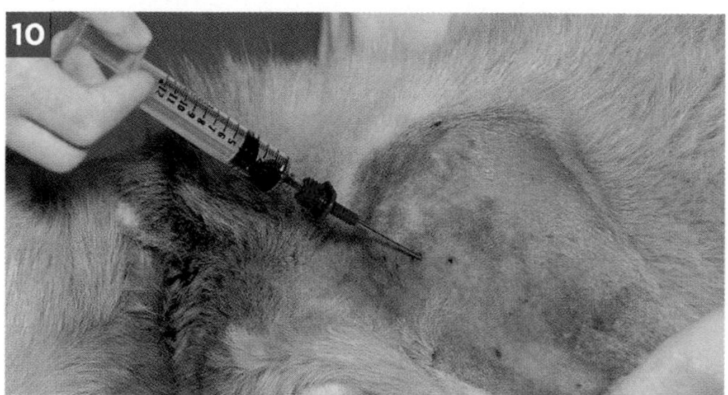

Bone marrow aspiration.

11. As soon as blood is seen in the needle hub, discontinue suction to minimize hemodilution of the sample.
12. Quickly disconnect the syringe from the needle and prepare slides for examination as outlined following.

PROCEDURE 12-1 Bone Marrow Aspiration—cont'd

TECHNIQUE: ILIAC CREST

1. With this approach, the needle is inserted into the widest portion of the dorsal iliac spine and directed caudally and ventrally into the marrow cavity.

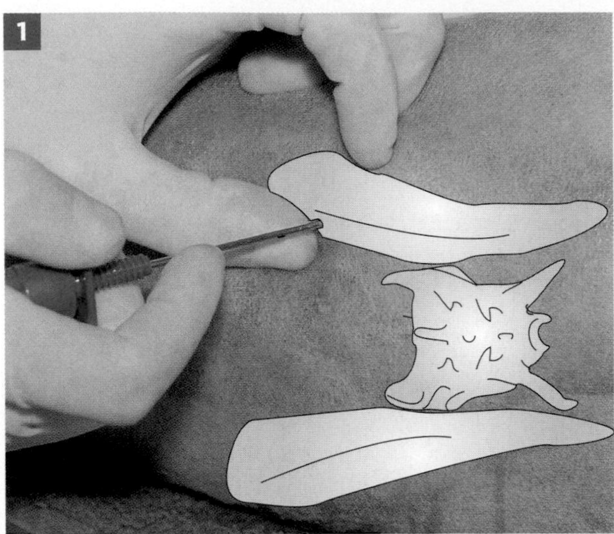

Anatomic overlay showing a bone marrow needle properly positioned for insertion.

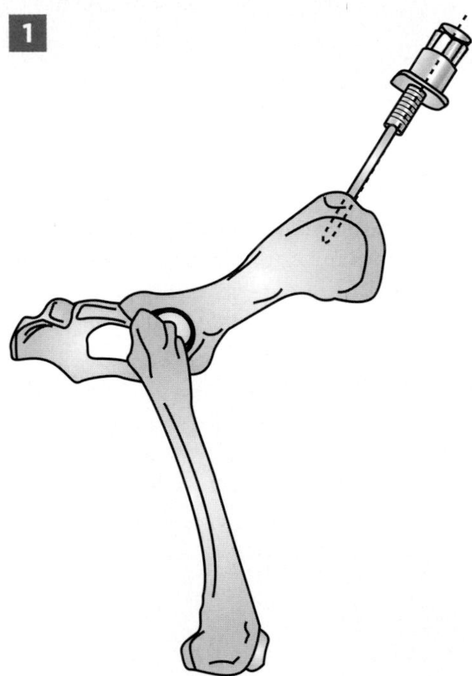

The pelvis showing landmarks for needle insertion.

2. Restrain the animal in lateral recumbency. Alternatively, the patient can be placed in sternal recumbency with the hind limbs under its body to maximize protrusion of the iliac crests.
3. Clip and surgically prep the skin in the region of the iliac crest.
4. The site of needle entry is the widest and most dorsal aspect of the wing of the ilium. Inject lidocaine blocking solution to block the skin and underlying tissues down to the bone at this site.
5. Use a scalpel blade (#11) to make a stab incision in the skin.
6. Palpate and locate the prominence of the iliac crest, placing a finger on either side of the bone. The needle should enter the widest and most dorsal aspect of the wing of the ilium.
7. Insert the needle through the hole in the skin until the cortex of the ilium is encountered. The long axis of the needle should be parallel to the long axis of the wing of the ilium, with the tip directed caudally and ventrally into the ilium.

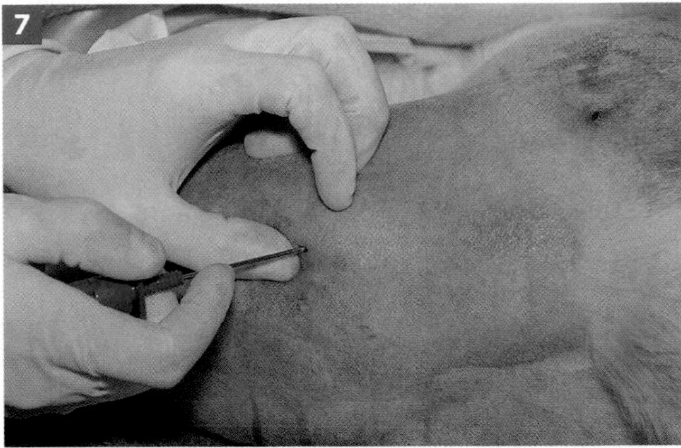

The needle enters the widest and most dorsal aspect of the wing of the ilium and is directed caudally and ventrally into the marrow cavity.

8. While moderate pressure is applied to the needle with the stylet in place, the needle should be rotated with short, alternating clockwise movements until it becomes firmly seated in the bone. Once the needle is firmly seated, it is usually within the marrow cavity.

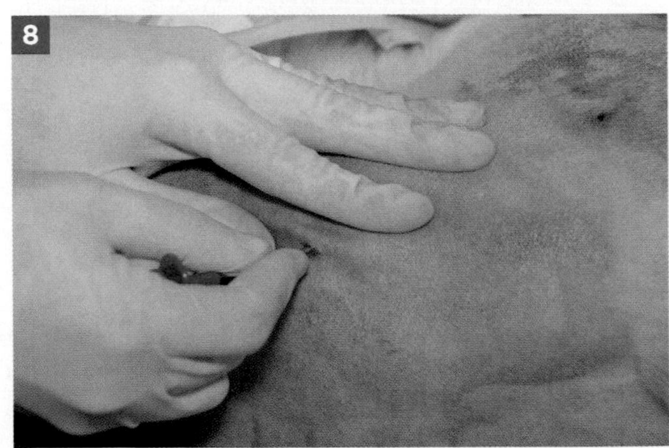

Pressure is applied as the needle is advanced by rotation into the bone.

9. Remove the cap and the stylet.

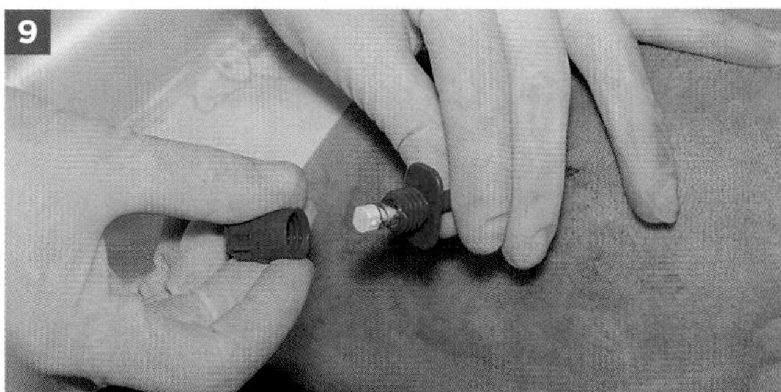

The cap is removed.

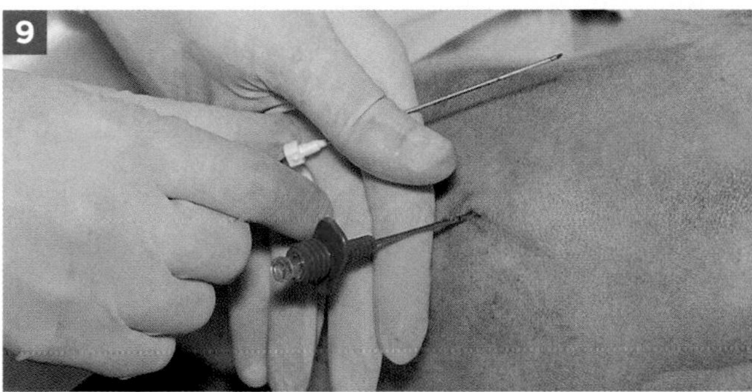

The stylet is removed.

10. Attach a 12-mL syringe and withdraw the syringe plunger, applying full negative pressure (6 to 8 mL) rapidly and vigorously until blood enters the hub of the needle.

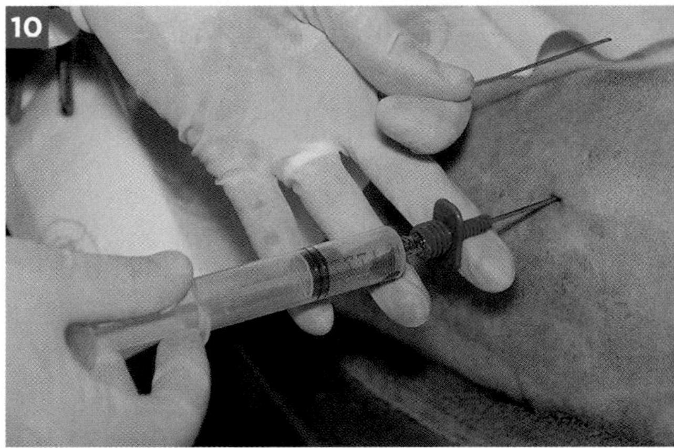

Suction is applied until bone marrow appears in the hub of the needle.

11. As soon as blood is seen in the needle hub, discontinue suction to minimize hemodilution of the sample.

12. Quickly disconnect the syringe from the needle and prepare slides for examination as outlined following.

SAMPLE HANDLING

Equipment

- Numerous clean glass slides
- Small plastic Petri dish
- 2% to 3% EDTA (ethylenediaminetetraacetic acid) solution
- Thumb forceps

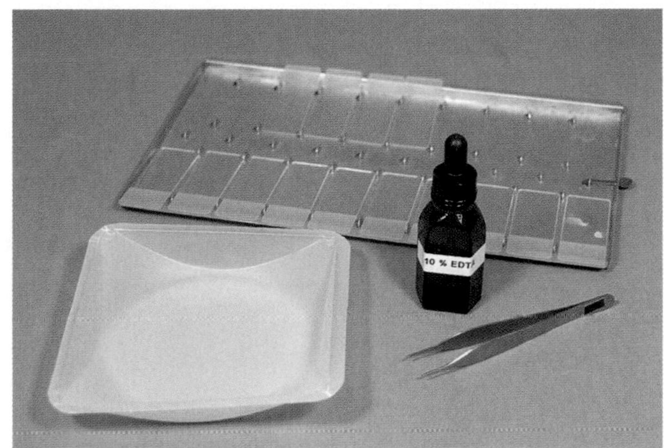

The equipment required for preparation of slides from bone marrow aspiration.

Technique

1. If bone marrow is collected without using EDTA for anticoagulation, then immediately after disconnecting the syringe from the needle, one drop of the material collected is placed on each of 10 to 12 waiting slides and smears are made. Smears must be made very rapidly because marrow clots quickly. If the material collected is very bloody, some of the excess blood can be removed by tilting the slide to the side to allow excess peripheral blood to roll away and then gently placing a second clean slide over the top of the remaining bone marrow on the first slide, and pulling the slides apart.

PROCEDURE 12-1 Bone Marrow Aspiration—cont'd

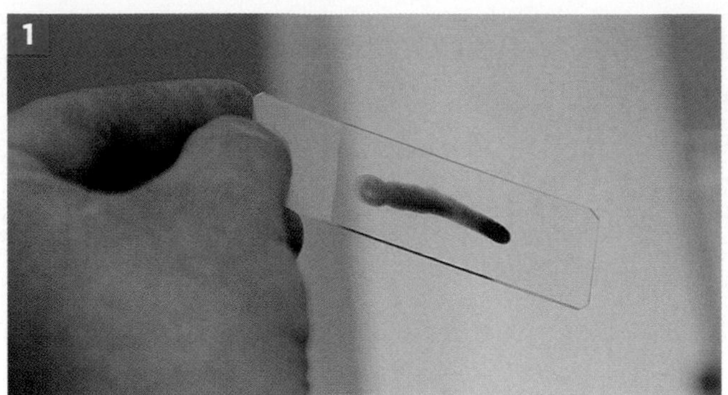

A drop of marrow is placed on a slide, and the slide is tilted to allow excess blood to roll away.

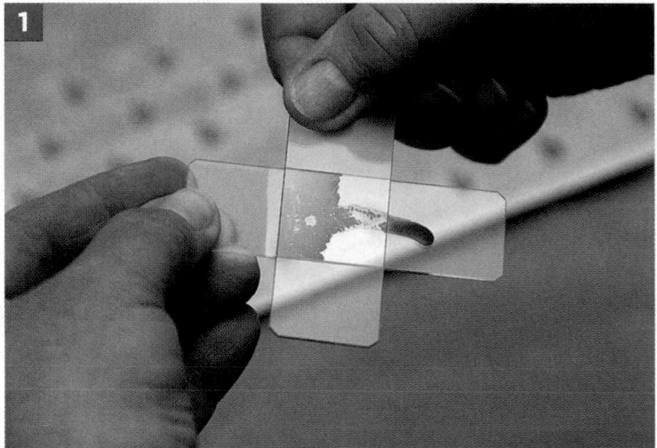

A second slide is used to gently compress the drop of marrow.

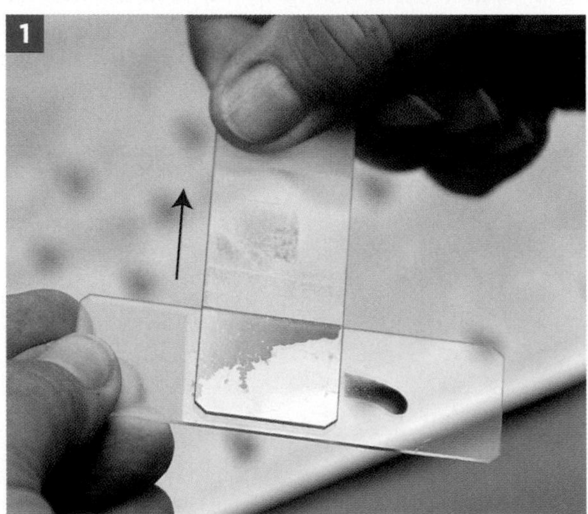

The top slide is pulled away, smearing the bone marrow sample on the second slide.

2. When EDTA is used, more care can be taken in making the slides. After detaching the syringe from the bone marrow needle, squirt the contents of the syringe into a chilled plastic Petri dish containing 1 or 2 drops of 10% EDTA, and swirl to mix. Once the anticoagulated sample is within the Petri dish, tilt the dish so that free blood flows to the side, leaving pale yellow glistening marrow particles visible on the bottom. Attempt to distinguish light opaque, slightly granular bone marrow spicules (which will be very cellular) from fat globules (which will be poorly cellular). Use forceps or a needle to collect the visible marrow particles and put them on a microscope slide. Gently place a second slide perpendicular to the first slide over the top of the marrow particle, and then pull the slides apart.

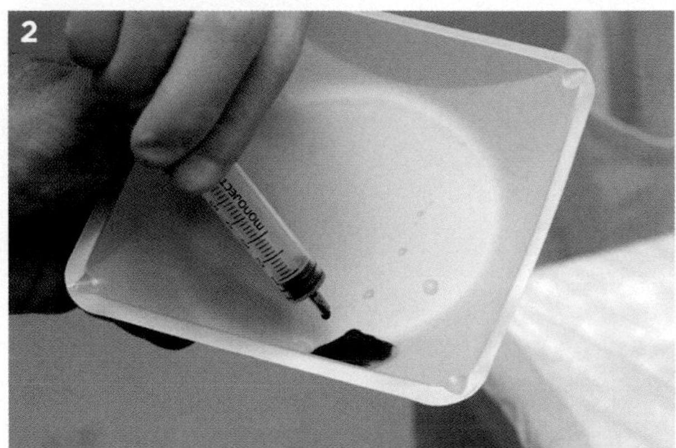

Bone marrow can be placed into a chilled plastic Petri dish containing 1 or 2 drops of 10% EDTA and swirled to mix.

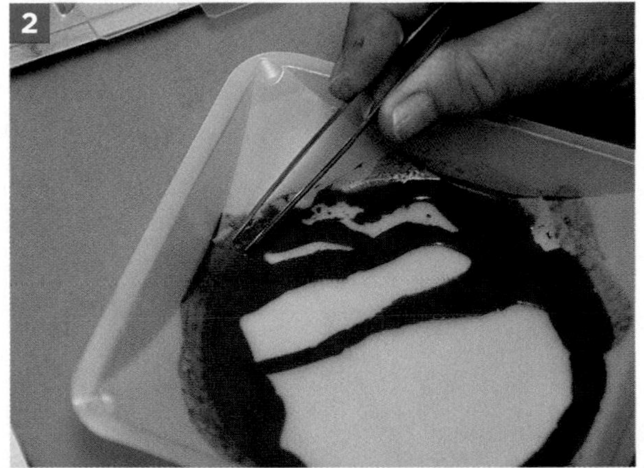

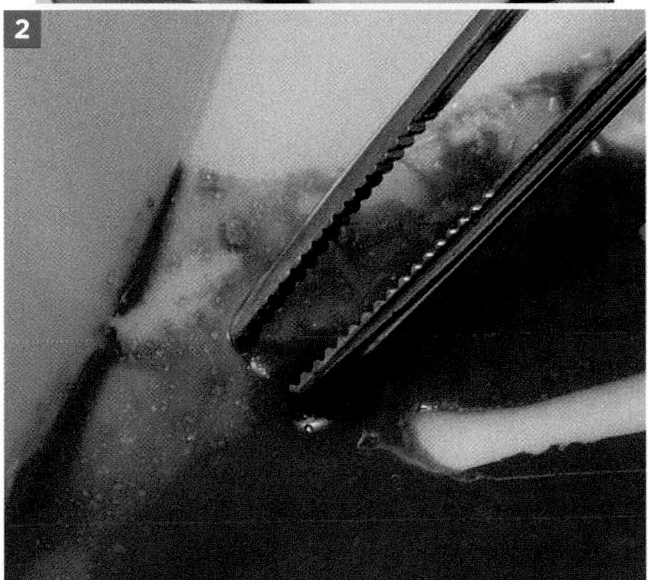

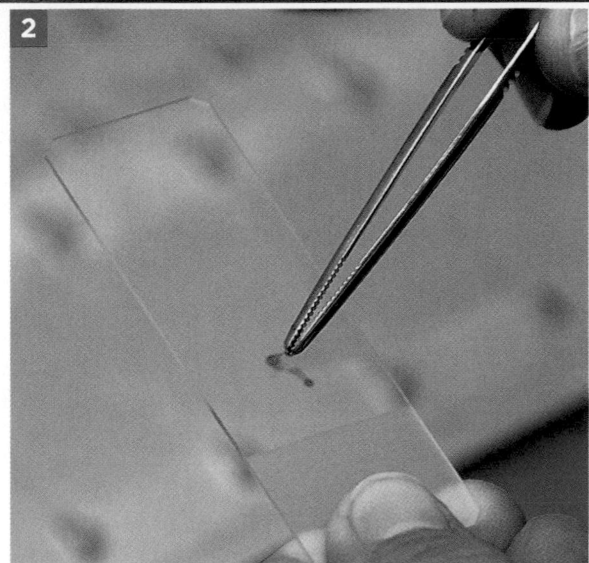

Granular bone marrow spicules are grasped with a forceps and transferred to a slide.

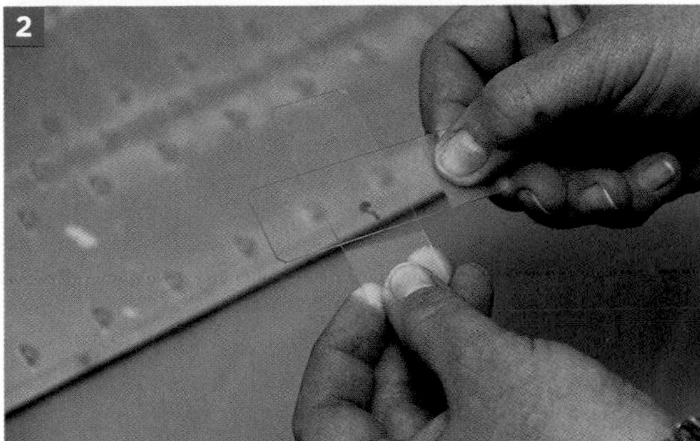

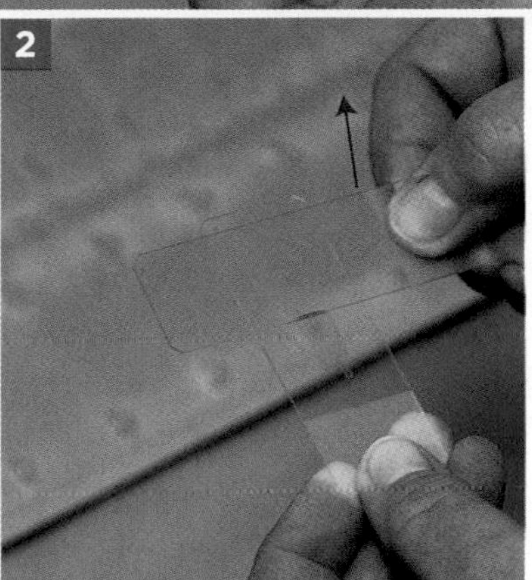

Gently place a second slide perpendicular to the first slide over the top of the marrow particle, and then pull the slides apart.

3. Dry slides quickly (hair dryer or rapid air dry), and submit at least four unstained slides to the laboratory
4. If desired, to assess the adequacy of the sample, one slide can be stained immediately with Diff-Quick stain. Spicules should stain dark blue, and be surrounded microscopically by a monolayer of hematopoietic cells.

Results

When performing a complete evaluation, smears must be examined in a systematic manner, and the following components should be analyzed:

1. Bone marrow cellularity
2. Iron stores
3. Megakaryocyte numbers and sequence of maturation. Mature forms normally exceed immature forms.
4. Erythroid lineage and sequence of maturation
5. Myeloid lineage and sequence of maturation
6. Myeloid to erythroid ratio (M:E)—this is normally 1:1 to 2:1
7. Differential count, presence of blast cells

PROCEDURE 12-2

Bone Marrow Core

PURPOSE

To collect a core of bone marrow tissue for evaluation

INDICATIONS

1. All indications as for bone marrow aspirate
2. Bone marrow core examination allows assessment of the architecture of the bone marrow, and the cellularity of the sample without interference by hemodilution.
3. Bone marrow core samples may be superior to bone marrow aspirates for diagnosis of marrow neoplasia, myelofibrosis, and necrosis.
4. Any patient in whom an inadequate sample was obtained during bone marrow aspiration
5. Focal lytic or proliferative bone lesions (for bone biopsy)

CONTRAINDICATIONS AND COMPLICATIONS

1. None. Even patients with severe thrombocytopenia or severe coagulopathy are unlikely to bleed excessively from this procedure.
2. It is important to submit a current CBC and blood smear and a bone marrow aspirate to facilitate interpretation of bone marrow core. Architecture is best assessed in the core sample, whereas cellular detail is better assessed using bone marrow aspirate cytology.

RESTRAINT

1. Sedation and local anesthesia are adequate in most cases.
2. To obtain a core from the ilium, place the animal in lateral recumbency or else sternal recumbency with the hind limbs under its body to maximize protrusion of the iliac crests.
3. To obtain a core from the proximal humerus, place the animal in lateral recumbency.
4. Lidocaine blocking solution (2% lidocaine mixed 9:1 with 8.4% sodium bicarbonate) can be used to block the skin, subcutaneous tissues, and periosteum. The addition of bicarbonate decreases the sting of injection and speeds the local analgesic effect of the lidocaine.

EQUIPMENT

- Jamshidi 3½-inch-long bone marrow biopsy needle with stylet (13-gauge for small dogs and cats, 11-gauge for larger dogs). This needle has a uniform external diameter and tubular construction except for the tapered distal portion. The distal tip is beveled and has a sharp cutting edge. The distal end is radically tapered toward the cutting tip to help retain the sample within the needle bore and prevent compression of the sample. To remove the biopsy sample, a crooked wire is inserted retrograde into the needle to push the core out through the wider proximal end.
- Sterile gloves
- Lidocaine blocking solution (2% lidocaine mixed 9:1 with 8.4% sodium bicarbonate)
- #11 scalpel blade
- Clean glass slides
- Formalin jar

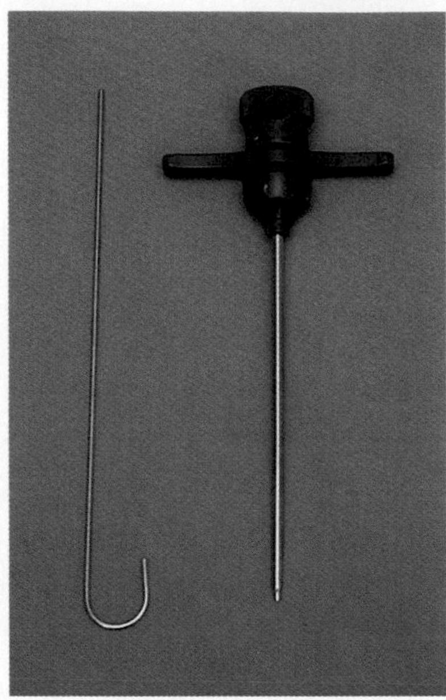

A Jamshidi bone marrow biopsy needle with stylet and crooked wire used to push the core out through the wider proximal end.

SPECIAL ANATOMY

Bone marrow core samples can be taken from the same bone as bone marrow aspirates, requiring shaving and preparation of only one site. The core collection site should be a few millimeters away from the aspiration site. Core samples are most often collected from the ilium (through-and-through sample from the wing of the ilium) or the proximal humerus.

PREPARATION

1. Clip and surgically prep the region. Bone marrow core collection should be performed as a sterile procedure.

TECHNIQUE: ILIUM

1. Core samples can be obtained as a through-and-through core from the dorsal aspect of the wing of the ilium.

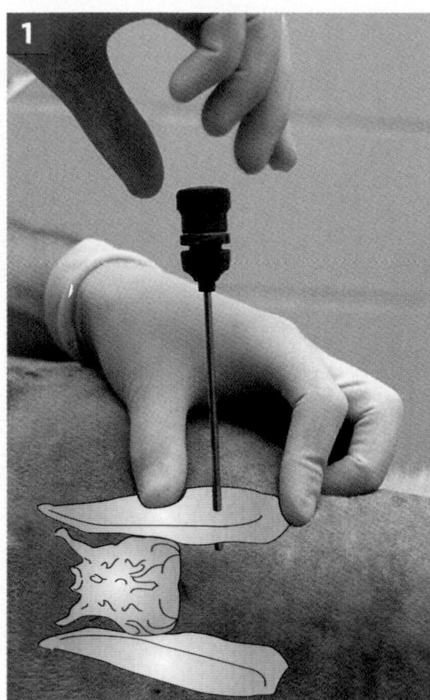

Needle in place for bone marrow core sample from the wing of the ilium.

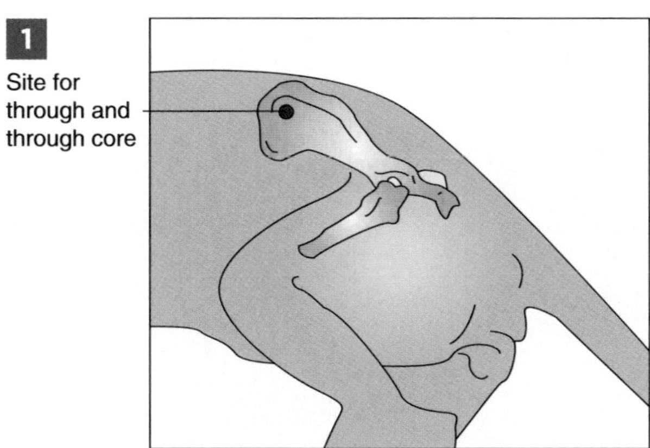

Anatomic landmarks for obtaining bone marrow core biopsy from the wing of the ilium.

2. Restrain the patient in lateral recumbency.
3. Palpate and locate the prominence of the iliac crest.

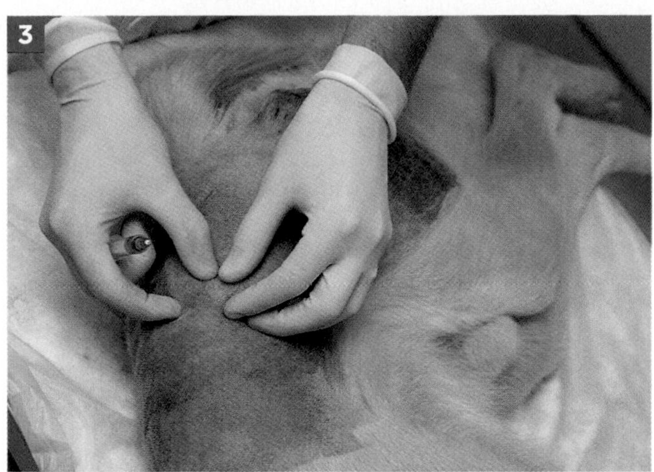

Palpating the prominence of the iliac crest.

4. The sample will be obtained as a through-and-through core from lateral to medial through the dorsal aspect of the wing of the ilium.
5. Inject lidocaine blocking solution to block the skin and subcutaneous tissues down to the periosteum.

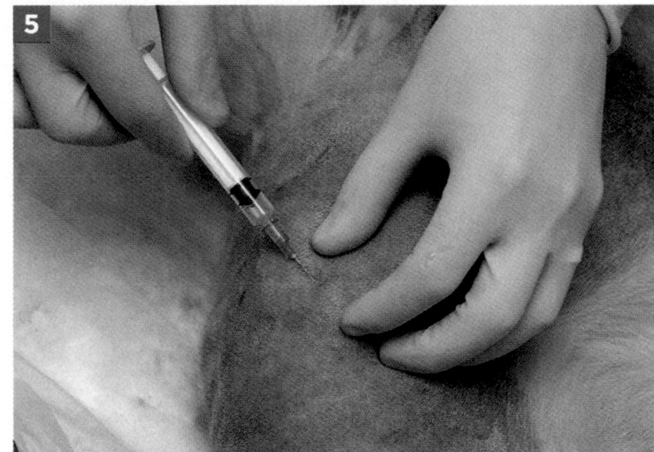

Lidocaine blocking solution is injected to block the skin and subcutaneous tissues down to the periosteum.

PROCEDURE 12-2 Bone Marrow Core—cont'd

6. Use a scalpel blade (#11) to make a stab incision in the skin.

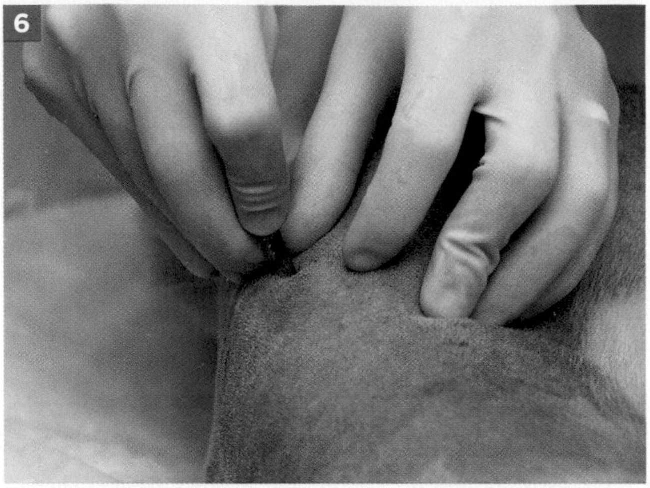

A # 11 scalpel blade is used to make a stab incision in the skin.

7. Insert the needle through the hole in the skin and advance it toward the bone, perpendicular to the ilium until the cortex is encountered.

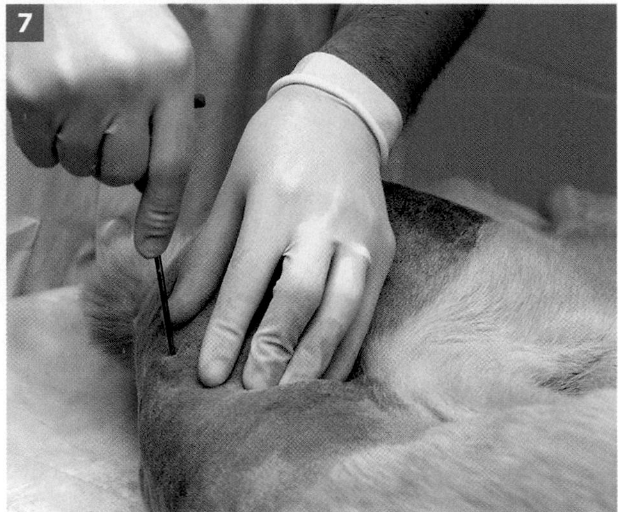

The needle is advanced toward the bone, perpendicular to the ilium until the cortex is encountered.

8. Remove the stylet.

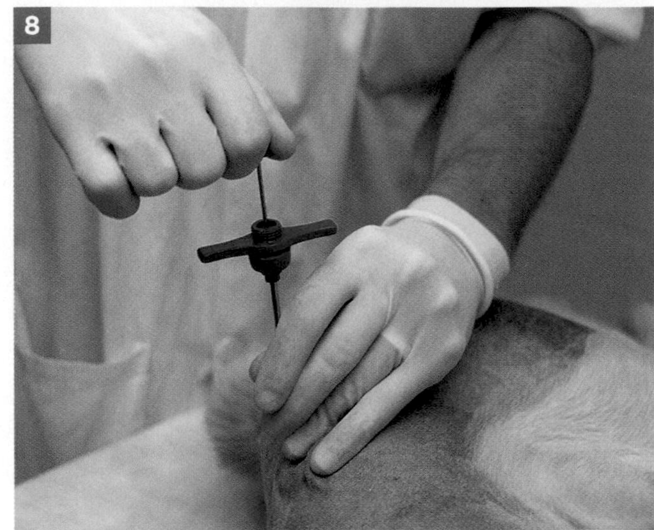

The stylet is removed.

9. Advance the needle into the canal with a twisting motion and forward pressure. Continue until the opposite cortex is encountered and penetrated.

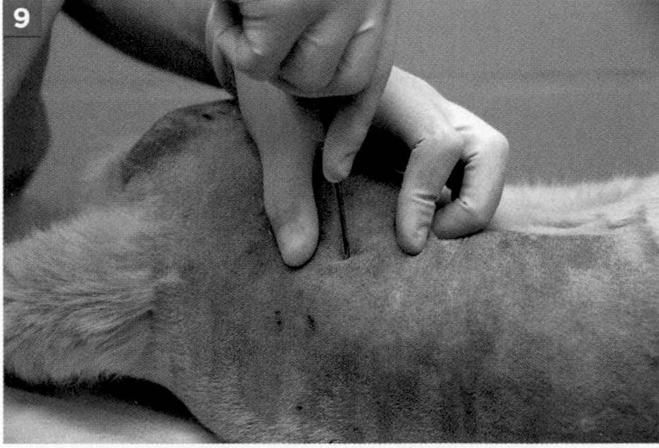

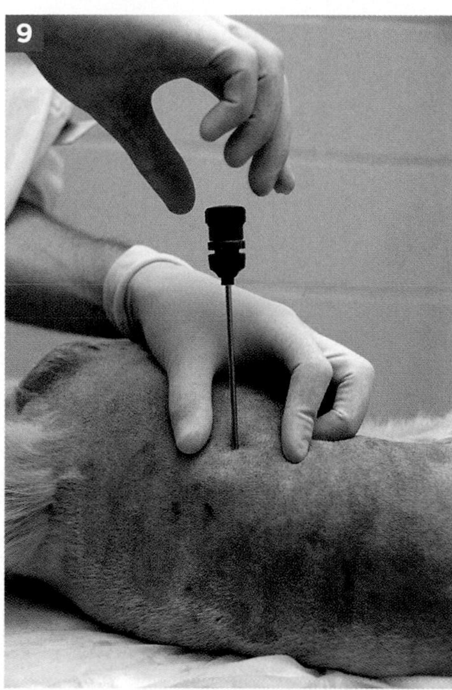

The needle is advanced through the wing of the ilium with a twisting motion and forward pressure until the opposite cortex is encountered and penetrated.

10. Rock the needle back and forth and "stir" the needle along its long axis to loosen the core.

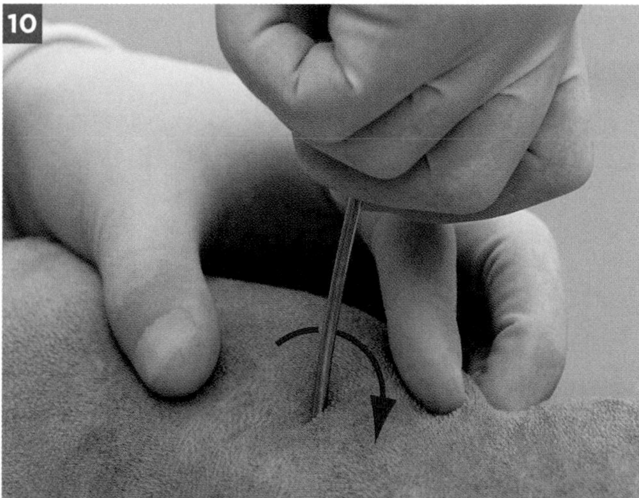

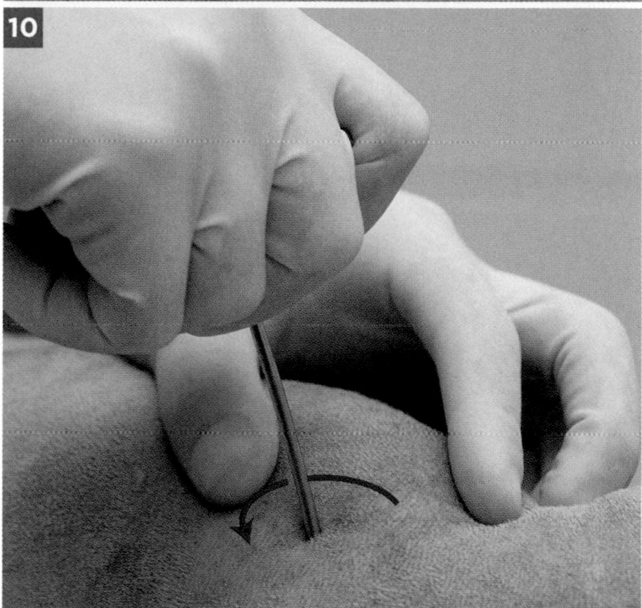

The needle is rocked back and forth in a stirring motion to loosen the core of bone.

11. Withdraw the needle from the bone with a twisting motion in one direction (clockwise or counterclockwise).

PROCEDURE 12-2 Bone Marrow Core—cont'd

TECHNIQUE: HUMERUS

1. Core samples can be obtained from the medullary cavity of the humerus, using the same landmarks as used for the angle approach for bone marrow aspiration from the proximal humerus.
2. Restrain the patient in lateral recumbency.
3. Grasp the elbow to stabilize the limb and flex the shoulder so that the humerus is parallel to the body wall.
4. Palpate the flat region on the craniolateral humerus, just distal to the greater tubercle. This will be the site of needle entry.

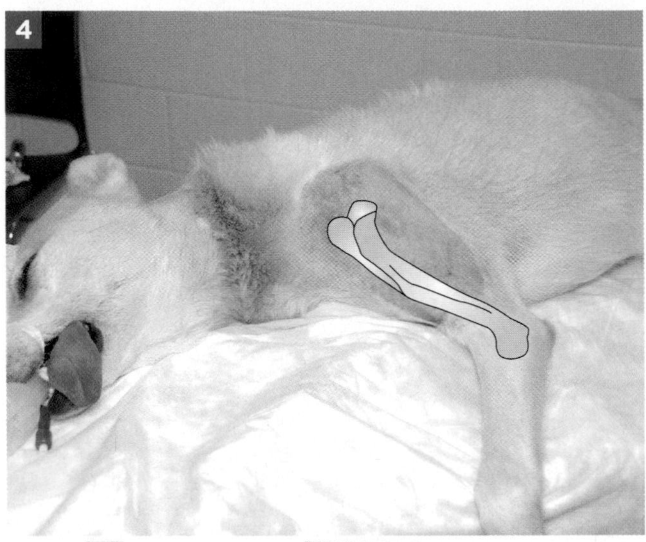

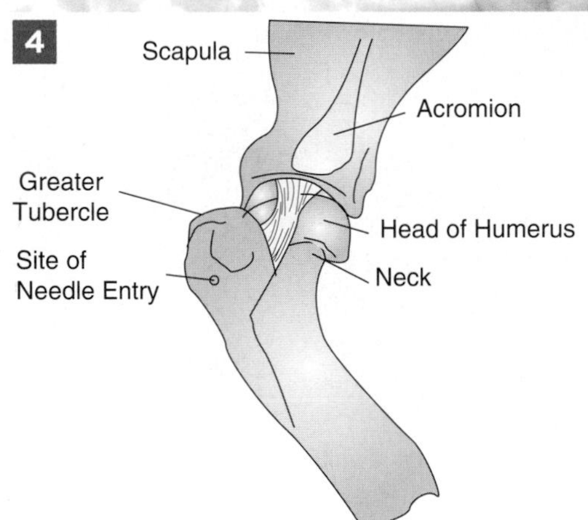

Needle entry is on the flat region on the craniolateral humerus, just distal to the greater tubercle.

5. Inject lidocaine blocking solution to block the skin and subcutaneous tissues down to the bone.
6. Use a scalpel blade to make a stab incision over the biopsy site.
7. Insert the needle through the stab incision, just distal to the greater tubercle, and direct the needle tip distally toward the elbow, at an angle 45 degrees from the long axis of the humerus.

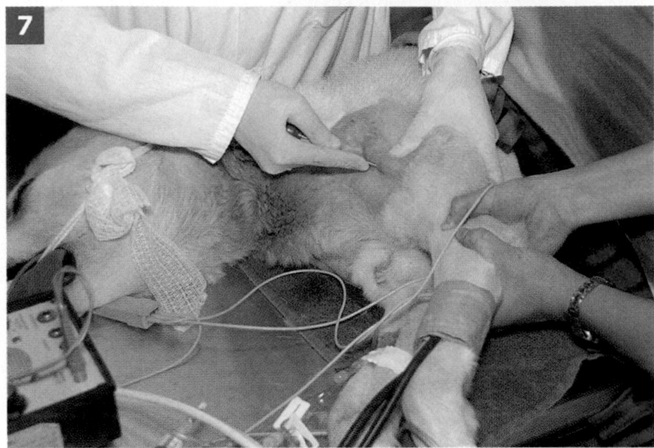

The needle tip should be directed distally toward the elbow.

8. Remove the stylet once the cortex has been penetrated.

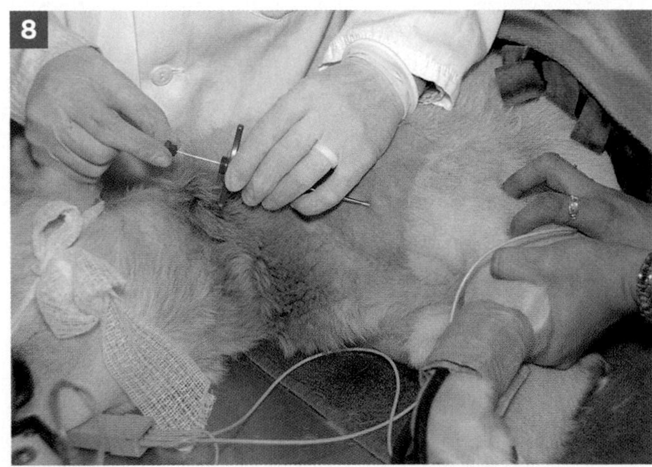

Remove the stylet once the cortex has been penetrated.

9. Forcefully advance the needle down the canal with a twisting motion and forward pressure until it is firmly seated.

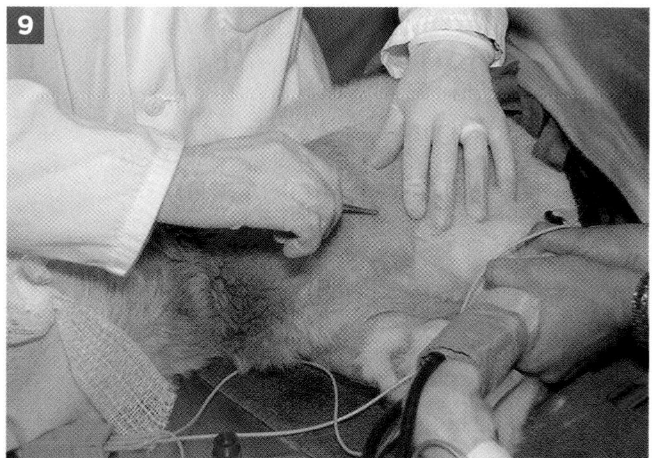

Advance the needle forcefully down the canal with a twisting motion and forward pressure until it is firmly seated.

10. Rock the needle back and forth and "stir" the needle along its long axis to loosen the core.

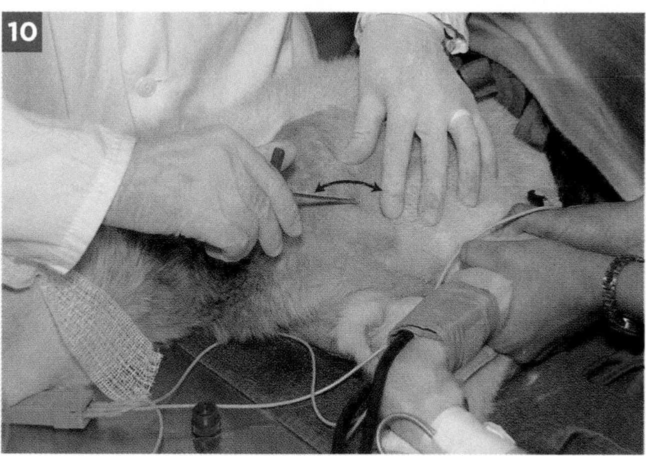

Stir the needle along its long axis to loosen the core.

11. Slightly retract the needle, redirect, and advance the needle again to cut a core of tissue.
12. Withdraw the needle from the bone with a twisting motion in one direction (clockwise or counterclockwise).

SAMPLE HANDLING

1. Use the stylet or a guidewire to expel the sample through the proximal hub of the needle onto a slide.

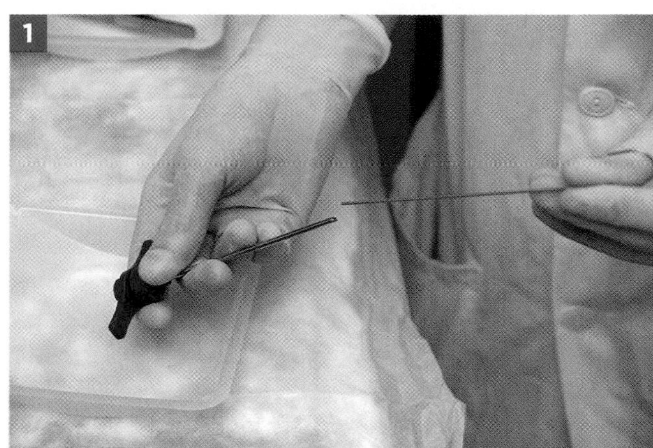

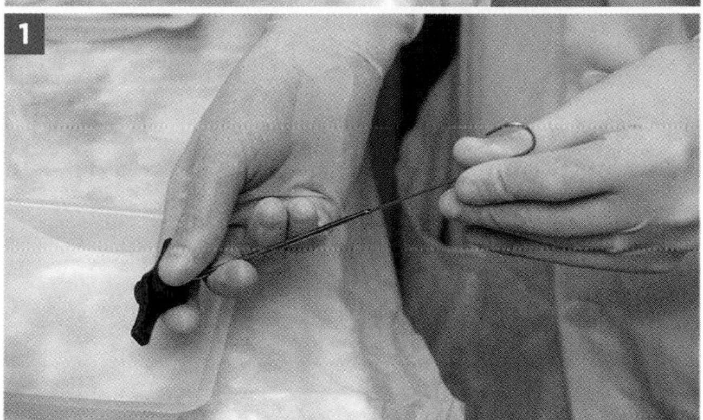

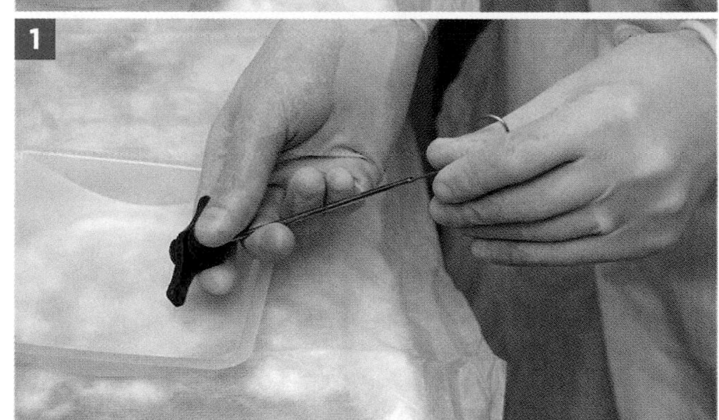

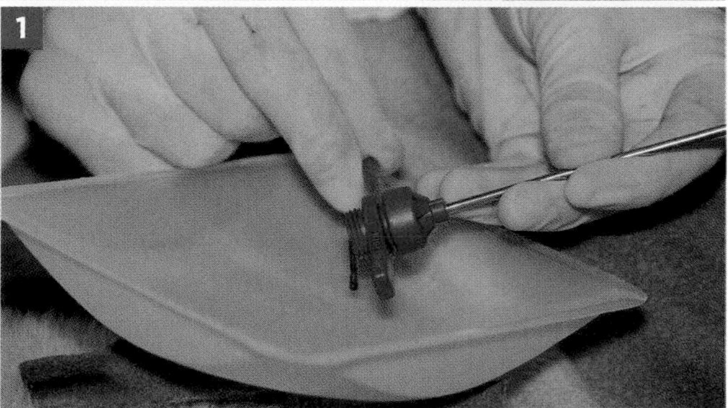

Use the crooked guidewire to expel the sample through the proximal hub of the needle onto a slide.

PROCEDURE 12-2 Bone Marrow Core—cont'd

2. Core samples typically appear as a pink or red core of tissue adjacent to a white piece of bone cortex.

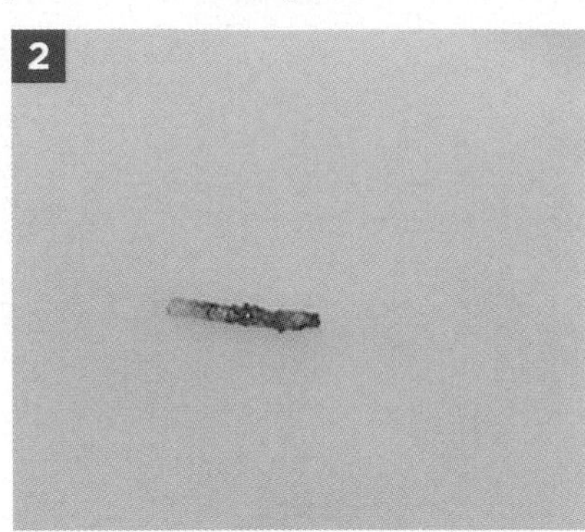

3. Gently roll the core on a slide to submit for cytologic evaluation.

4. Place the core in formalin.

5. Ideally repeat and obtain two or three cores for evaluation.

Note: Never place formalin jars or samples near cytology smears because the formalin fumes will interfere with staining of the cytology slides.

Arthrocentesis 13

PROCEDURE 13-1
Arthrocentesis

PURPOSE

To collect synovial fluid for analysis

INDICATIONS

1. Any dog or cat with joint swelling or joint pain in one or multiple joints
2. Dogs or cats with a shifting leg lameness or a "walking on eggshells" gait.
3. Dogs with fever of unknown origin (FUO). Polyarthritis is one of the most common causes of FUO in dogs.
4. Dogs with inflammatory bloodwork (leukocytosis, hyperglobulinemia) with no known site of infection or inflammation
5. Whenever a dog is evaluated for polyarthritis, it is important to tap at least five joints. The small joints (carpi and hocks) are most likely to be affected with immune-mediated disease.

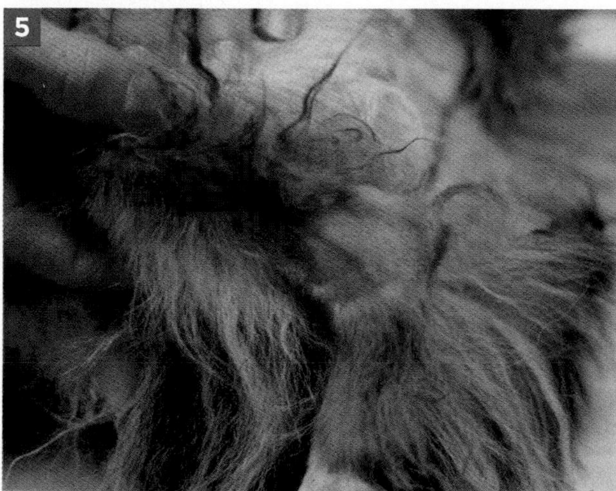

Swollen hock in a Shetland Sheepdog with immune-mediated polyarthritis. This dog was unwilling to walk due to pain and was referred for suspected paralysis.

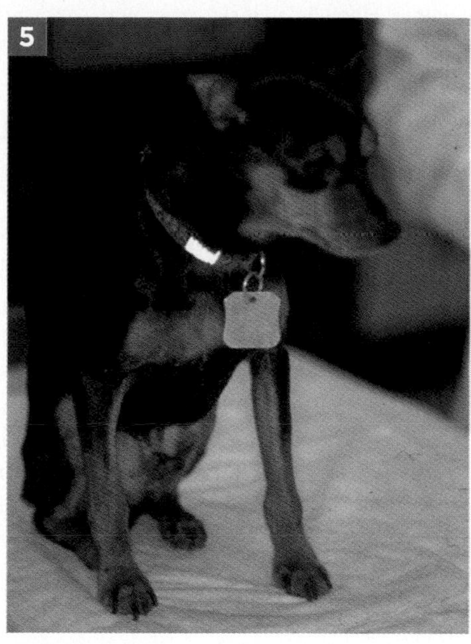

Swollen carpis in a Miniature Pinscher with immune-mediated polyarthritis.

PROCEDURE 13-1 Arthrocentesis—cont'd

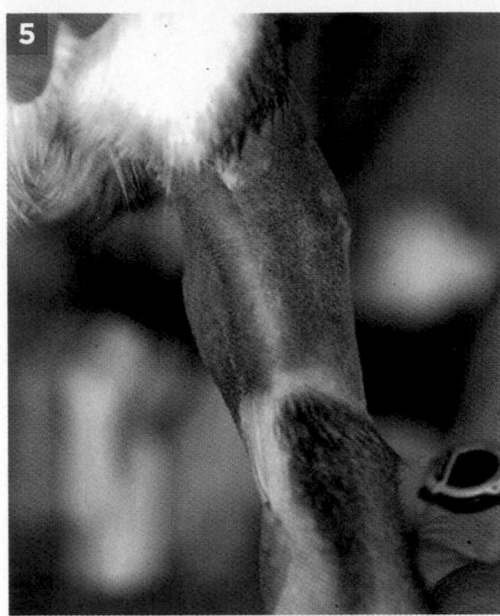

Swollen and painful elbow in a Husky-cross with septic arthritis caused by migration of a porcupine quill into the joint.

CONTRAINDICATIONS AND WARNINGS

Significant coagulopathy

POSITIONING AND RESTRAINT

1. Restrain the patient and administer sedation to prevent movement. Collection of fluid from carpi, hocks, and stifles causes minimal discomfort in a relaxed patient, whereas tapping elbows, shoulders, and hips requires more analgesia and sedation. It is very important to avoid patient movement, which can cause blood contamination of the sample.
2. Adequate sedation and analgesia for arthrocentesis can usually be obtained using injectable acepromazine and hydromorphone. General anesthesia is recommended for tapping the hip.

EQUIPMENT

- 25-gauge needles
- 22-gauge, 1½-inch needles
- 3-mL syringes
- Glass microscope slides
- Blood culture bottle

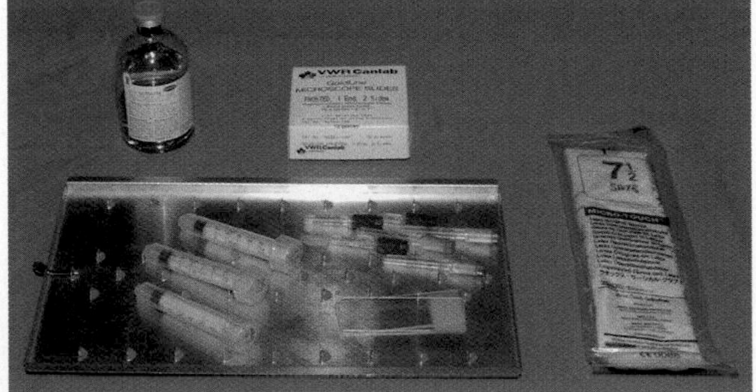

Equipment required to collect synovial fluid in dogs and cats.

GENERAL TECHNIQUE

1. Clip and aseptically prepare the site, and wear sterile gloves.
2. Have an assistant hold the limb and flex and extend the joint as directed.
3. Palpate the joint, manipulating it so that the joint spaces and landmarks can be appreciated. Examine a skeleton if necessary to become familiar with the anatomic landmarks.
4. Attach a needle to a 3-mL syringe. The size of needle will depend on the size of the dog and the joint being aspirated. The carpi and hocks of all dogs and cats can be accessed with a 25-gauge needle, as can the larger joints in small dogs. Once a dog exceeds 10 kg (22 lb), a longer and sturdier 22-gauge needle is necessary to tap the stifle, elbow, and shoulder. In large dogs a spinal needle may be required to tap the hip joint.
5. Insert the needle into the joint space, and apply gentle suction.

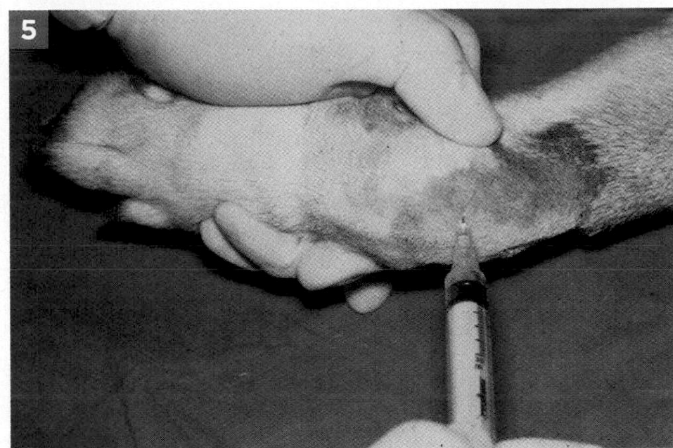

Gentle suction is applied once the needle is inserted into the joint space.

6. As soon as one drop of joint fluid is visible in the hub of the needle, release suction and withdraw the needle from the joint and the skin. Only a very small amount of joint fluid (1 to 3 drops) is necessary for analysis—the risk of blood contamination increases if additional joint fluid is removed. Also, failure to release suction before needle withdrawal may cause blood contamination of the sample from cutaneous vessels.

7. Disconnect the needle from the syringe, place air in the syringe, then reattach the needle.

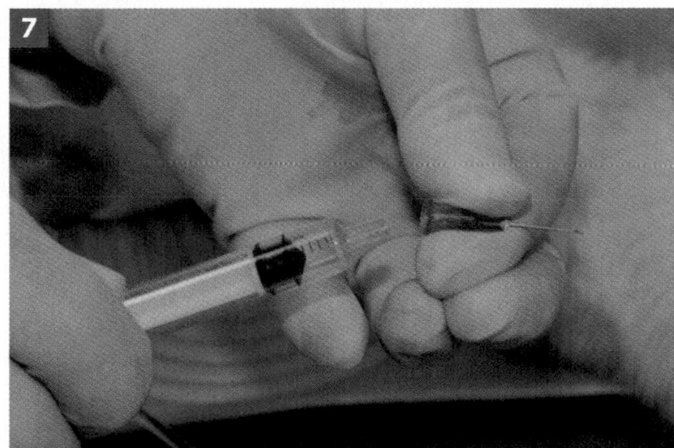

The needle is disconnected, air is placed in the syringe, and the needle is reconnected.

8. Expel a drop of synovial fluid onto a microscope slide. Assess the color, clarity, and viscosity of the fluid.

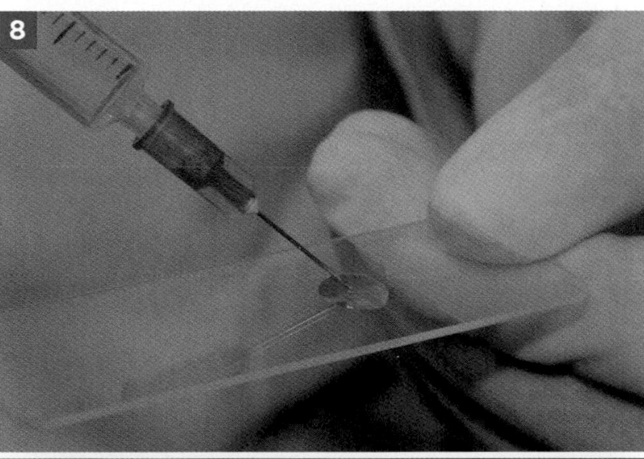

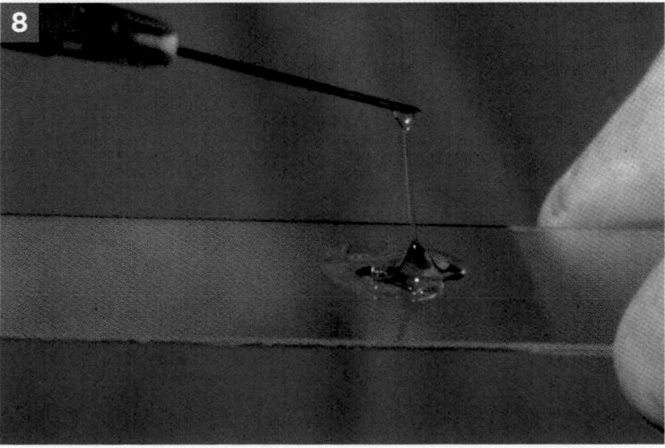

Expelling a drop of synovial fluid onto a microscope slide and assessing color, clarity, and viscosity.

9. Gently place a second microscope slide on top of the first, compressing the drop of joint fluid, and pull the two slides apart to make a smear. Let this dry, then stain to evaluate cytology.

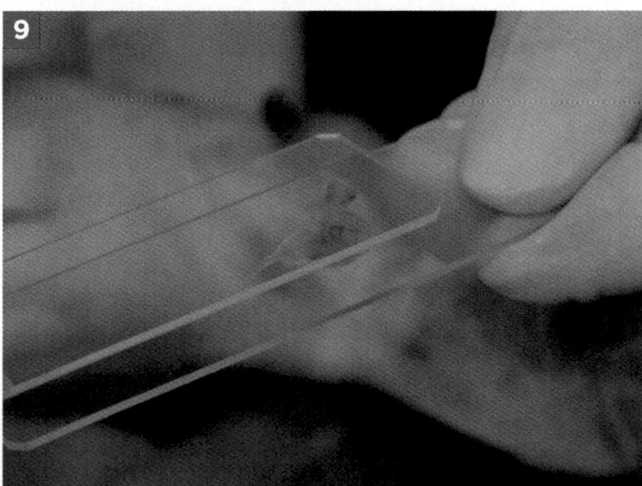

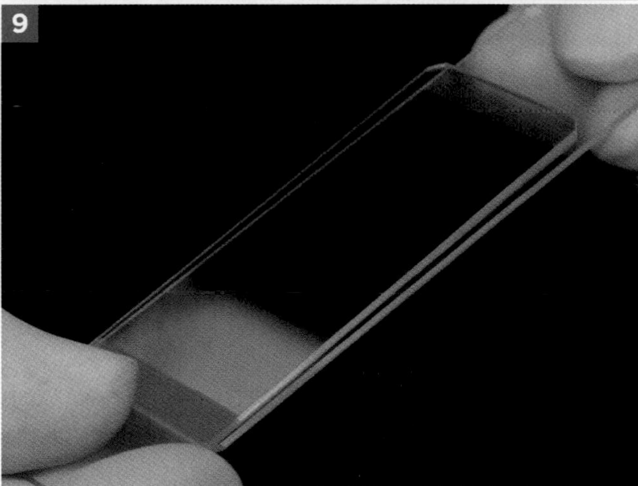

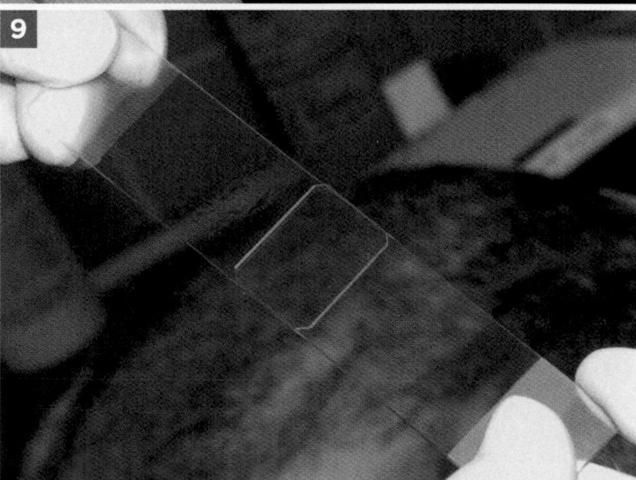

A second microscope slide is placed on top of the first, compressing the drop of joint fluid, and the two slides are pulled apart, smearing the joint fluid.

PROCEDURE 13-1 Arthrocentesis—cont'd

10. After all the joints have been tapped for cytologic evaluation, re-tap a joint to obtain 0.5 to 1 mL for bacteriologic culture. Inoculate this sample into a blood culture bottle and incubate at body temperature for 24 hours before plating for culture. This increases the likelihood of positive culture in an infected joint.

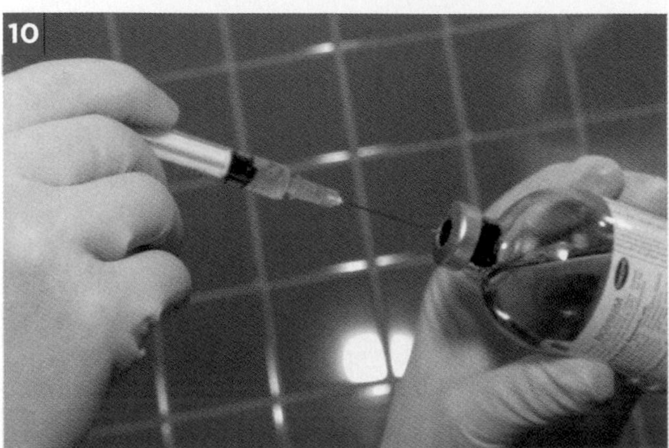

Synovial fluid for culture is inoculated into a blood culture bottle.

RESULTS

1. Normal joint fluid is clear and colorless.

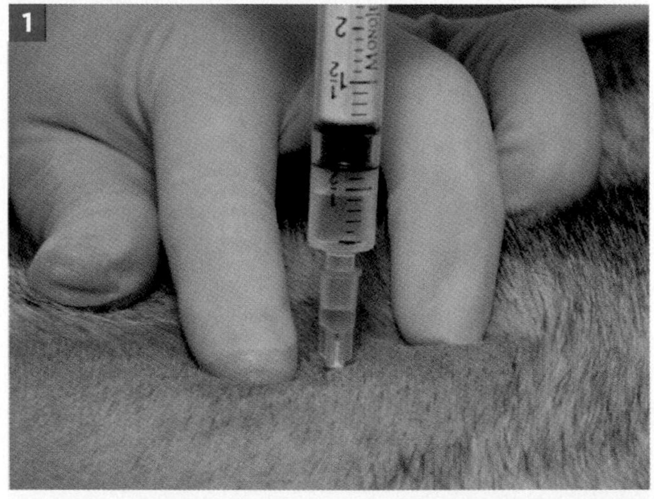

Normal joint fluid is clear and colorless.

2. Normal joint fluid is also very viscous (stringy) due to a high content of hyaluronic acid. Inflammation and infection decrease joint fluid viscosity, making it appear more watery.

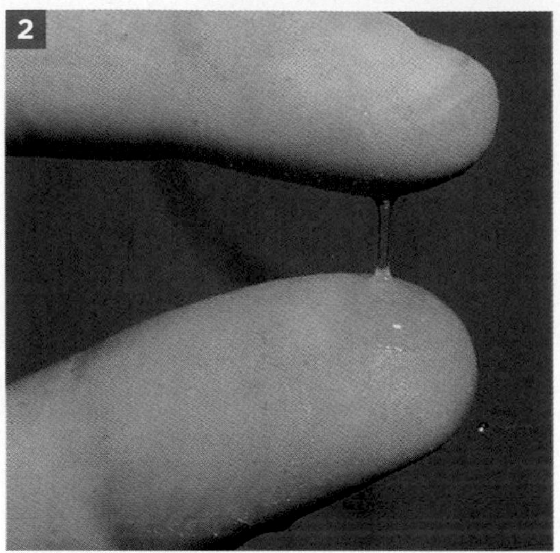

Normal joint fluid is viscous.

3. Normal joint fluid has a high protein content (stippled background) and contains no neutrophils and only a few mononuclear cells (<3000/μL; 1-5/HPF).

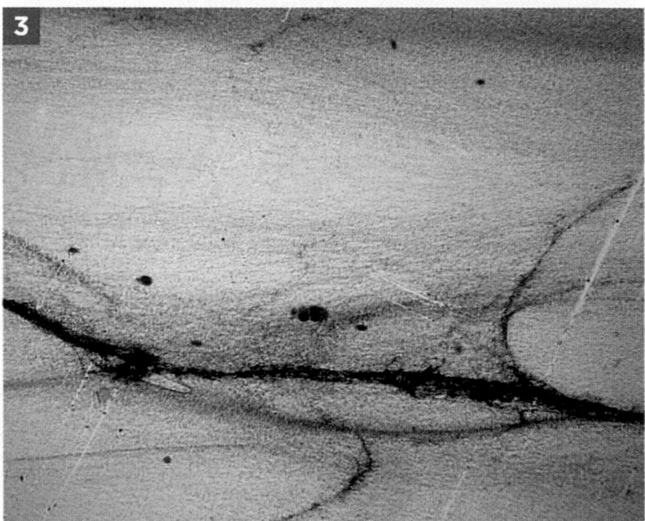

A smear of normal joint fluid has a stippled background and low cellularity.

4. Inflammatory joint fluid (increased neutrophils) can be seen in dogs with infectious or immune-mediated diseases affecting the joints.

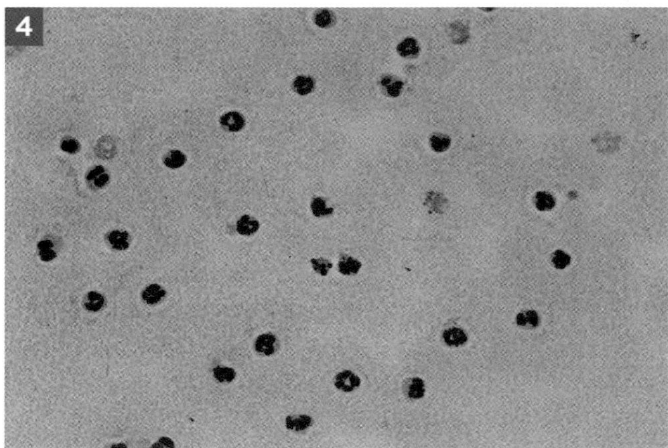

Joint fluid from a dog with polyarthritis contains many neutrophils.

5. Synovial fluid from some dogs with polyarthritis contains neutrophils that have ingested opsonized nuclear material. These cells are lupus erythematosus (LE) cells, and their presence suggests that the dog may have systemic lupus erythematosus (SLE).

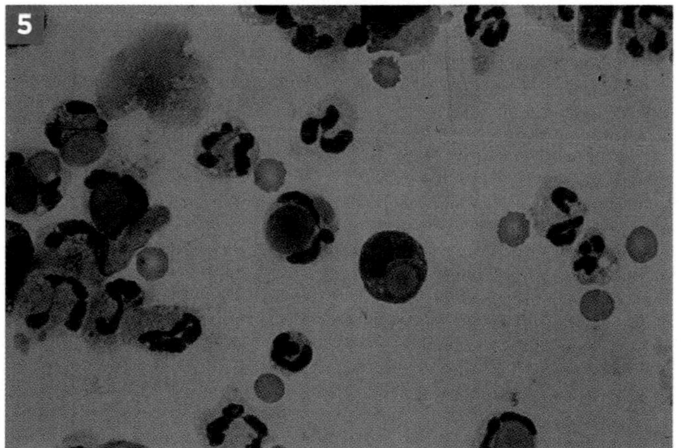

LE cells are neutrophils that have ingested opsonized nuclear material. Their presence in synovial fluid suggests a diagnosis of systemic lupus erythematosus (SLE).

SPECIFIC TECHNIQUE: CARPUS

1. Joint fluid can be collected from the radiocarpal or the intercarpal joint in the carpus. The radiocarpal is the easier joint to palpate and is the most common location for arthrocentesis.

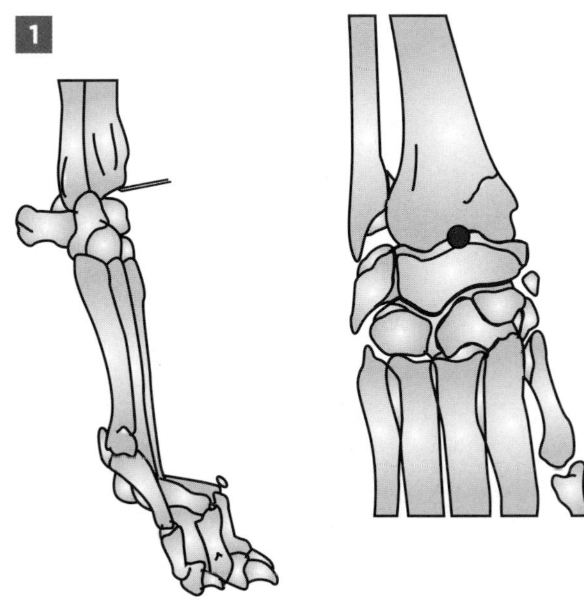

2. Partially flex the joint, palpating and inserting the needle in the radiocarpal space—the anteromedial aspect is usually best.

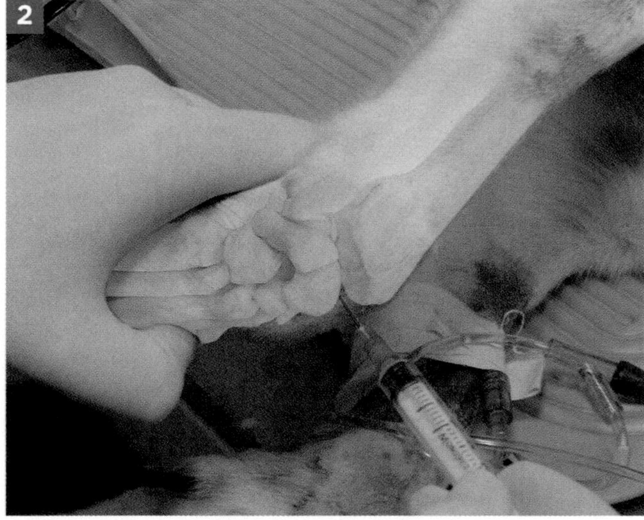

PROCEDURE 13-1 Arthrocentesis—cont'd

3. The distal radius has a complex contour, with bony prominences projecting into the joint space, occasionally making it impossible to advance the needle even when the space feels clear on external palpation. If your needle hits bone, try another site.
4. Once the needle enters the joint space, apply gentle suction.

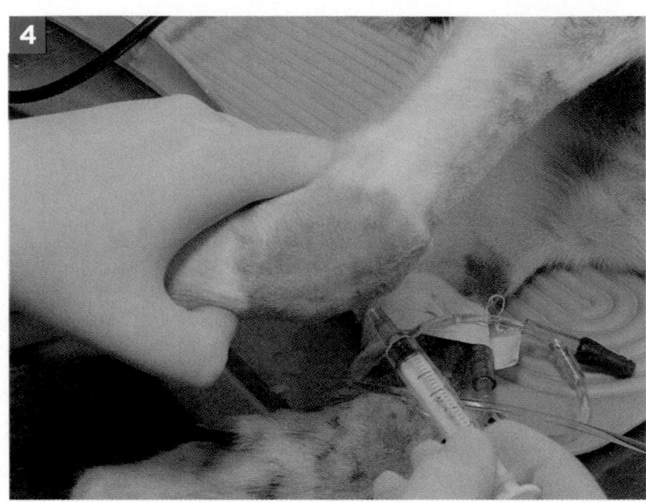

Synovial fluid collection from the anteromedial radiocarpal space.

5. The radiocarpal joint does not communicate with the other carpal joints—if blood contamination occurs during fluid collection from the radiocarpal joint, try tapping the intercarpal joint to obtain a sample. The intercarpal and carpometacarpal joints communicate.

SPECIFIC TECHNIQUE: HOCK

There are three different approaches to tapping the hock (tarsal) joint. Each is effective, so operator preference is the major reason for selecting one approach over another.

Anterior Approach

1. Alternately flex and extend the joint to palpate the landmarks.
2. Palpate the space between the distal tibia and the tibiotarsal bone on the anterolateral surface of the joint.

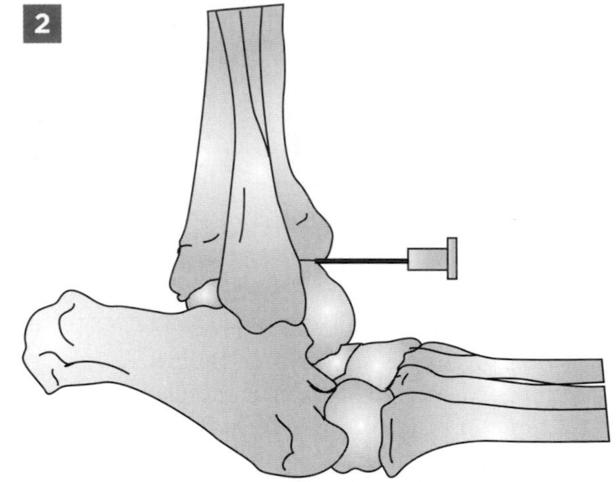

3. Hold the joint in extreme full extension so that the distal tibia is palpable as a ridge of bone.

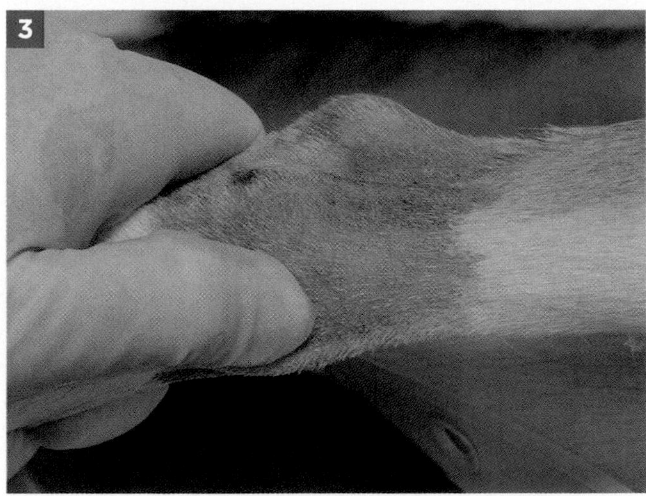

4. Insert the needle just distal to this ridge. The needle will hit bone almost immediately. Apply gentle suction.

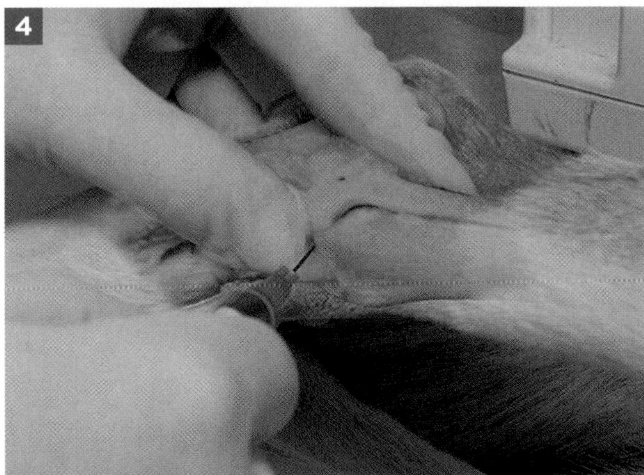

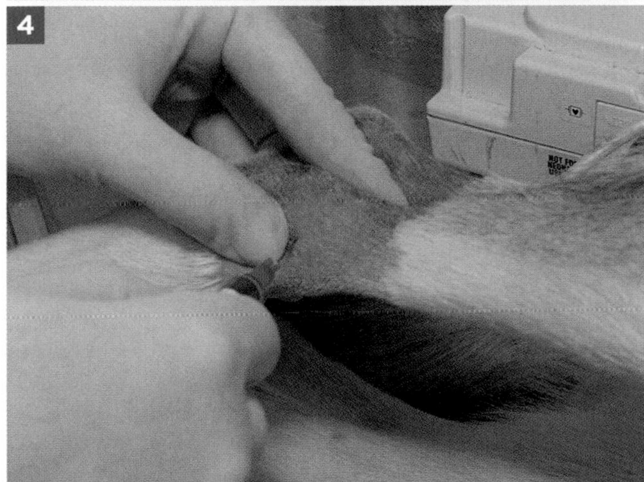

5. The needle will hit bone almost immediately. Apply gentle suction.

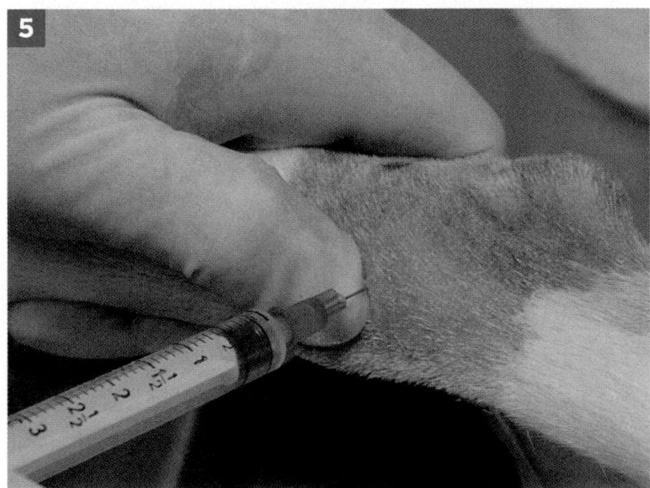

The anterior approach for synovial fluid collection from the hock involves passing the needle between the distal tibia and the tibiotarsal bone on the anterolateral surface of the joint.

Lateral Approach

1. The lateral approach is often used to collect joint fluid from the hock.

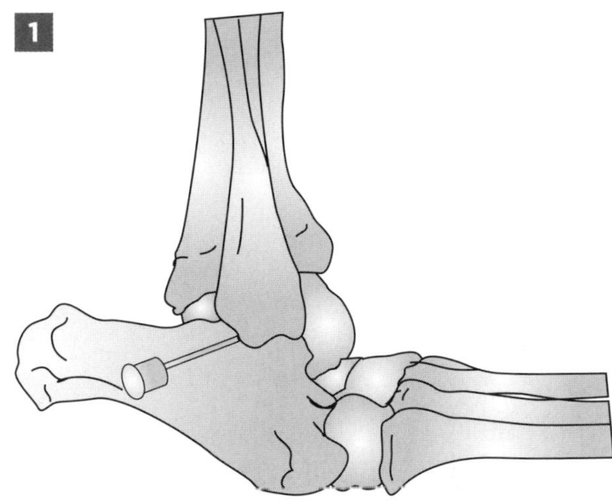

2. Hold the joint in partial flexion and palpate the lateral malleolus of the fibula.

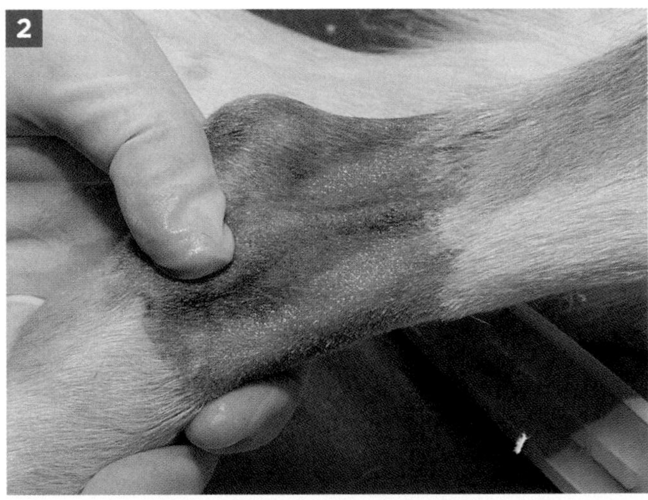

PROCEDURE 13-1 Arthrocentesis—cont'd

3. Insert the tip of the needle into the skin at the distal aspect of the lateral malleolus of the fibula.

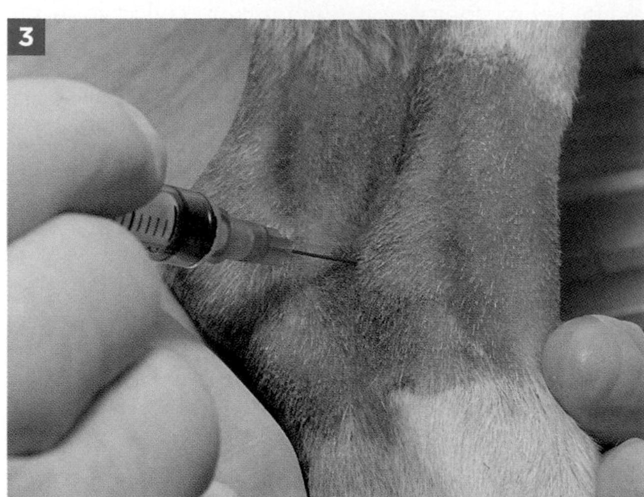

4. Use the needle in the skin to push the skin caudally (together with the caudal branch of the saphenous vein).
5. Once the skin has been shifted caudally, advance the needle to enter the joint just distal and caudal to the malleolus, directing the needle tip medially, slightly cranially, and slightly proximally. This may require "walking off the bone" until the joint space is identified.

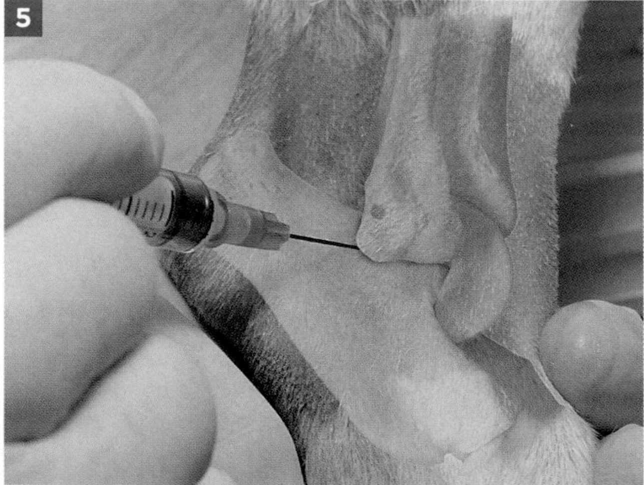

During the lateral approach to the hock the needle is inserted just distal and caudal to the malleolus of the fibula and directed medially and slightly proximally.

6. Apply gentle suction.

Caudal Approach

1. Flex and extend the joint to feel the movement of the tibia relative to the trochlea of the talus caudally. It is at this junction where the tip of the needle will be inserted.

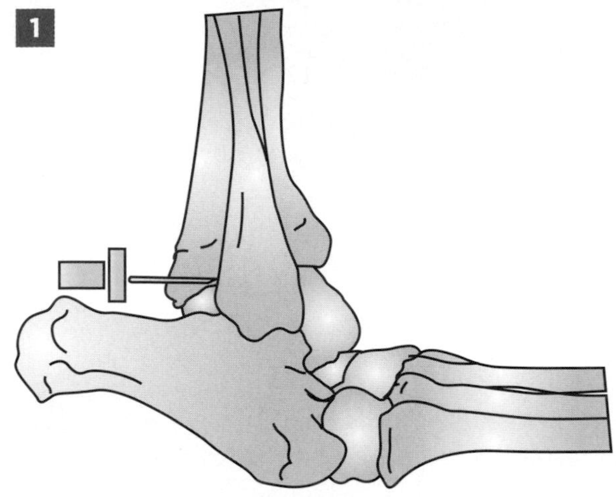

2. Hold the joint in partial flexion.
3. Insert the tip of the needle in the skin caudal to the fibula at the level of the joint.
4. Direct the needle anteriorly, sliding medial to the lateral malleolus of the fibula.

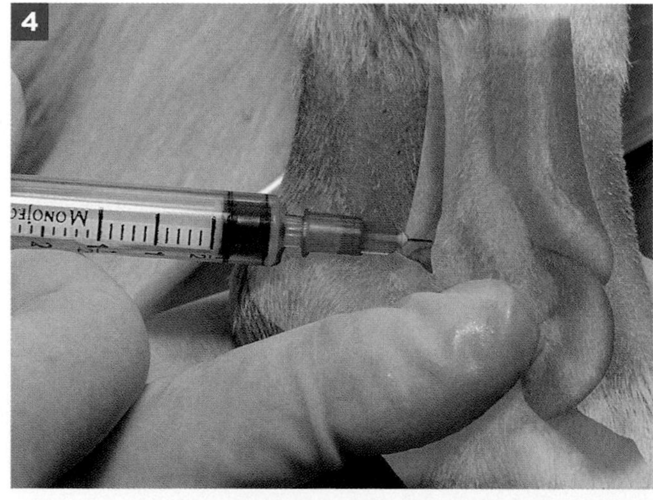

5. Apply gentle suction.

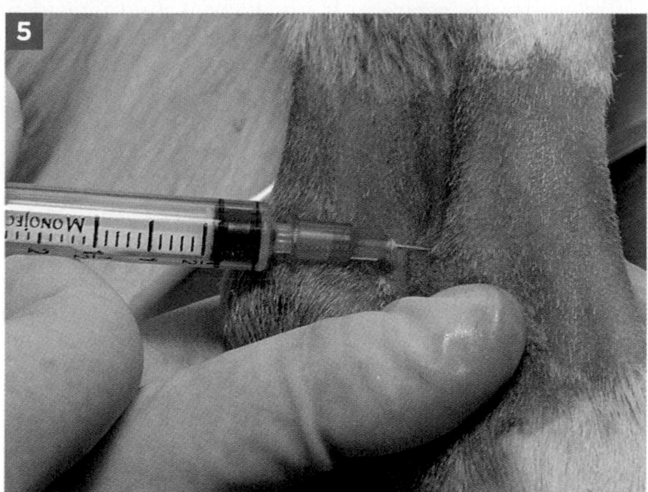

The caudal approach for synovial fluid collection from the hock involves passing the needle into the palpable joint space between the tibia and the trochlea of the talus caudal and medial to the lateral malleolus of the fibula.

SPECIFIC TECHNIQUE: ELBOW JOINT

1. Hold the elbow in partial flexion.
2. Direct the needle just above the dorsal edge of the olecranon, and maintain the needle parallel to the dorsal edge of the olecranon.

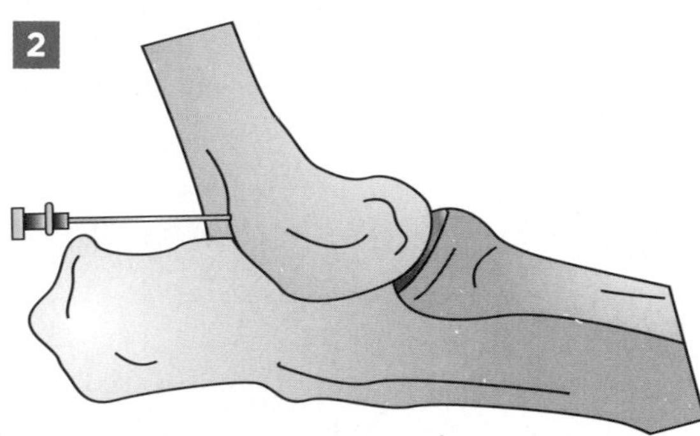

3. The needle tip should enter the skin just behind the lateral epicondyle of the humerus.

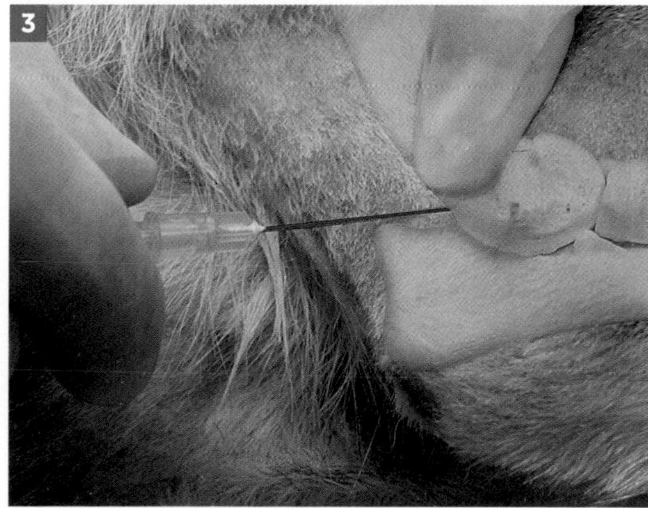

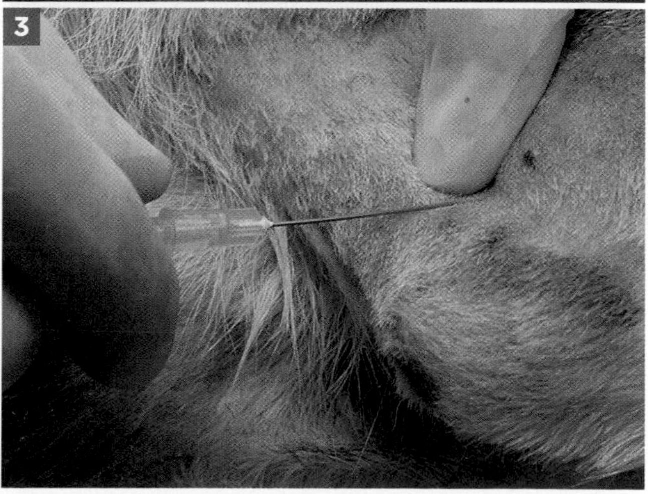

PROCEDURE 13-1 Arthrocentesis—cont'd

4. The needle tip will need to end up just medial to the lateral epicondylar ridge of the distal humerus. This is a wide ridge of bone, so to accomplish this it is necessary (once the needle is through the skin) to apply downward (medial) pressure on the shaft of the needle with the thumb while it is advanced toward the joint space. This is necessary in order to maintain the needle's caudal to cranial orientation parallel to the olecrenon and straight into the joint. The needle tip should not be directed medially.

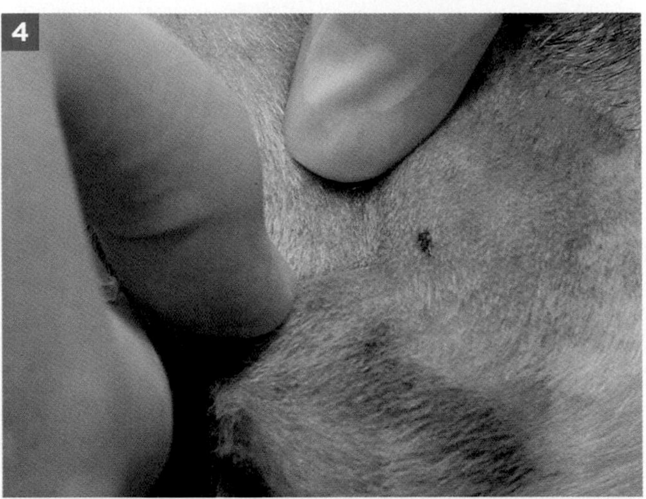

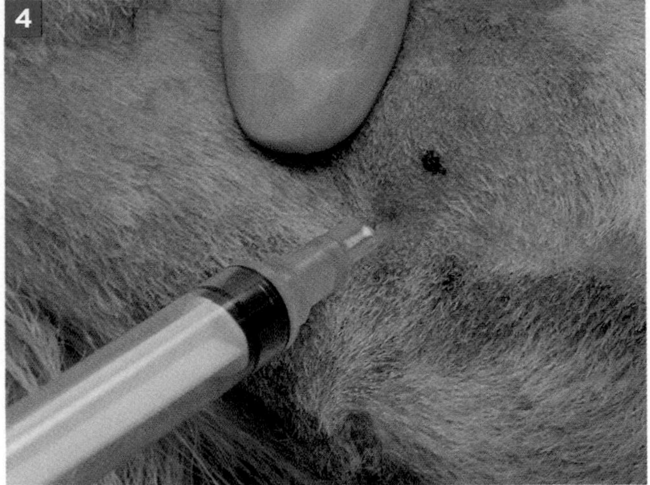

Downward (medial) pressure on the shaft of the needle during insertion is necessary to direct the needle medial to the thick lateral epicondyle of the humerus into the joint space.

5. If the needle advances some distance, but will not advance farther, gently aspirate. If no synovial fluid is evident, attempt to advance the needle farther while the elbow is extended. In most cases the needle needs to be deeply inserted into the joint before joint fluid can be aspirated.

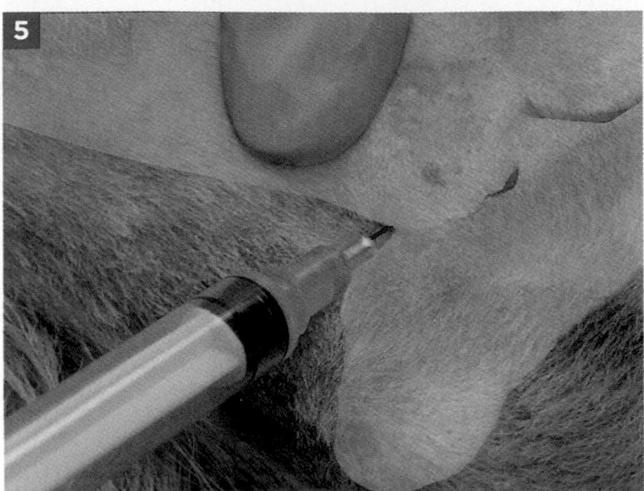

When collecting synovial fluid from the elbow, the needle should be directed parallel to the dorsal edge of the olecranon, with the needle tip inserted just medial to the lateral epicondylar ridge of the humerus.

6. Apply gentle suction.

SPECIFIC TECHNIQUE: SHOULDER JOINT

1. The dog should be in lateral recumbency.
2. Hold the shoulder joint in partial flexion, and maintain the limb parallel to the table as if the dog was standing and weight bearing.

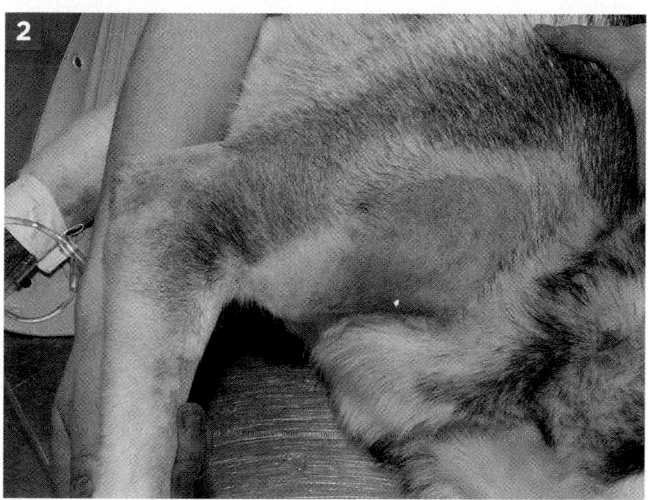

3. Enter the joint just cranial to the glenohumeral ligament, barely distal to the acromion process of the scapula.

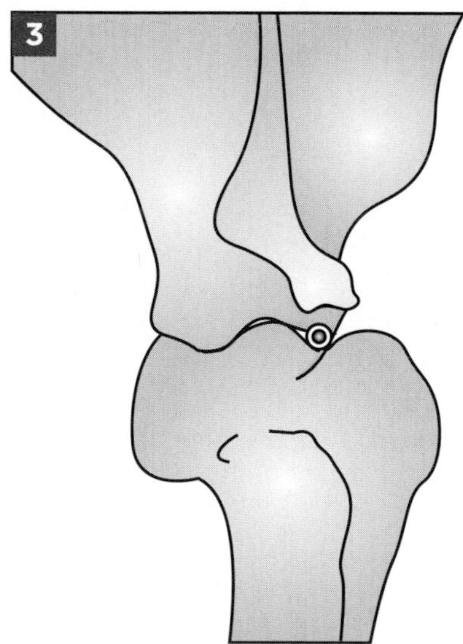

4. Direct the needle medially (straight in).

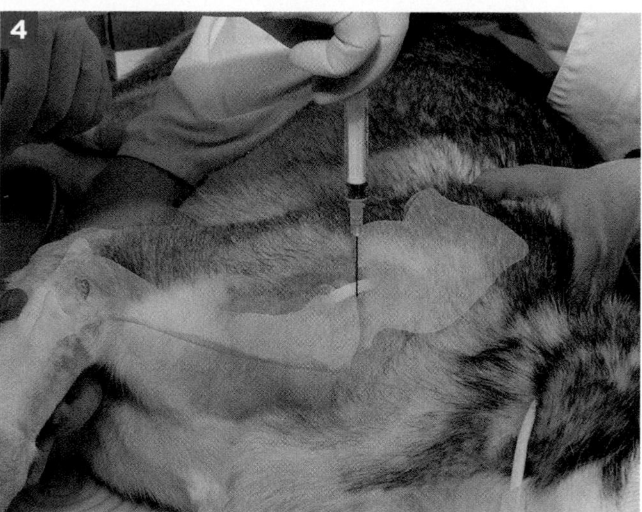

5. If bone is encountered, assess whether the needle is hitting the distal scapula or the proximal humerus, withdraw the needle to the level of the skin, and redirect.
6. Once the needle is deeply inserted, apply gentle suction.

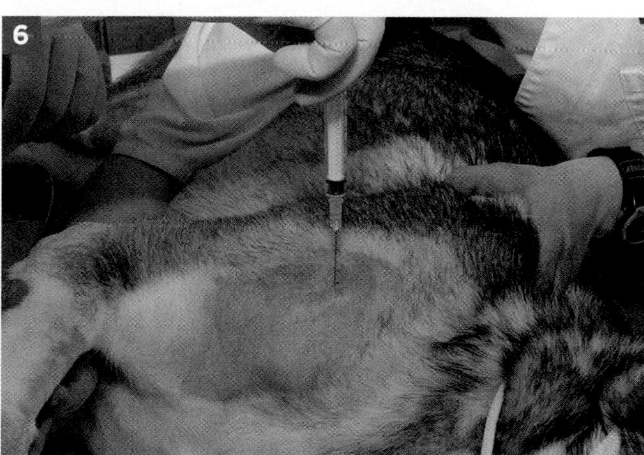

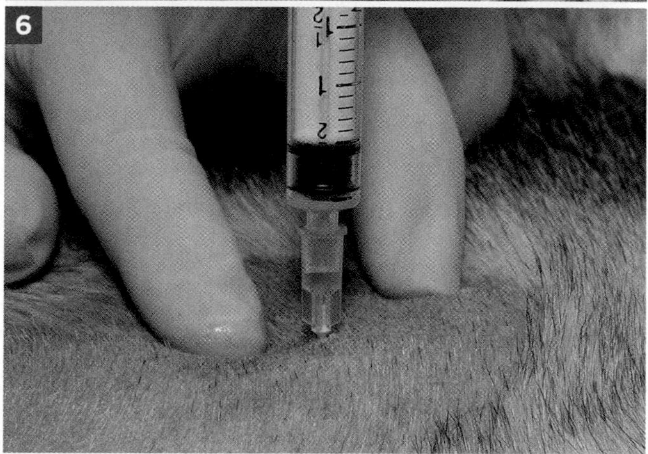

Synovial fluid can be collected from the shoulder joint by inserting the needle medially just cranial to the glenohumeral ligament, barely distal to the acromion process of the scapula.

PROCEDURE 13-1 Arthrocentesis—cont'd

SPECIFIC TECHNIQUE: STIFLE JOINT

1. Flex and extend the joint, palpating to identify the center of the joint—this is where the tip of the needle needs to be during fluid collection.
2. Flex the joint slightly.
3. Identify the midpoint of the length of the "free" patellar tendon between the distal patella and the tibial tuberosity. Insert the needle at that point, just barely lateral to the patellar tendon halfway between the patella and the proximal tibia.

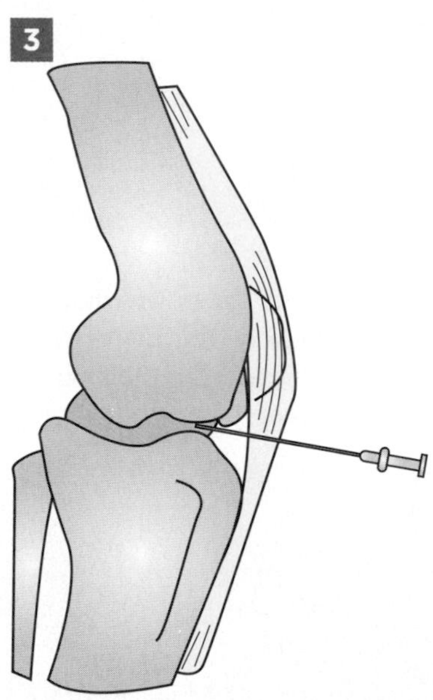

4. Direct the needle tip very slightly medially as the needle is inserted caudally towards the center of the joint.

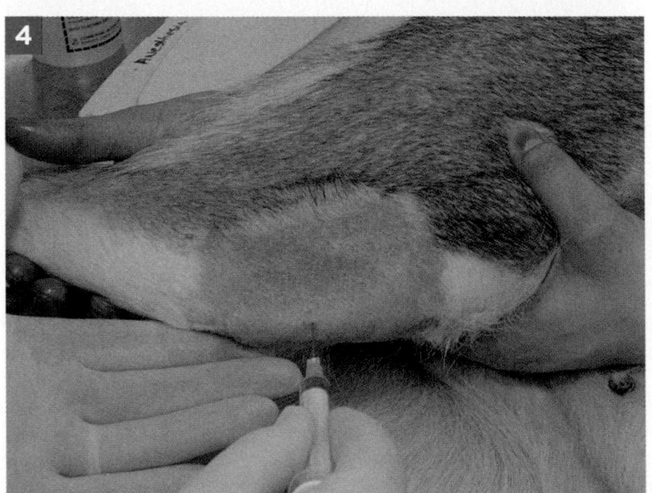

5. The needle should advance without difficulty until the tip is in the center of the joint.

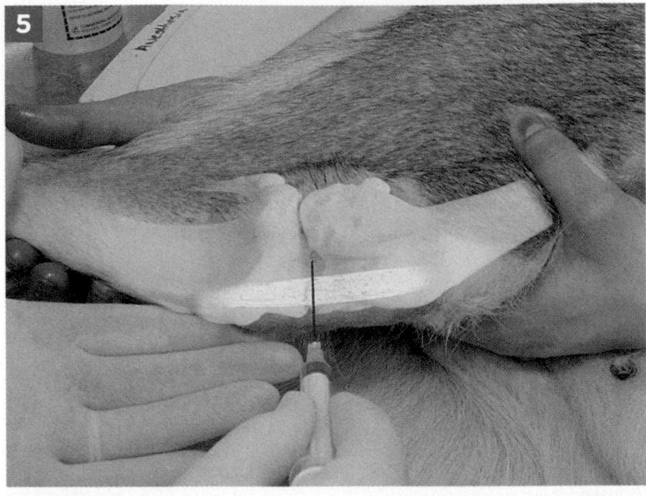

6. Apply gentle suction.

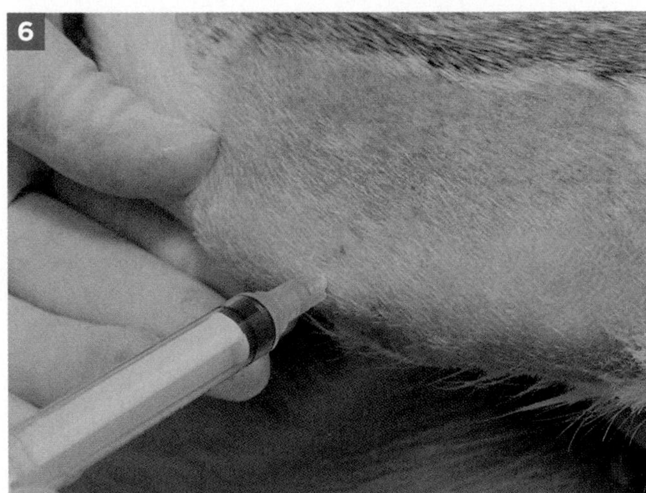

To collect synovial fluid from the stifle joint, the needle is inserted barely lateral to the midpoint of the length of the free patellar tendon toward the center of the joint.

7. The medial and lateral joint spaces communicate.

SPECIFIC TECHNIQUE: HIP JOINT

1. Arthrocentesis of the hip joint usually requires general anesthesia.

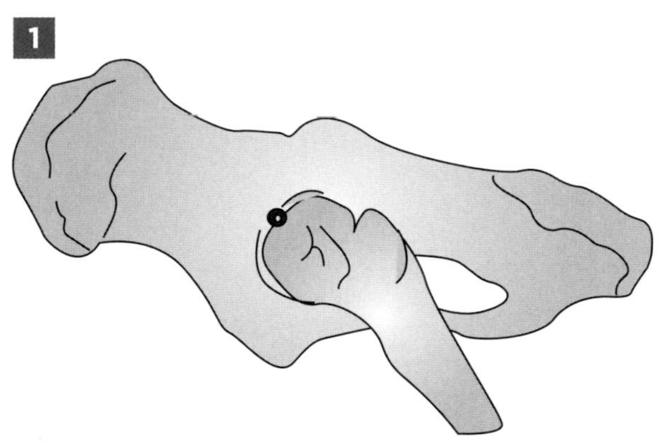

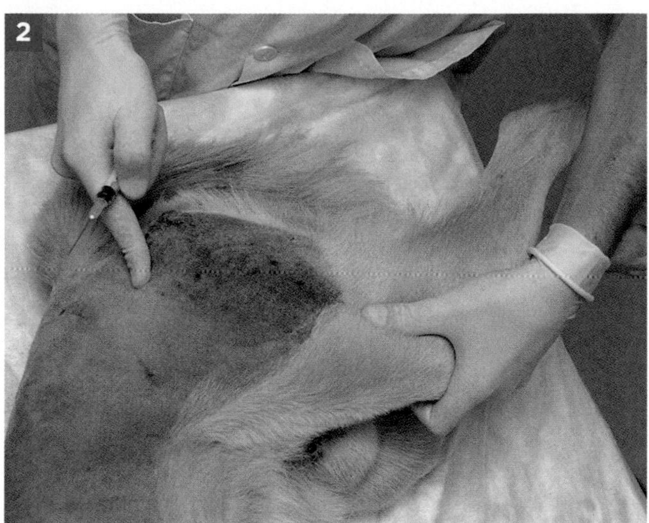

2. Position the animal in lateral recumbency, with the rear limb supported parallel to the table as though the patient were standing, and palpate the greater trochanter of the femur.

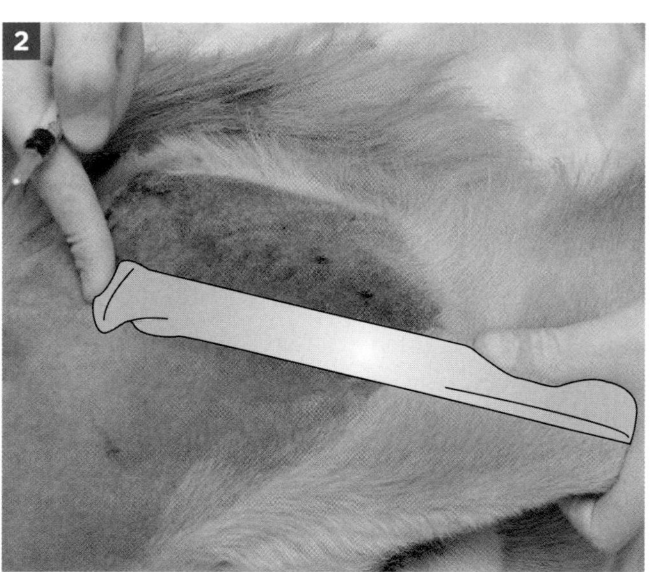

3. Insert the needle straight in medially, perpendicular to the table just barely dorsal to the anterior (cranial) edge of the greater trochanter until bone is encountered.

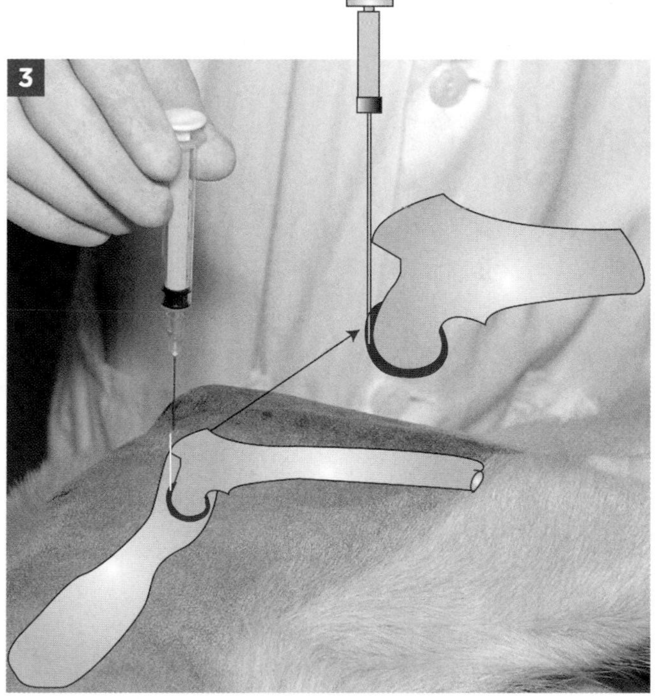

PROCEDURE 13-1 Arthrocentesis—cont'd

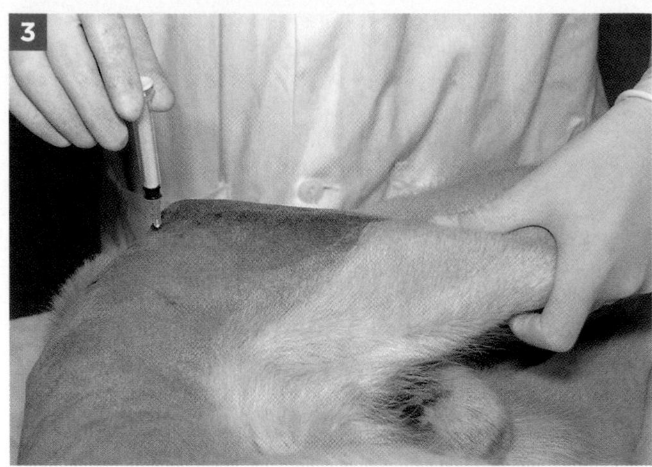

4. Abduct and medially rotate limb the limb while advancing the needle slightly ventrally and cranially into the joint space.

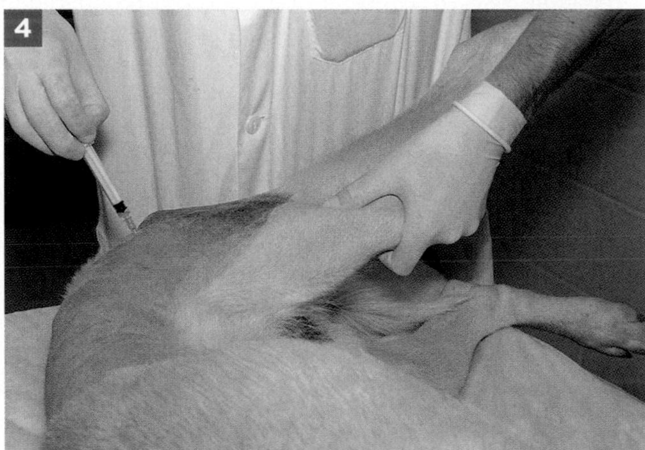

To collect synovial fluid from the hip joint the needle is inserted just dorsal to the anterior edge of the greater trochanter until bone is encountered, and then it is advanced ventrally and cranially while the limb is abducted and medially rotated.

5. Be aware that the sciatic nerve lies deep to the gluteal muscles dorsal to the greater trochanter of the femur and then passes caudal to the greater trochanter before coursing distally in the limb behind the shaft of the femur between the biceps femoris and the semitendinosus muscle.

Cerebrospinal Fluid Collection

14

PROCEDURE 14-1

Cerebrospinal Fluid Collection

PURPOSE

To collect cerebrospinal fluid (CSF) for analysis

INDICATIONS

1. Animals with progressive brain or spinal cord disease
2. Animals with fever and neck pain
3. Any animal before injection of radiographic contrast media into the spinal subarachnoid space for myelography

CONTRAINDICATIONS AND CONCERNS

1. CSF collection requires general anesthesia, so is contraindicated in animals that present a serious anesthetic risk.
2. CSF collection should be avoided in animals with severe coagulopathy.
3. When increased intracranial pressure is suspected, measures should be taken to decrease intracranial pressure before anesthesia for CSF collection in order to decrease the risk of brain herniation (Box 14-1, page 204).
4. Care must be taken to advance the needle slowly during cisternal CSF collection to decrease the risk of needle puncture of the parenchyma because neurologic damage at this site can be fatal.

SPECIAL ANATOMY

1. Cerebrospinal fluid is a clear, colorless fluid contained within the ventricular system of the brain and the subarachnoid spaces of the brain and spinal cord.

1

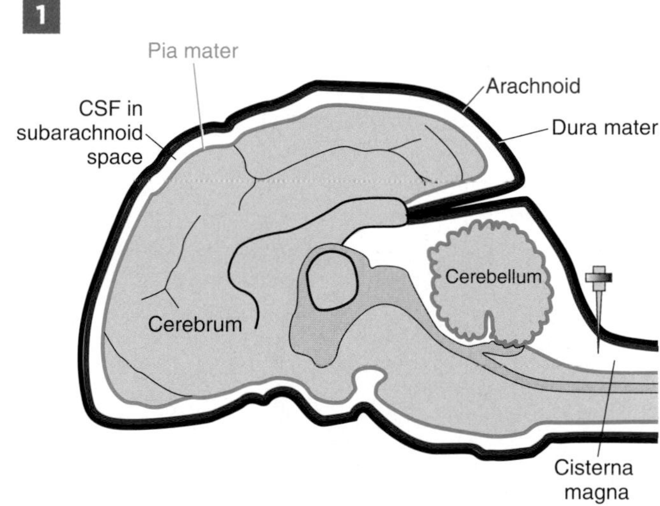

Cerebrospinal fluid (CSF) is contained within the ventricular system of the brain and the subarachnoid spaces of the brain and spinal cord.

2. The brain and spinal cord are surrounded by three layers of meninges. The thin inner layer, the pia mater, is intimately attached to the underlying nervous system tissues. The subarachnoid space is the CSF-filled space between the pia mater and the next layer of the meninges, the arachnoid mater. The arachnoid mater is attached to the thick outer membrane—the dura mater, which is attached to the skull and to the bones of the vertebral canal.

PROCEDURE 14-1 Cerebrospinal Fluid Collection—cont'd

BOX 14-1

Signs Suggesting Increased Intracranial Pressure

Depressed mentation or abnormal behavior
Constricted, dilated or unresponsive pupils
Bradycardia
Increased arterial blood pressure
Altered breathing pattern

Treatment Steps to Decrease Intracranial Pressure

Oxygenate
Administer 20% mannitol: 1 g/kg IV over 15 minutes
Administer furosemide: 1 mg/kg IV

Anesthesia of Patients Suspected to Have Increased Intracranial Pressure

Rapid induction: intubate and ventilate to maintain $Paco_2$ 30 to 40 mm Hg

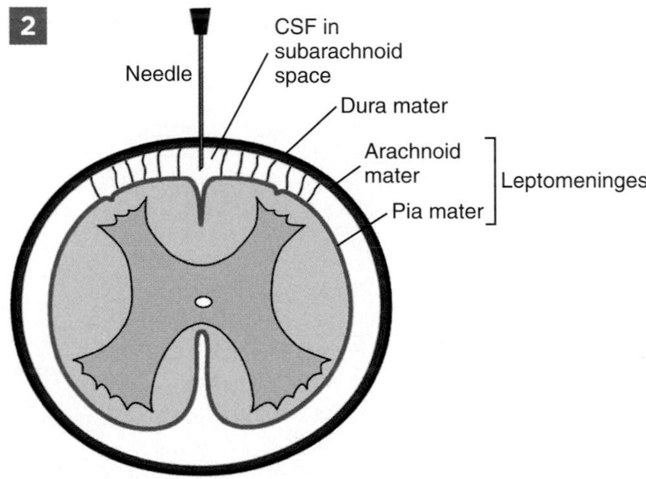

Diagram showing the relationship between the meninges and the CSF surrounding the spinal cord.

CHOOSING THE SITE

In dogs and cats the most reliable source of uncontaminated CSF for analysis is the cerebellomedullary cistern (cisterna magna). Although it is often stated that cisternal CSF best reflects intracranial disease and lumbar CSF reflects spinal cord disease, diagnostically samples from the two sites are not very different. Collection of CSF from the lumbar site is more difficult, and blood contamination is more frequent.

EQUIPMENT

- 20- or 22-gauge, 1½- or 3-inch (3.75 to 7.5 cm) spinal needle with stylet
- Sterile gloves
- EDTA (ethylenediaminetetraacetic acid) and red-top tube for collection of fluid

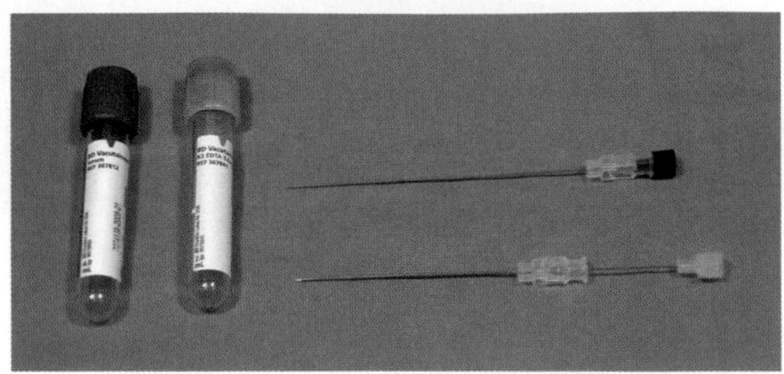

Equipment required for CSF collection.

TECHNIQUE: CISTERNAL CSF COLLECTION

1. The animal should be placed under general anesthesia with a noncollapsing endotracheal tube in place to avoid occluding airflow during positioning for the procedure.
2. Shave a rectangular area on the back of the neck centered over the needle insertion site. The region shaved should extend from 2 cm rostral to the external occipital protuberance to 2 cm caudal to the cranial aspect of the wings of the atlas. Laterally the clipped region should include the most lateral aspects of the wings of the atlas. The entire clipped region should be prepared as for surgery.
3. The person holding the animal's head should stand across the table from the person collecting the sample. If the clinician is right-handed, the animal should be placed in right lateral recumbency with its cervical spine at the edge of the table. The neck should be flexed so that the median axis of the head is perpendicular to the spine. The patient's nose should be elevated slightly so that its midline is parallel to the surface of the table.

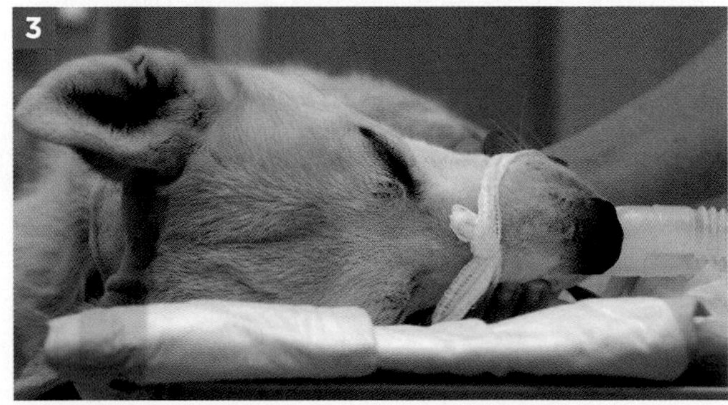

For cisternal CSF collection the neck is flexed so that the median axis of the head is perpendicular to the spine and the patient's nose is elevated slightly so that its midline is parallel to the surface of the table.

4. The person performing the CSF tap should kneel on the floor or sit in a chair so that the point of needle insertion is at eye level.

5. Wearing sterile gloves, the person performing the CSF collection should palpate the site and be certain that the positioning is correct and symmetric. Sometimes padding needs to be inserted underneath the scapula to ensure that a line connecting the most cranial aspect of the left and right wings of the atlas (C1) is perpendicular to the table and to the spine. Taking the time to establish proper positioning is an important step in successful CSF collection.

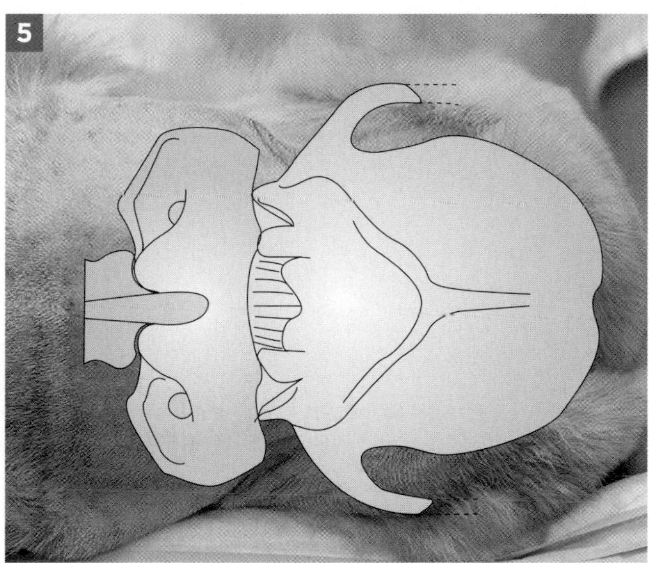

Positioning is correct and symmetric, with a line connecting the most cranial aspect of the left and right wings of the atlas (C1) perpendicular to the table and to the spine.

6. With the thumb and third finger of the left hand, the clinician should palpate the cranial edges of the wings of the atlas and draw an imaginary line at their most cranial aspect.

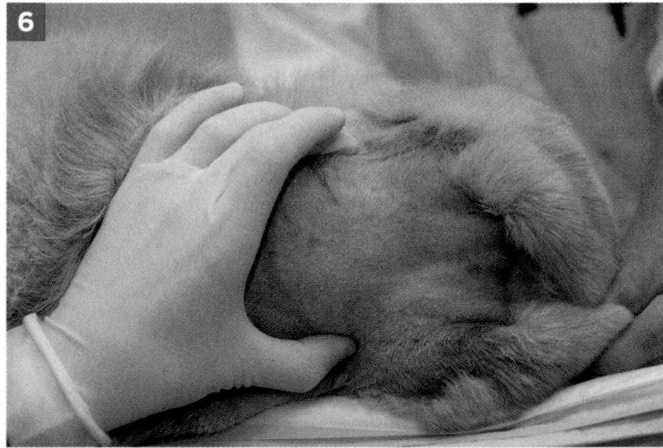

With the thumb and third finger of the left hand, the clinician palpates the cranial edges of the wings of the atlas and draws an imaginary line at their most cranial aspect.

7. The examiner can then use the left index finger to palpate the external occipital protuberance and draw a second imaginary line caudally from that site along the dorsal midline. The needle is inserted where the two imaginary lines intersect.

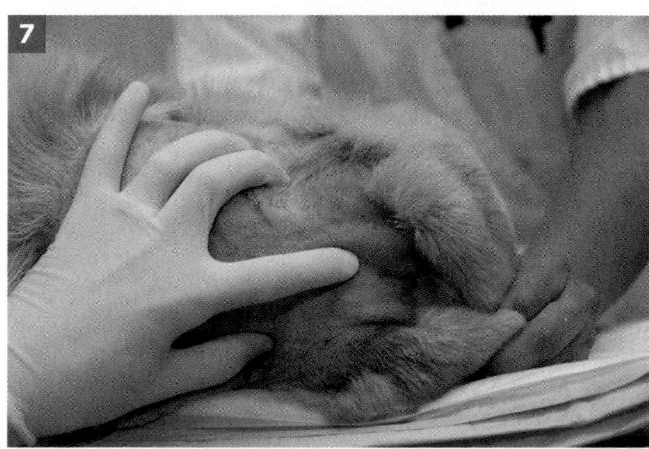

The external occipital protuberance is identified.

PROCEDURE 14-1 Cerebrospinal Fluid Collection—cont'd

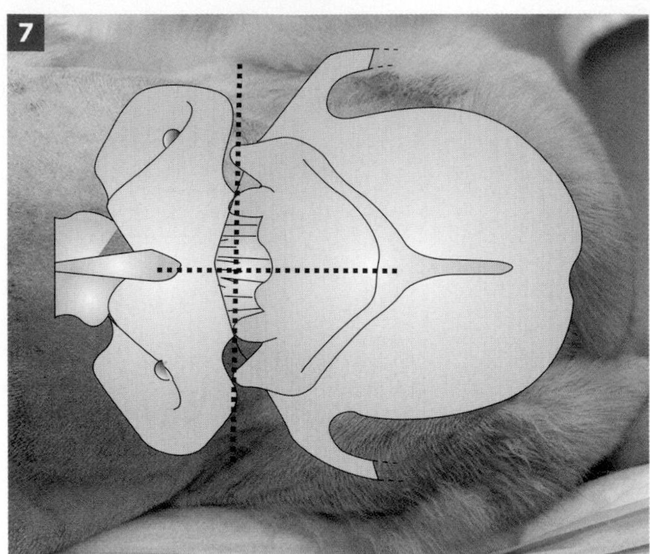

The needle is inserted where an imaginary line connecting the most cranial aspects of the wings of the atlas intersects a line running down midline caudally from the occipital protuberance.

8. While the landmarks are palpated with the left hand, the needle is inserted with the right hand. During needle insertion the right hand should be rested on the animal's head or the table edge for added stability. The spinal needle with stylet in place is directed straight in through the skin, perpendicular to the spine, and into the underlying tissues. For CSF collection in patients with brain disease, the bevel of the needle is directed cranially and for those with suspected spinal cord disease, the bevel is directed caudally.

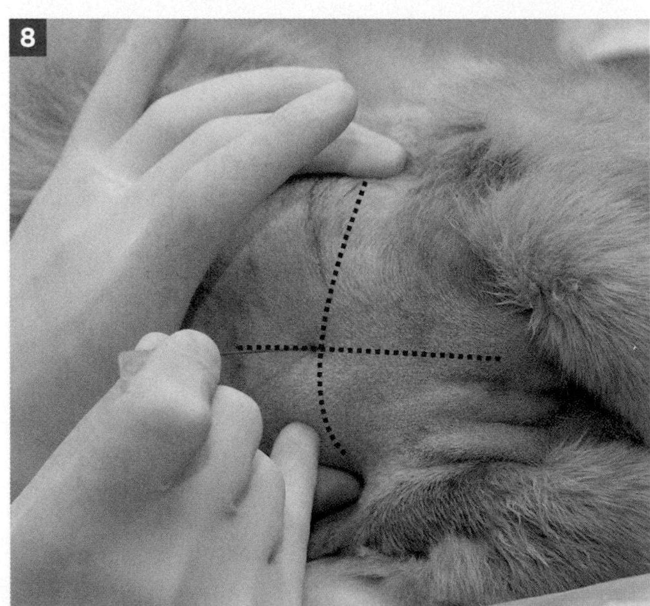

While the landmarks are palpated with the left hand, the needle is inserted at the intersection of the two imaginary lines.

9. Once the needle tip is through the skin, the needle is slowly advanced through the underlying tissues. Varying resistance is noted as different fascial and muscle planes are encountered. Advance the needle only a few millimeters at a time, then remove the stylet to look for CSF. The thumb and first finger of the left hand, which is rested against the spine for support, should grasp and stabilize the needle while the right hand is used to remove the stylet.

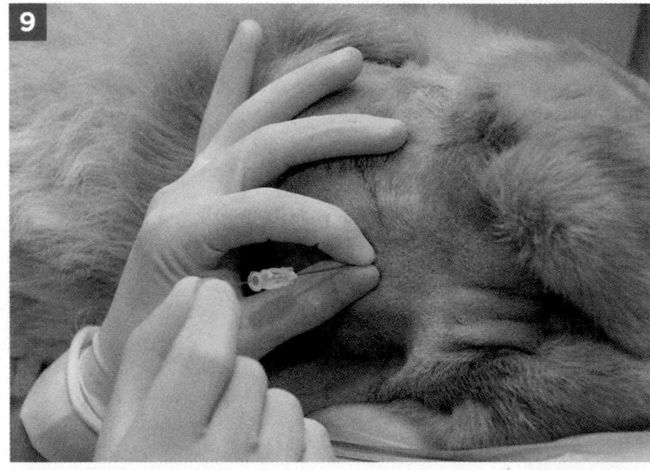

When removing the stylet to look for CSF, the thumb and first finger of the left hand, which is rested against the spine for support, grasp and stabilize the needle.

10. If there is no fluid seen, the stylet should be reinserted and the needle advanced a few millimeters again.

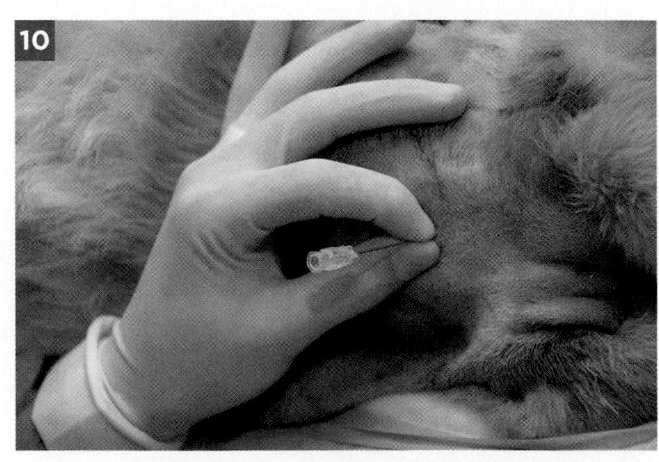

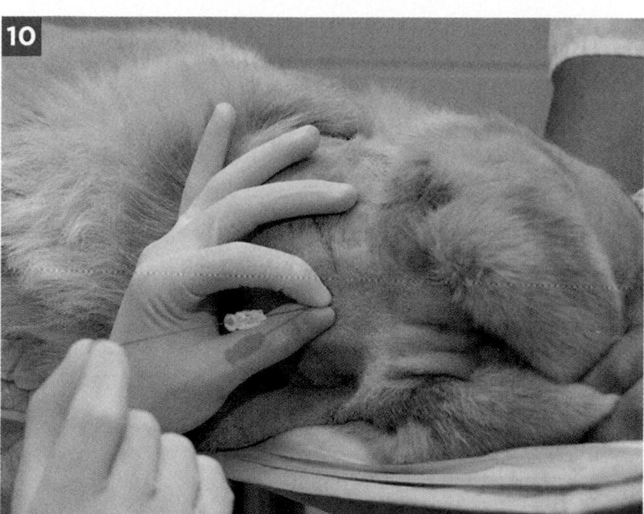
If there is no fluid seen, the stylet is reinserted and the needle advanced a few millimeters before checking again for CSF.

11. Each time the needle is advanced a few millimeters the needle should be stabilized and the stylet removed to check for the flow of CSF. If none is seen, the stylet is reinserted and the needle is advanced a few millimeters more before checking for CSF.
12. A "pop" may be felt as the dorsal atlantooccipital membrane and the dura mater and arachnoid mater are penetrated. This is not a reliable sign, however, and the level at which the subarachnoid space is reached varies greatly with the breed and individual animal. It is often very close to the skin surface in toy breeds and some cats.
13. If the needle strikes bone, it should be withdrawn, patient position and landmarks reassessed, and the procedure repeated with a new needle.
14. If dark venous blood appears in the spinal needle, the needle should be withdrawn and the procedure repeated with another sterile needle. It is most likely that venous structures lateral to midline and external to the dura mater were punctured, so the CSF should be uncontaminated.
15. When CSF is observed, the fluid should be allowed to drip directly from the needle into a tube.

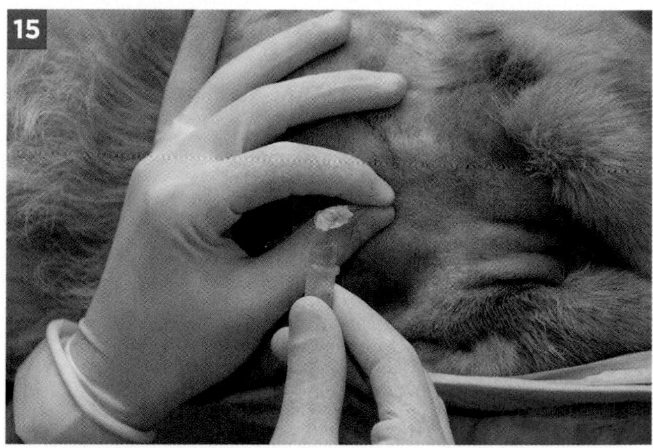
CSF is allowed to drip directly from the needle into a tube.

16. Withdraw the needle after CSF collection, without replacing the stylet. CSF from inside the needle can then be dripped into a second tube for additional testing.

TECHNIQUE: LUMBAR PUNCTURE FOR CSF COLLECTION

1. Place the animal under general anesthesia or heavy sedation.
2. Hold the animal in lateral recumbency with its trunk flexed. Towels are placed between its limbs and beneath the lumbar region as needed to achieve true lateral positioning, with the spine parallel to the tabletop.

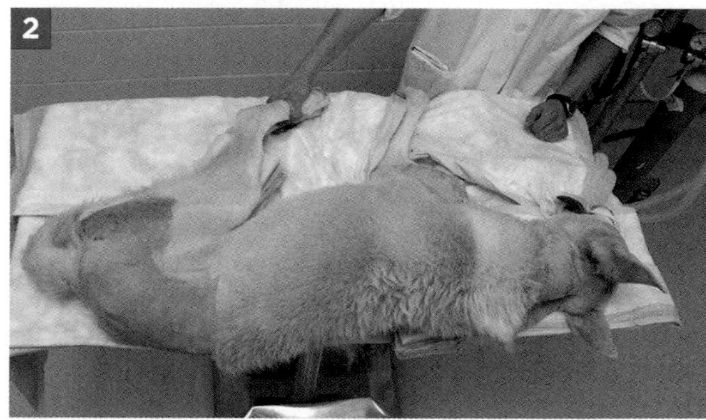
For lumbar puncture the animal is positioned in lateral recumbency with a flexed trunk.

PROCEDURE 14-1 Cerebrospinal Fluid Collection—cont'd

3. Widely clip and surgically prepare the skin over the dorsal lower lumbar and lumbosacral spine. Wear surgical gloves.
4. Have an assistant who is standing on the animal's sternal side flex the lumbar spine by bringing the animal's front and rear legs together.
5. The small dorsal spinous process of L7 lies between the wings of the ilium, and the larger L6 dorsal process is more easily palpable just cranial to that site. Lumbar collection is usually from the L5-6 or L4-5 site in dogs, and the L6-7 site in cats.

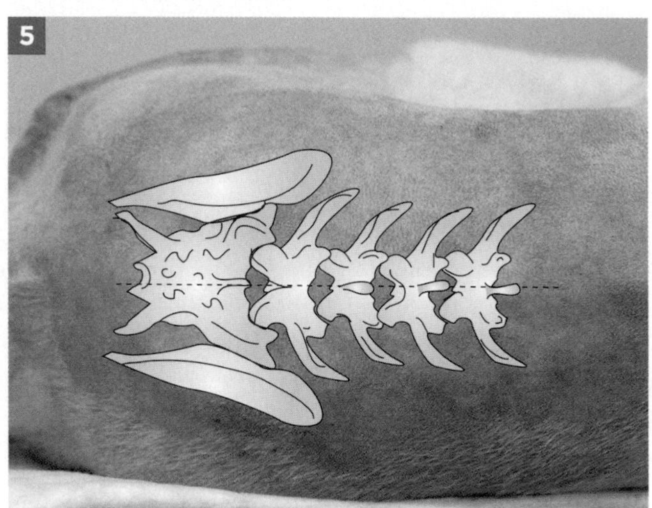

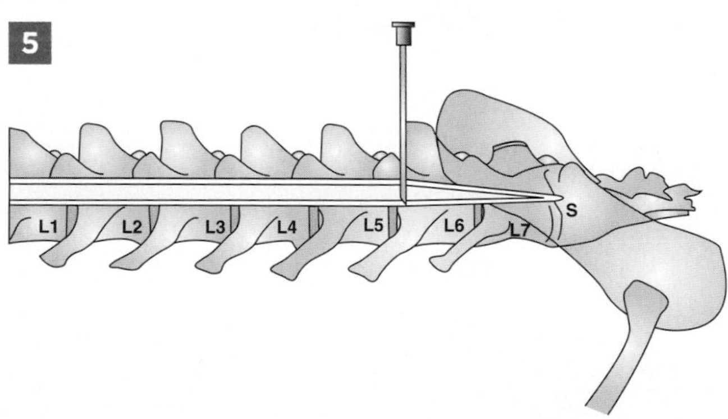

Landmarks for lumbar CSF collection from the L5-6 site.

6. Palpate and identify the dorsal process of L7 between the wings of the ilium.

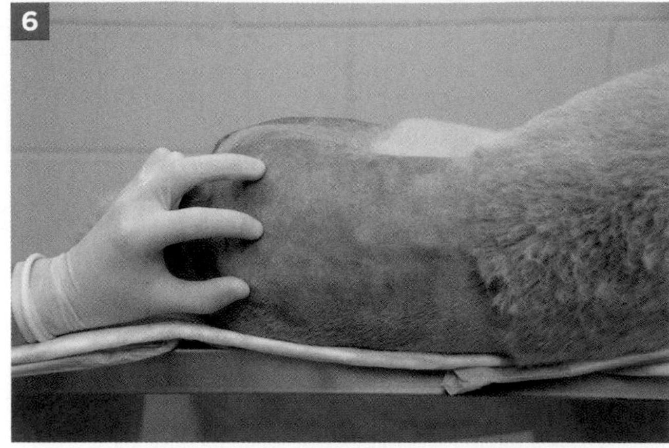

The small dorsal spinous process of L7 can be palpated between the wings of the ilium.

7. For lumbar puncture at L5-6, palpate the dorsal spinous process of L6. Entry is just cranial to this dorsal spinal process on midline.

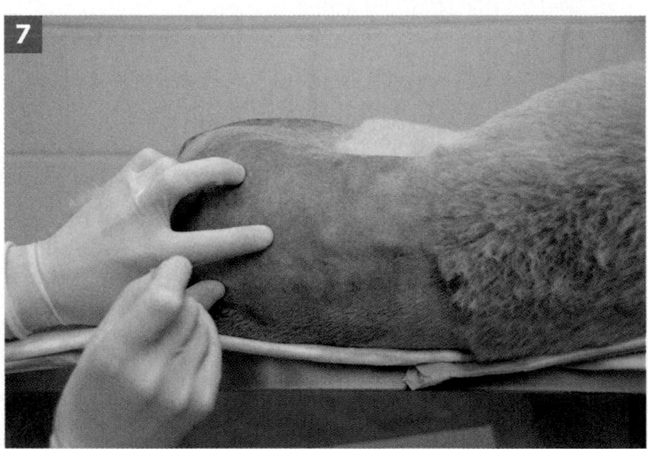

For lumbar puncture at L5-6, needle entry is just cranial to the dorsal spinous process of L6 on midline.

8. Insert a spinal needle through the skin on midline at the cranial aspect of the dorsal spinal process at the desired site. Advance the needle vertically until the dorsal lamina of the spine is encountered and then walk the needle tip slightly cranially to the ligamentum flavum at the intervertebral space.

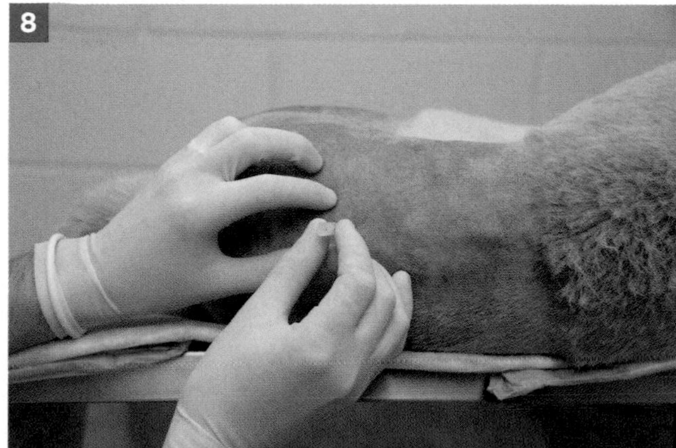

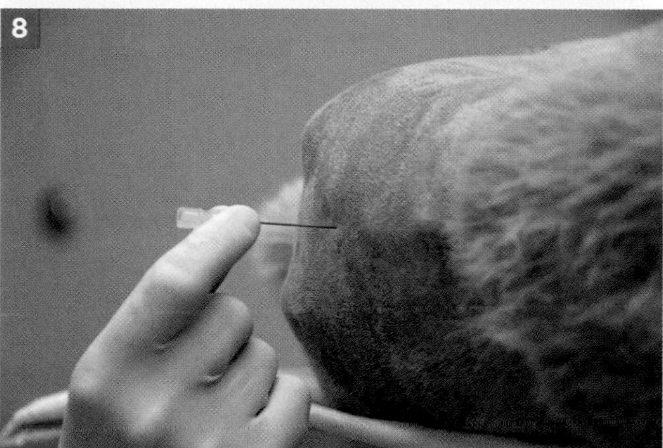

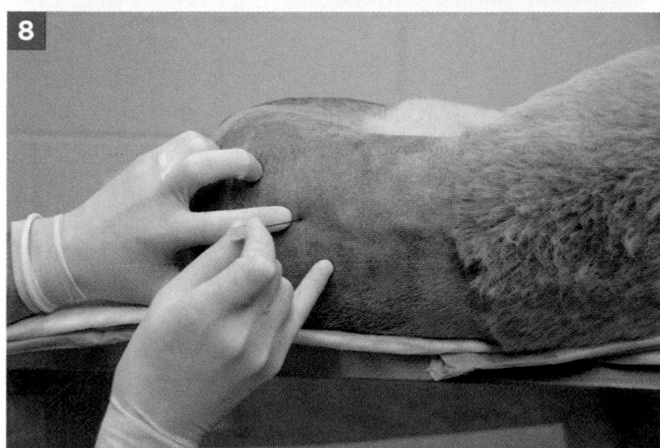

The spinal needle is advanced toward the spine just cranial to the dorsal spinal process of L6, and when the dorsal lamina is encountered, the needle tip is walked slightly cranially to penetrate the ligamentum flavum at the intervertebral space.

9. The ligamentum flavum in the intervertebral space can be tough, but is not hard like bone. There will be considerable resistance to passage of the needle. Advance the needle in a smooth motion through the neurologic tissues to the floor of the spinal canal. A slight twitch of the tail or legs may be seen as the cauda equina is penetrated. Once the bony floor of the spinal canal is encountered, remove the stylet. If there is no CSF flow, carefully withdraw the needle 1 to 2 mm to obtain fluid flow.

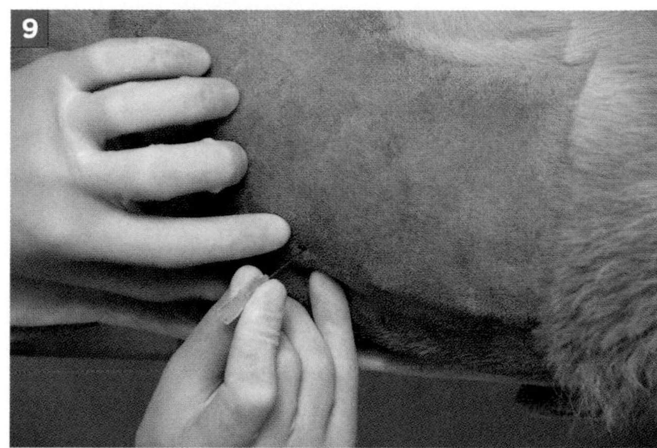

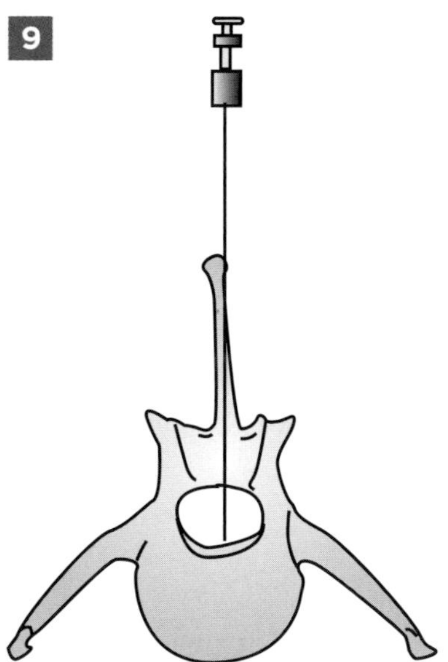

PROCEDURE 14-1 Cerebrospinal Fluid Collection—cont'd

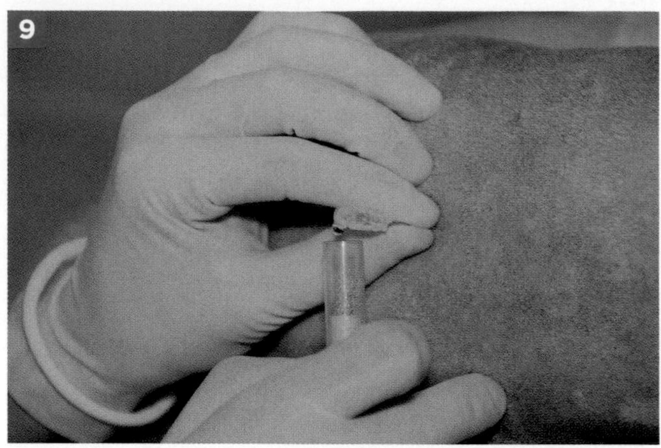

The needle is advanced through the neurologic tissues to the floor of the spinal canal and then withdrawn 1 to 2 mm to obtain flow of CSF.

10. When CSF is observed, the fluid should be allowed to drip directly from the needle into a tube.
11. Withdraw the needle after CSF collection, without replacing the stylet. CSF from inside the needle can be dripped into a second tube for additional testing.

SAMPLE COLLECTION AND HANDLING

1. The amount of CSF collected ranges from 0.5 to 3 mL (no more than 1 mL/5 kg body weight), depending on the size of the animal. Simultaneous jugular vein compression hastens flow from a cisternal tap but transiently increases intracranial pressure.
2. CSF is routinely collected into a sterile tube that is empty or that contains EDTA. The clinician should check with the laboratory to determine the tube preferred.
3. Blood within the CSF may be the result of disease or may be tap-induced. Mild CSF contamination with hemorrhage (<500 red blood cells/μL) will not substantially alter CSF protein and leukocyte determinations. Grossly hemorrhagic CSF should always be collected into a tube containing EDTA to prevent clotting.

RESULTS

1. Normal CSF is clear and colorless and has very low cellularity (<5 cells/μL).

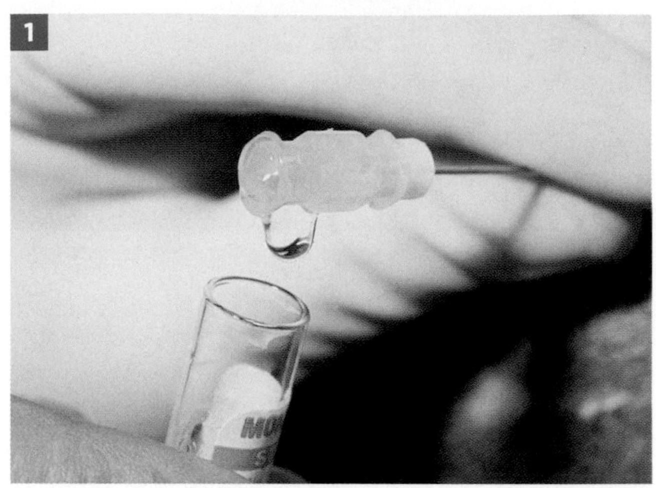

Normal CSF is clear and colorless.

2. Cells within CSF deteriorate rapidly, so cell count and cytologic preparations should be prepared quickly. When the sample must be stored for longer than 1 hour before analysis, refrigeration is advised.
3. Adding autologous serum (0.1 mL for each 0.9 mL of CSF) preserves cytology in refrigerated CSF for 24 to 48 hours after collection, but a separate sample must be saved for protein analysis.
4. One drop of buffered 10% formalin added for each 0.25 mL of CSF also preserves cytologic features without significantly altering protein measurement.
5. Most of the cells in normal CSF are small well-differentiated lymphocytes and large mononuclear phagocytes. A concentration procedure is usually required to obtain sufficient cells for cytologic assessment.

6. A specific cytologic diagnosis is rarely obtained, but typical CSF findings have been established for a number of neoplastic, infectious, and noninfectious inflammatory conditions in dogs and cats.

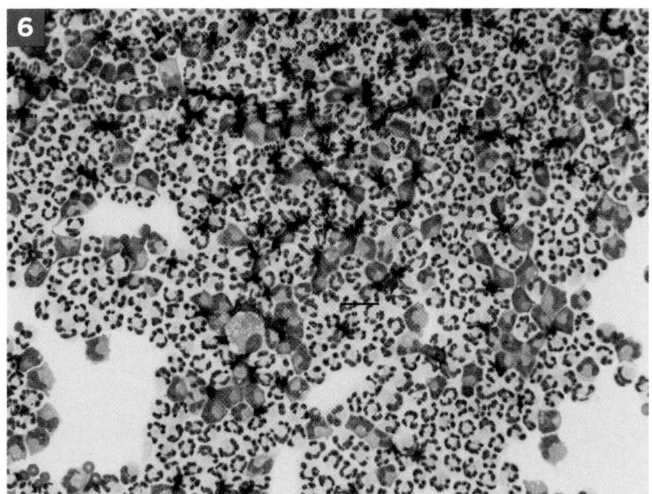

CSF from a 14-month-old female Boxer with neck pain and fever. The nucleated cell count is high (7330 white blood cells/μL) with a predominantly neutrophilic pleocytosis. This dog had aseptic meningitis.

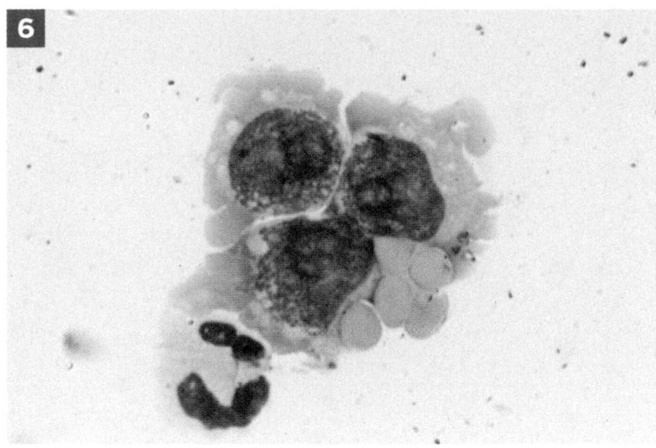

Atypical lymphocytes are identified in this CSF from a 2-year-old cat with progressive rear limb paresis due to spinal lymphoma.

Index

Page numbers followed by *f* denotes figures, *t* denotes tables, and *b* denotes boxes.

T

Reinforce topics from the text with this *interactive* review tool!

This **companion CD** included with the textbook demonstrates clinical techniques in small animal procedures in vivid detail, enabling you to review essential concepts in class or independently!

Master clinical techniques with:

- **Narrated video, photos, and drawings** that walk you through proper practices.
- **Visual guidance and explanations** detailing over 25 small animal procedures.

COMPANION CD

Small Animal **Clinical Techniques**

SAUNDERS
ELSEVIER

TAYLOR

WIN/MAC

999605750X

Start using your CD now!

TR/KB SL90665